Respiratory Tract Mucus

The Ciba Foundation for the promotion of international cooperation in medical and chemical research is a scientific and educational charity established by CIBA Limited – now CIBA-GEIGY Limited – of Basle. The Foundation operates independently in London under English trust law.

Ciba Foundation Symposia are published in collaboration with Elsevier Scientific Publishing Company / Excerpta Medica / North-Holland Publishing Company in Amsterdam

Elsevier / Excerpta Medica / North-Holland, P.O. Box 211, Amsterdam

Respiratory Tract Mucus

Ciba Foundation Symposium 54 (new series)

1978

Elsevier · Excerpta Medica · North-Holland

Amsterdam · Oxford · New York

ISBN 0-444-90016-0

Published in January 1978 by Elsevier/Excerpta Medica/North-Holland, P.O. Box 211, Amsterdam and Elsevier/North-Holland Inc., 52 Vanderbilt Avenue, New York, N.Y. 10017.

Suggested series entry for library catalogues: Ciba Foundation Symposia.
Suggested publisher's entry for library catalogues: Elsevier/Excerpta Medica/North-Holland

Ciba Foundation Symposium 54 (new series)

342 pages, 79 figures, 22 tables

Library of Congress Cataloging in Publication Data

Symposium on Respiratory Tract Mucus, London, 1977.
Respiratory tract mucus.

(Ciba Foundation symposium; new ser., 54)
"Symposium ... held at the Ciba Foundation, London, 22–24 March 1977."
Includes bibliographies and index.
1. Mucus–Congresses. 2. Respiratory organs–Congresses. I. Title. II. Series: Ciba Foundation. Symposium; new ser., 54.
DNLM: 1. Mucus–Congresses. 2. Respiratory system–Physiology–Congresses. 3. Respiratory tract diseases–Physiopathology–Congresses.
W3 C161F v. 54 / WF102 R441
QP215.S95 1975 559'.01'2 77–16019
ISBN 0-444-90016-0

Printed in The Netherlands by Casparie, Alkmaar

Contents

Participants

Symposium on Respiratory Tract Mucus held at the Ciba Foundation, London, 22–24 March 1977

A. C. ALLISON *(Chairman)* Division of Cell Pathology, MRC Clinical Research Centre, Watford Road, Harrow, Middlesex HA1 3UJ, UK

I. CARLSTEDT Department of Physiological Chemistry, Faculty of Medicine, University of Lund, PO Box 750, S-220 07 Lund 7, Sweden

G. CUMMING Midhurst Medical Research Institute, Midhurst, Sussex GU29 0BL, UK

B. DAVIS School of Medicine Cardiovascular Research Institute, University of California, San Francisco, California 94122, USA

K. W. DONALD Nant-Y-Celyn, Cloddiau, Welshpool SY21 9JE, Powys, Wales, UK

W. W. DOUGLAS Department of Pharmacology, Sterling Hall of Medicine, Yale University School of Medicine, 333 Cedar Street, New Haven, Conn. 06510, USA

R. C. GODFREY Western Hospital, Oakley Road, Mill Brook, Southampton SO9 4WQ, UK

A. GUZ Department of Medicine, Charing Cross Hospital, Fulham Palace Road, London W6 9HH, UK

J. IRAVANI Institut für Anatomie Lehrstuhl für Anatomie II, Postfach 102148/MA6/148, Ruhr-Universität Bochum, Universitätsstrasse 150, 4630 Bochum 1, West Germany

P. K. JEFFERY Basic Medical Sciences Group, Department of Physiology, Chelsea College, University of London, Manresa Road, London SW3 6LX, UK

J. G. JONES Division of Anaesthesia, MRC Clinical Research Centre, Watford Road, Harrow, Middlesex HA1 3UJ, UK

R. JONES Department of Pathology, Children's Hospital Medical Center, 300 Longwood Avenue, Boston, Massachusetts 02115, USA

P. W. KENT Glycoprotein Research Unit, Science Laboratories, University of Durham, South Road, Durham DH1 3LE, UK

M. F. KRAMER Department of Histology and Cell Biology, Rijksuniversiteit Utrecht, Nic. Beetsstraat 22, Utrecht 2501, The Netherlands

J. A. NADEL School of Medicine Cardiovascular Research Institute, University of California, San Francisco, California 94122, USA

C. F. PHELPS Department of Biological Sciences, University of Lancaster, Lancaster LA1 4YQ, UK

D. F. PROCTOR Department of Otolaryngology, The Johns Hopkins Hospital, Baltimore, Maryland 21205, USA

L. REID Department of Pathology, Children's Hospital Medical Center, 300 Longwood Avenue, Boston, Massachusetts 02115, USA

P. S. RICHARDSON Department of Physiology, St George's Hospital Medical School, Tooting, London SW17 0QT, UK

P. SADOUL INSERM U 14, Case officielle no. 10, 54500 Vandœuvre-les-Nancy, France

A. SILBERBERG Polymer Department, Weizmann Institute of Science, Rehovot, Israel

W. M. THURLBECK Department of Pathology, Health Sciences Centre, The University of Manitoba, 700 William Avenue, Winnipeg, Manitoba, Canada R3E OZ3

J. G. WIDDICOMBE Department of Physiology, St George's Hospital Medical School, Tooting, London SW17 0QT, UK

Editors: Ruth Porter *(Organizer)*, John Rivers and Maeve O'Connor

Chairman's opening remarks

A. C. ALLISON

Division of Cell Pathology, MRC Clinical Research Centre, Harrow, Middlesex

Many of you will be wondering why I am here, and I wonder more than you do; but it is a long-established British tradition to have non-experts participating in everything from local dispensation of justice to hospital administration.

I suggest that we approach this whole subject from the point of view of cell biologists and look at respiratory tract mucus in the way in which I was originally taught by Sir Howard (later Lord) Florey. He was one of the first to point out that mucus is not just gubbins but an interesting substance which performs important and distinct functions in different places. When Florey was active, very little was known about the chemistry of mucus. Now we are able to use established techniques to discover the structure both of mucus from different sites and of related substances such as synovial fluid, and to compare structure with mechanical and other properties. Synovial fluid has interesting rheological properties, for example non-Newtonian viscosity, a property associated with joint lubrication which would be disastrous if it existed in respiratory tract mucus. One of the features of mucus is that it acts as the mechanical link between the energy provided by ciliary beats and translocation of particles. Professor Silberberg, who has been a pioneer in this field, has done a lot to associate the rheological properties and chemistry of mucus. This link is important not only in the respiratory tract but also, for example, in the female genital tract. Mucus is associated with translocation of the ovum down the Fallopian tube, the probability of fertilization and, in the uterus itself, with the site of implantation and the allowing of implantation. There, hormonal influences are strong and one of the main ways in which the contraceptive pill works is by changing the properties of mucus in the genital tract.

We should like to know the structure of mucus and how it is related to particular functions. The old concept of a uniform blanket of mucus now seems to be disappearing in favour of the concept of isolated patches. We shall also hear a good deal about the chemical structure and I regret that Dr Pierre Masson cannot be with us, because one of the points which he has made is that instead of rather long protein chains—with carbohydrate side chains, which is true of proteoglycan in synovial fluid—there may be uniform units of protein which are quite short, with a molecular weight of about 30 000 daltons on the basis of published N-terminal determinations and more recent C-terminal determinations (Masson 1973). Because of the larger sizes of the units observed and their properties there is the interesting possibility that the subunits may be cross-linked by carbohydrate chains. So I hope that the chemists here will address themselves to the questions: what is the basic structure of respiratory tract mucus? is Masson's model correct? and what would be the properties of material of this kind in contrast to other proteoglycans with which we are all familiar?

In synovial fluid there are specific interactions between proteoglycan and hyaluronic acid, mediated by specific bonds, and these interactions determine the properties of the material. Although hyaluronic acid is absent, there may be other constituents of respiratory tract mucus which interact in a specific way with proteoglycan to generate particular behavioural properties. For example, calcium and magnesium ions may interact with the carbohydrate side chains and with the cell coat. It may be possible to generate, from combinations of different secretions, material which behaves differently from the original secretions themselves. Professor Silberberg makes the point that the behaviour of this material is quite evanescent and that if fresh mucus is isolated its mechanical properties are different from those of material that has been frozen and then thawed. Such material is convenient for biochemical analysis but its mechanical properties may in fact be greatly changed. So we want to know what the constituents are, how they change, whether they are changed by enzymic action, by cross-linking, or by degradation of either the carbohydrate units or the protein units of which they are composed, and whether any changes result from interaction of different components.

The anatomical basis of mucus secretion is itself quite complex. We were taught that there are in respiratory tract epithelium three cell types—an undifferentiated cell, a ciliated cell and a goblet cell. Now we are told that there are many cell types—11 according to Dr Jeffery, who will be describing their properties—and during the meeting we shall want to look at the changes which occur in these cell types. Can a serous cell be transformed into a mucus-secreting cell and if so in what circumstances? What induces the differentiation of these relatively undifferentiated cells into cells of particular types, and is the process reversible? We know, for example, that in the development of the blood system there is a series of stem cells; the early ones are multipotential, but at each stage of development the potentialities are further restricted. One starts with cells which can become lymphocytes, erythrocytes or granulocytes. At later stages they are committed, for example, to the erythrocyte series of differentiation or to the granulocyte–monocyte series, and cells in the latter series can become either monocytes, neutrophils or eosinophils. Particular local factors, some of which are now defined, determine which pathway of differentiation these cells will follow. We know very little about analogous processes in the respiratory tract but these are questions to which we should address ourselves, not looking at structure just from a static viewpoint but trying to bear in mind how cells can follow one pathway of differentiation or another.

Again, very little is known about the control of mucus secretion. We know a great deal about the mechanisms underlying secretion in other cells, particularly the role of calcium, the relationship to microtubules, microfilaments, membrane fusion and so on. Professor Douglas, who is one of the experts in that field, will remind us of the general background and I think it would be appropriate in the near future to apply to respiratory tract mucus the general principles and information which have emerged from other systems. We know very little about whether the control is determined by local mediators: interesting possibilities are emerging about the role of prostaglandins with the use of indomethacin and other drugs to inhibit the formation of prostaglandins or divert their metabolism along particular pathways. From studies of inflammation it is already clear that this is a very complicated process. For example, it is not usually the final stages of prostaglandins, the E and F series, which are so easily obtained and analysed, that are particularly important in inflammation, but rather the transient intermediates—prostaglandin A and the thromboxanes. We don't know the relative importance of local humoral factors and nervous control of respiratory tract mucus secretion. There is an intimate structural relationship between nerves and the cells of the respiratory tract epithelium and we suspect that reflex stimulation may be important; interesting examples have been studied in frogs and other experimental animals. We know a great deal more about the new neurotransmitters and how to block transmission, and there is now good opportunity for applying accumulated physiological or cytopharmacological knowledge to the respiratory tract.

I hope, then, that we shall try to apply the principles of cell biology and developmental biology to our subject so as to provide the scientific background for the discussions of the clinical aspects which will follow. It will be more appropriate to discuss general points, such as the nature of the linkages between polypeptide and carbohydrate chains, rather than go into enormous detail on the actual amino-acid and sugar sequences which are involved, unless they have some bearing on general structural problems. In the same way I am sure we don't want elaborate descriptions of the different cell types in several species of animals.

Finally, we can already see from the contributions to this meeting how much there is to be learnt from other fields. For example, Dr Nadel will be reminding us of the application to the respiratory tract of the basic work on the toad bladder, which yielded a great deal of information about ion movements across membranes, and of the micropuncture techniques which were used so successfully in kidney physiology. Dr Kramer will be describing the beautiful work which has been done in cell biology on finding out the sites of synthesis of proteins and carbohydrates in different cell types—work which was pioneered by Leblond, Jamieson and Palade and is now applied to mucus secretion. Many special disciplines impose in an interesting way on the subject of this meeting and I am sure that we shall have fruitful discussions.

Reference

MASSON, P. L. (1973) Carbohydrate component of cervical mucus, in *Cervical Mucus in Human Reproduction* (Elstein, M. *et al.*, eds.), p. 82, Scriptor, Copenhagen

Structure and function of mucus-secreting cells of cat and goose airway epithelium

PETER K. JEFFERY

Chelsea College and St George's Hospital Medical School, London

Abstract In the cat and goose, studies have been undertaken to determine the ultrastructure of airway epithelia, the concentration and distribution of the secretory cells which produce respiratory tract mucus, and the histochemistry of mucins located within cells and on their luminal surfaces. By electron microscopy all the 11 cell types so far described can be found in the airways of the cat but not the goose. Both goblet cells and submucosal glands are abundant in the cat whereas the trachea of the goose lacks the latter, having instead abundant goblet cells many of which form 'intraepithelial glands'. Histochemically, the goblet cells of the cat and goose are similar in that they contain mucins with a predominance of sulphate esters. A surface mucosubstance can be demonstrated which, histochemically, is similar to that described in dog and man. Interestingly, this surface layer may be sloughed in response to an inhaled irritant such as ammonia and thereby contribute to the respiratory tract mucus recovered experimentally. Incorporation into macromolecules of radioactively labelled mucin precursors is assessed by autoradiography of tissue sections, and preliminary results of experiments designed to test the response of mucus-secreting cells to airway irritation and the parasympathomimetic drug, pilocarpine, are also presented.

The airways which supply the respiratory portion of the lung are responsible for the clearance of inhaled particulate and gaseous pollutants deposited on their mucosal lining. To this end, the lining mucosa produces a mucous secretion in which pollutants become dissolved or entangled, and which is then moved by cilia to the pharynx, where it is normally swallowed. The mucous secretion so produced (normally between 10 and 100 ml/day) is a complex mixture of about 95% water and 5% carbohydrate, protein, lipid and inorganic material—usually in the form of a number of different glycoproteins, each differing in the ratio of its protein to carbohydrate component and its degree of acidification. The physical (i.e. viscoelastic) properties of the secretion are largely due to these glycoproteins which are produced by a variety of cell types comprising the airway wall.

In man, respiratory mucus may come from two anatomical sources—the secretory cells of the surface epithelium and those of the submucosal glands (Reid 1954; McCarthy & Reid 1964). This is also true of the respiratory tract of the rat, dog and pig, three animals which have been used as experimental animal 'models' for mucous studies (Reid 1963; Chakrin & Saunders 1974; Jones *et al.* 1975). More recently, both the cat and the goose have been used in studies of the control of mucin secreted in a tracheal segment isolated *in situ* in the anaesthetized animal (Gallagher *et al.* 1975; Phipps *et al.* 1977). Whereas the fine structural anatomy of the airway mucosal linings of the human, rat, dog and pig have been well described (Rhodin 1966; Jeffery & Reid 1975; Frasca *et al.* 1968; Baskerville 1970), those of the cat and goose have not. In particular, the goose may be a useful animal to study in that its airways, like those of other species of birds, have an abundance of epithelial goblet cells but no submucosal glands, thus allowing mucin from a purely epithelial source to be investigated (Cover 1953; Purcell 1971; Walsh & McLelland 1974).

The work presented here is the result of new studies we have undertaken to determine, in the cat and goose, the ultrastructure of airway epithelia, the concentration and distribution of the secretory cells which produce the respiratory tract mucus found in these two species, and the histochemistry of the mucin, whether it be located within cells or on their surfaces. Preliminary results on the histology of tracheal 'segments' taken from cats or geese which have been stimulated (by neural or pharmacological means) to increase their output of tracheal mucin will also be given.

ULTRASTRUCTURE OF THE EPITHELIUM

As reviews of the ultrastructure and diversity of cell types which make up the airway epithelium of different species have recently been published (see Breeze *et al.* 1976; Jeffery & Reid 1977), this section will give only a general survey of the cell types which have now been found in the airways of the cat and goose.

Up to 11 distinct cell types (nine epithelial and two migratory) have been described in airway epithelia, depending upon the species studied and the anatomical location of the respiratory tract examined (Fig. 1). Except for the cat, each species is deficient in one or more of the 11 cell types (Table 1). The cat airway epithelium has the full complement of cell types as well as the occasional mast cell and neutrophil (polymorphonuclear leucocyte) (Jeffery

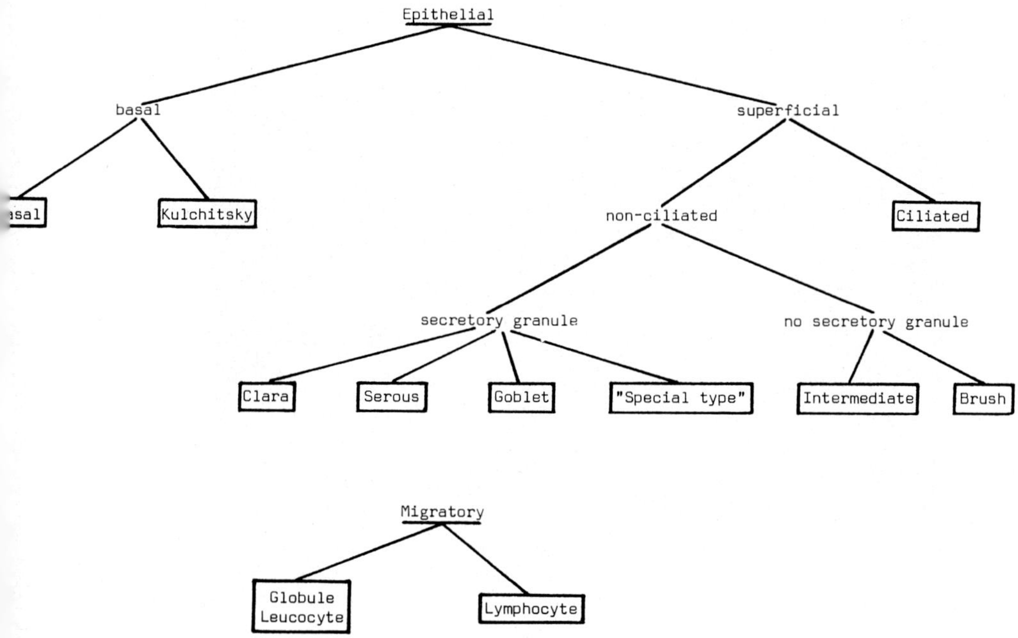

FIG. 1. Epithelial cell types described by electron microscopy.

TABLE 1

Epithelial cell types identified by electron microscopy in various species

	Man	*Monkey*	*Dog*	*Cat*	*Pig*	*Cow*	*Rat*	*Mouse*	*Hamster*	*Rabbit*	*Certain birds*
Ciliated	+	+	+	+	+	+	+	+	+	+	+
Goblet (lucent granule)	+	+	+	+	+	—	+	+	+	+	+
Serous (dense granule)	+	—	—	+	—	—	+	—	—	—	+
'Special type'	+	—	+	+	—	—	—	—	—	—	—
Clara	+	+	—	+	+	—	+	+	?	+	—
Intermediate	+	—	—	+	+	—	+	—	—	—	+
Brush	?	—	—	+	+	—	+	—	—	?	—
Basal	+	+	+	+	+	+	+	+	+	+	+
Kulchitsky	+	—	—	+	—	—	+	+	—	+	+
Globule leucocyte	—	'migratory'	+	+	—	—	+	—	—	—	—
Lymphocyte	+	'migratory'	—	+	—	—	+	—	—	—	—
Intraepithelial nerve	+	—	—	+	—	—	+	+	—	+	+

+ identified; — not yet identified; ? unconfirmed.

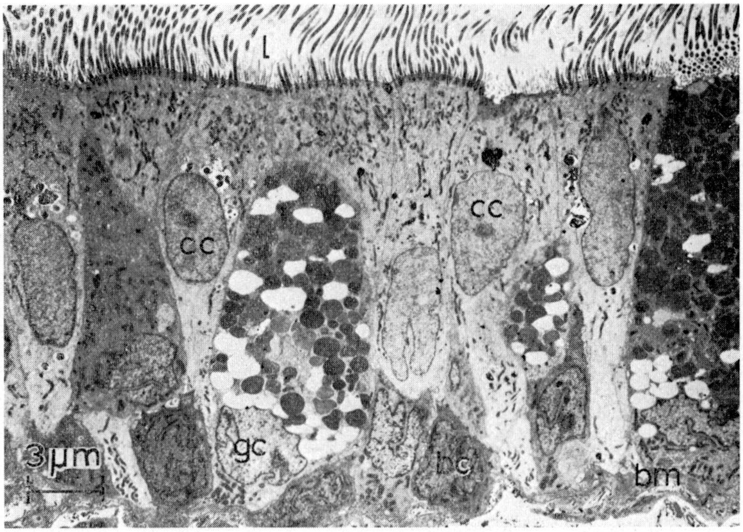

FIG. 2. An electron micrograph of cat tracheal epithelium showing goblet (gc), ciliated (cc) and basal cells (bc). Goblet cells contain a mixture of electron-lucent and electron-dense secretory granules. Airway lumen (l) and basement membrane (bm). Glutaraldehyde and osmium tetroxide: uranyl acetate and lead citrate. × 3000

& Das 1977). In particular, the cat has all four secretory cell types, i.e. goblet cells, 'epithelial serous cells' (Jeffery & Reid 1975), Clara cells (most frequent in bronchioli), and 'special type cells', which have also been described in the airways of dog and man (Frasca *et al.* 1968).

Fig. 2 shows cat tracheal epithelium. The most frequent type of secretory cell is the goblet cell, which in the cat constitutes between 7 and 15% of all epithelial cells, depending on the location of the airway examined. Unlike the rat, many goblet cells of the cat contain a mixture of electron-lucent and electron-dense granules within the same cell, which suggests that there is a mixture of distinct glycoproteins within the same cell (see below). The 'epithelial serous cell' and 'special type cell' are infrequently found. Fig. 3 shows gosling tracheal epithelium. Goblet and 'epithelial serous' cells have been identified, the latter being found infrequently (Phipps *et al.* 1977). The goblet cells are unique in containing electron-lucent secretory granules each of which is 'speckled' with electron-dense areas. This morphological heterogeneity suggests that within each granule there may be two or more distinct types of glycoprotein. Goblet cells of the trachea are present as 12% of the epithelial cells. The intrapulmonary airways of the goose have not yet been examined histologically.

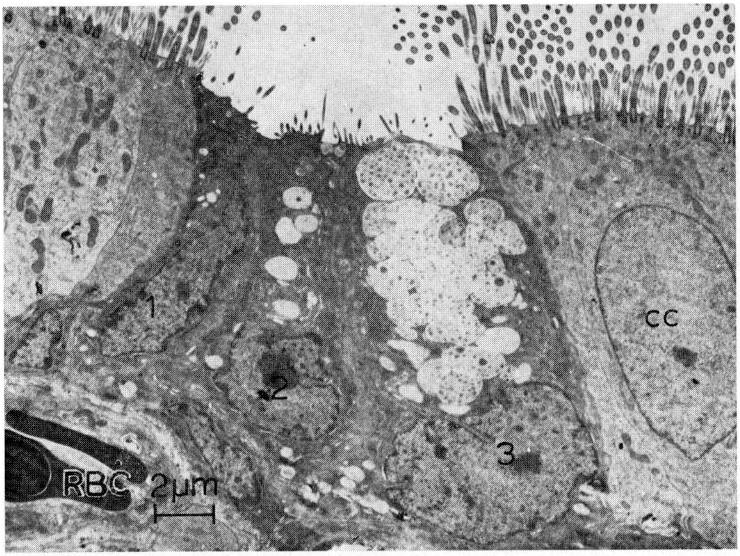

FIG. 3. Gosling tracheal epithelium showing goblet cells in various stages of synthesizing mucus (1, 2, & 3). A nucleated red blood cell (RBC) is seen in the lamina propria. Ciliated cell (cc). Glutaraldehyde and osmium tetroxide: uranyl acetate and lead citrate. × 4300

CONCENTRATION AND DISTRIBUTION OF GOBLET CELLS AND SUBMUCOSAL GLANDS

(1) Goblet cells

In the cat, the goblet cells of surface epithelium were abundant in all airways which had cartilage in their walls. This means that goblet cells were still frequently found deep in the lung, i.e. in bronchi of 0.5 mm in diameter. In nine normal cats, the mean number of goblet cells per high power field (i.e. per 0.44 mm length of epithelium) was 20, 34 and 29 in the trachea, hilum and distal airway respectively. Most of these cells were filled with secretion from apex to base (Fig. 4).

In the gosling trachea, goblet cells were distributed uniformly along its entire length, whereas in the adult they were often bunched together in shallow depressions as intraepithelial glands (Fig. 5). Goblet cells were numerous. In the gosling trachea, there were 20 goblet cells per 0.44 mm length of epithelium, 65% of the total number being full of secretion with the remaining 35% having secretion limited to their apices. The concentration of goblet cells in the trachea of both the goose and cat is therefore similar.

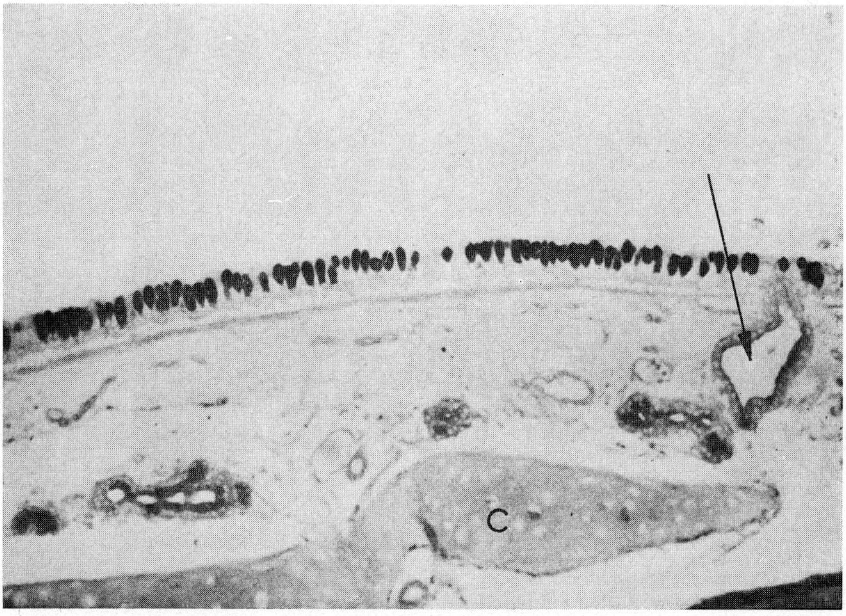

FIG. 4. Light microscopic appearance of tracheal epithelium stained with periodic acid-Schiff (PAS) for the carbohydrate component of mucus. Goblet cells are abundant and filled with intracellular secretion. Gland duct (arrow) and cartilage (c). × 130

(2) Submucosal glands

In the cat, submucosal glands occupied a significant proportion of the tracheal and hilar airway walls and submucosal glands were still found in the distal airway, albeit to a lesser extent. The Reid index, i.e. mean gland to wall ratio, in the tracheas of five 'conventional' cats was 0.75, and in four clean or 'specific pathogen-free' cats it was 0.65. Both values are considerably higher than 0.33, the value for normal adult man (Reid 1960). By point counting, Lamb (see Gallagher *et al.* 1975) has shown that the submucosal glands of the cat trachea form between 61 and 94% of the total secretory cell volume (i.e. goblet cells and glands) of which the greater part (up to 80%) is composed of serous cells.

HISTOCHEMISTRY

(1) Goblet cells

The histochemical characteristics of the goblet cells of the cat airway have

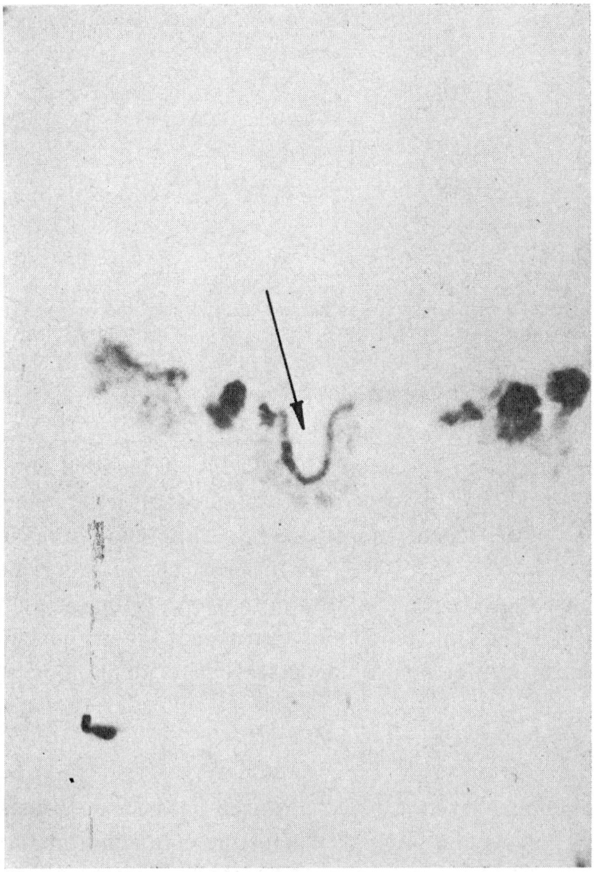

FIG. 5. Photomicrograph of goose epithelium to show shallow epithelial depressions in which goblet cells are grouped to form 'intraepithelial' glands (arrow). Alcian blue/PAS. × 650

been described qualitatively by Lamb (see Gallagher *et al.* 1975). The goblet cells contain mainly sulphated mucin but a proportion have sialomucin which is resistant to digestion by the enzyme sialidase (neuraminidase, EC 3.2.1.18). Some cells contain mixtures of sialomucin and sulphomucin.

In the goose trachea, a histochemical analysis of some 6000 goblet cells showed that, after they were stained with combined Alcian blue, pH 2.6/periodic acid Schiff (AB 2.6/PAS), most goblet cells stained blue—i.e. although both acid and neutral glycoproteins were present, the acid predominated and was present in more than 95% of goblet cells (Fig. 6). When the cells were stained with combined AB 1.0/PAS, more than 90% of goblet cells were

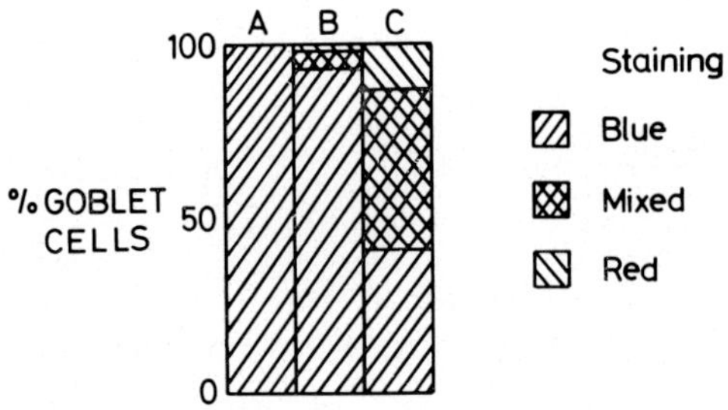

FIG. 6. The percentage of goblet cells in gosling epithelium staining either blue or red, or showing a mixture of these two colours after: (A) AB pH 2.6/PAS; (B) AB pH 1.0/PAS; (C) sialidase + AB pH 2.6/PAS.

shown to contain mucin with sulphate esters. Treatment of sections with sialidase demonstrated that 60% of goblet cells contained at least some sialomucin which was susceptible to enzyme digestion. After sialidase, AB stain was completely lost from only 10% of cells. In most cells, it was only the cell apex which retained the AB stain, indicating not only a mixture of sulphomucin and sialomucin in the same cell but also a tendency for sialomucin to be located in a supranuclear position beneath an 'apical cap' of sulphomucin.

(2) Surface 'mucosubstance'

In the airways of man and dog, a layer of 'mucosubstance' has been described which forms a surface layer along the luminal edge of the epithelium at the base of the cilia (Spicer *et al.* 1971). Histochemically, the mucosubstance is distinct from the intracellular mucin of neighbouring goblet cells, and also from the already secreted mucus that overlies the tips of cilia, in that it is a PAS-unreactive, sulphated mucosubstance with weak alcianophilia but with a strong affinity for aldehyde fuchsin and high iron diamine.

Such a surface layer of mucosubstance was also found in our studies of the cat and goose epithelia, and its appearance after various histochemical techniques is indicated in Table 2. From these results it would seem that the surface mucosubstances of cat and goose are similar to those of dog and man—i.e. PAS-unreactive yet sulphated.

At the ultrastructural level, a surface layer has also been demonstrated in the dog and rat (Spicer *et al.* 1973). When epithelia are stained with dialysed iron, the cilia, apical plasma membranes and (especially) the microvilli appear to be intimately coated by a layer of acid mucosubstance. Spicer *et al.* (1973) presume that the layer represents a non-motile component adherent to the

TABLE 2

Histochemistry of epithelial surface mucosubstance in the trachea

Stain[a]	*Species*	
	Cat	*Goose*
PAS alone	—[b]	?
AB2.6/PAS	+[c]	+ (slight)
AB1.0/PAS	+	+
AH/AB2.6/PAS	—	—
AH/AB1.0/PAS	?	+
Sialidase/AB2.6/PAS	+	+ (patchy)
AF/AB2.6	?	+ (AF)

[a] PAS = periodic acid-Schiff; AB = Alcian blue at given pH; AH = acid hydrolysis; AF = aldehyde fuchsin
[b] — unreactive; + reactive; ? untested
[c] not into ciliated duct of glands

cell, corresponding to the histochemically distinctive mucosubstance visible under the light microscope.

(3) Submucosal glands

In the cat submucosal glands, the mucous cells contain mainly mucin with sulphate esters. The histochemical results for serous cells are not clear but there are indications that they may also produce a sulphated glycoprotein (Gallagher *et al.* 1975).

AUTORADIOGRAPHY

We have recently studied, by autoradiography of tracheal sections, the uptake and incorporation into macromolecules of several radioactively labelled precursors of mucin (Table 3). The sections were taken from animals which earlier had had the radioactive precursor given directly into the tracheal lumen by a method described by Gallagher *et al.* (1975). Satisfactory labelling and localization was found after [^{3}H]glucose (0.1 mCi/ml), [^{35}S]sodium sulphate (0.25 mCi/ml) and [^{3}H]fucose (0.25 mCi/ml).

In the cat, [^{3}H]glucose was selectively taken up and incorporated into the surface mucosubstance, epithelial ciliated cells, submucosal glands and, rarely, the epithelial goblet cells, in that order of priority. [^{35}S]Sodium sulphate

TABLE 3

Uptake of mucin precursors by the tracheal mucosae of cat and goose

Labelled precursor	*Species/Site*[a]						
	Cat				*Goose*		
	Epithelium			*Glands*	*Epithelium*		
	SMS	*GC*	*Other*		*SMS*	*GC*	*Other*
[^{3}H]Glucose	++	—	+	+	—	+ (patchy)	+ (patchy)
[^{35}S]Sodium sulphate	+	—	+	++	+ (patchy)	+ (patchy)	+
[^{3}H]Fucose	—	—	+	+	?	?	?
[^{3}H]Glucosamine	—	—	—	—	—	—	—
[^{3}H]Leucine	?	?	?	?	—	+	++

[a]SMS = surface mucosubstance; GC = goblet cells; Other = mainly ciliated cells; + = equals AR grain concentration; — equals no AR grains.

showed a different pattern—submucosal glands took up the label most noticeably, and to a lesser extent so did the epithelial ciliated cells and surface mucosubstance. Once again the goblet cells were rarely labelled. [^{3}H]Fucose was taken up by epithelial ciliated cells and submucosal glands with a similar concentration of label in each; there was little incorporation of fucose into the surface mucosubstance. With the concentrations of precursors used here, by far the heaviest concentration of label found was in the surface mucosubstance after [^{3}H]glucose.

Unlike the cat, the epithelial goblet cells of the goose (and particularly those areas where goblet cells form intraepithelial glands) often incorporated both [^{3}H]glucose and [^{35}S]sodium sulphate. [^{3}H]Glucosamine, at the concentration used (0.25 mCi/ml), was not taken up well by either the goblet or the submucosal gland cells, in either the goose or the cat.

EXPERIMENTAL STUDIES

The application of these histological techniques to cat tracheal segments (see Gallagher *et al.* 1975) which have been stimulated to secrete mucus is just beginning, yet already there are some interesting preliminary findings.

(i) Tracheal segments taken for histology after either ammonia (1 part in 500) or tobacco smoke had been administered directly into the lumen of the segment have usually shown a marked decrease in goblet cell number (due to their discharge of intracellular mucin), with little observable effect on submucosal gland. For example, in a comparison made between part of the trachea (i.e. below the segment) not isolated for treatment and the ammonia-treated 'segment', the goblet cell number fell from a mean of 23.5 ± 2.2 per microscopic field to 1.6 ± 0.4 respectively. In another experiment, pilocarpine nitrate (a parasympathomimetic) was administered directly into the 'segment' at a concentration of 7 μg/ml. Histology showed that this had little effect on goblet cell number but submucosal glands were emptied of their intracellular secretion (Fig. 7).

(ii) In another experiment, *two* tracheal segments were isolated and each was labelled with [^{3}H]glucose. Ammonia was then administered into one of the segments, causing a marked increase in ^{3}H-labelled mucus recovered in the tracheal washings of that segment. Histology and autoradiography of sections from both the ammonia-treated and untreated segments showed that not only were goblet cells decreased in number in the ammonia-treated

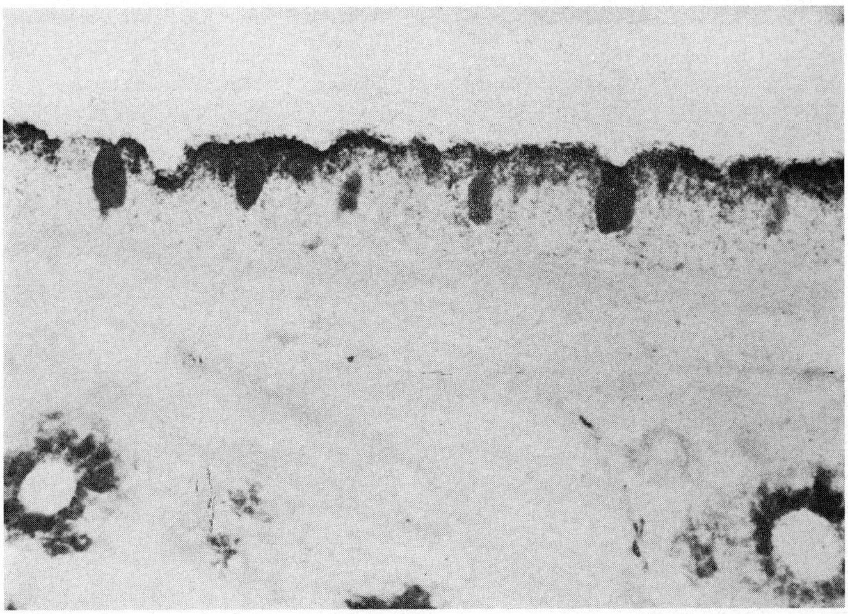

FIG. 7. Three photomicrographs of cat tracheal epithelia. In each case [^{3}H]glucose was incorporated into the tissue. After the experimental stimulus the tissue was then sectioned, prepared for autoradiography and stained with PAS:
(a) No stimulus (i.e. control) showing intracellular secretion within goblet and gland cells. The black line along the epithelial surface represents autoradiographic (AR) grains and hence localization of [^{3}H]glucose. $\times$ 300. Figs. 7*b* and 7*c*, see p. 16.

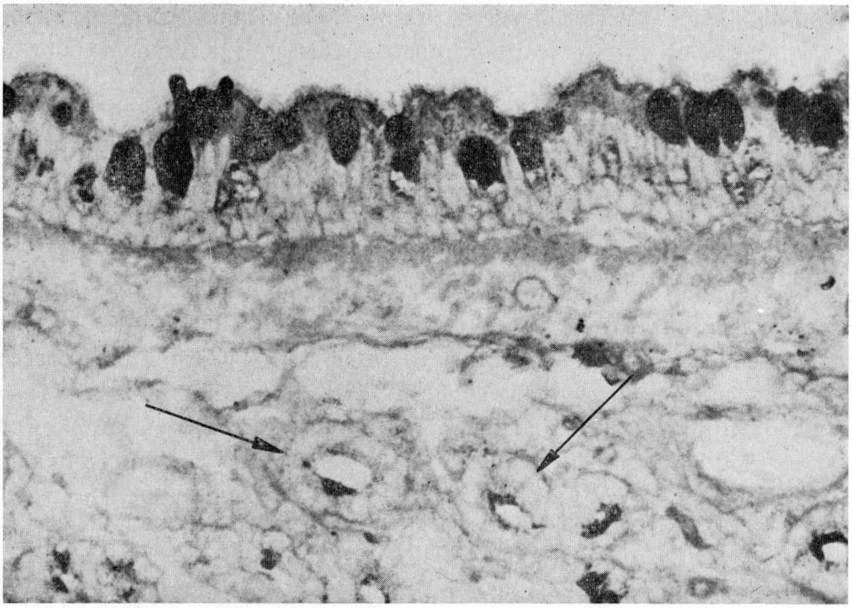

(b) After pilocarpine (into the airway lumen), there is discharge of mucus from submucosal gland acini (arrow), partial loss of surface mucosubstance, but no discharge of surface goblet cells. × 300

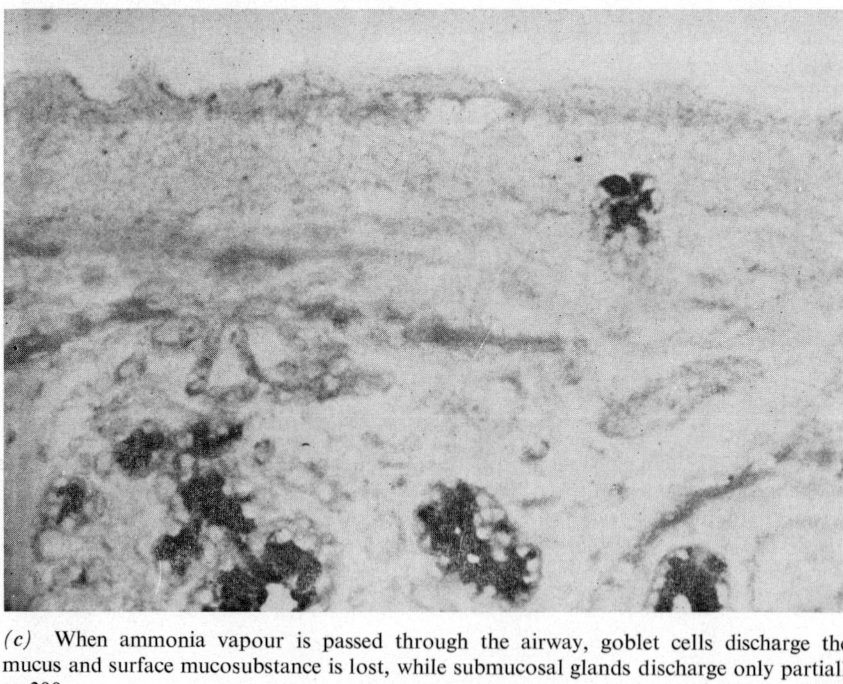

(c) When ammonia vapour is passed through the airway, goblet cells discharge their mucus and surface mucosubstance is lost, while submucosal glands discharge only partially. × 300

segment, but there was also a marked loss of labelled surface mucosubstance. This suggests that surface mucosubstance contributes to the increased ^{3}H-labelled mucus recovered from the segment treated with ammonia.

In a similar experiment where the stimulant for secretion was pilocarpine nitrate, the labelling of surface mucosubstance remained intact in spite of exhaustion of the submucosal glands by this parasympathomimetic drug.

SUMMARY AND CONCLUSIONS

(1) Species variation

It is clear from these and other histological studies that there is considerable inter-species variation in the mucus-producing cells of the respiratory tract.

In any airway, the number of goblet cells and the amount of gland varies. Notably the specific pathogen-free rat has a deficiency of goblet cells (less than 1% of cells are goblet) when compared to the cat, dog, goose and man (see Jeffery & Reid 1975). With regard to the amounts of submucosal glands cats have an abundance (by human criteria they would be considered bronchitic!), while the lack of submucosal glands in the goose makes it a useful animal for studies of pure epithelial secretion.

The variation in the electron microscopic appearance of the secretory granules of goblet cells suggests that there may be heterogeneity of glycoprotein composition both within a single secretory granule (e.g. goose) or between granules present in the same cell (e.g. cat). The latter suggestion is confirmed by the histochemical results.

Histochemically, the goblet cells of the cat, goose and dog are similar in that they contain a mucin with a predominance of sulphate esters. The normal rat differs in having goblet cells which in the main secrete a neutral glycoprotein (Jones *et al.* 1973). A surface mucosubstance has been demonstrated in the cat and goose which, histochemically, is similar to that described in the dog and human (Spicer *et al.* 1971). Far from being an integral and non-mobile part of the surface membrane of ciliated epithelial cells, it appears that the mucosubstance may be easily sloughed and may contribute to respiratory mucus.

(2) Structure and function

Histology may help to explain the results of some of the physiological experiments now in progress (Richardson *et al.*, this symposium, pp. 111–125), on the isolated, *in situ*, cat-tracheal preparation.

For example, in experiments where two radioactive precursors of mucin,

[^{35}S]sodium sulphate and [^{3}H]glucose, were given simultaneously into one tracheal segment, stimulation by pilocarpine nitrate resulted in an outflow of mucin which was heavily labelled with ^{35}S (with little ^{3}H), whereas when ammonia was given (after pilocarpine) a significantly higher proportion of the mucin was labelled with ^{3}H than with ^{35}S. Our histological and autoradiographic results suggest that, in the main, the ^{35}S-labelled mucin came from the epithelium and most probably from the layer of surface mucosubstance. The chemical analysis of each of these distinct fractions is now in progress.

Finally, after parasympathetic stimulation, secretion of mucus ensues. Histology shows that, although gland cells have discharged, surface goblet cells have not. Ultrastructural studies indicate why this may be so. With the electron microscope, the concentration and type of intraepithelial nerve fibre have been recently determined in airways of the cat (Das *et al.* 1977*a*). Although intraepithelial nerve fibres are often found, their lack of neurosecretory vesicles suggests that most are sensory in function. Examination of the cat submucosal gland, however, shows nerve fibres, each packed with neurosecretory vesicles (and therefore thought to be motor), lying adjacent to secretory (serous) cells. Furthermore, after unilateral infra-nodose vagotomy, most intraepithelial nerve fibres of the cat degenerate on the ipsilateral and vagotomized side (Das *et al.* 1977*b*). This procedure is designed to destroy vagal afferents selectively, leaving postganglionic parasympathetic motor fibres intact.

In the goose, where only surface goblet cells are present, stimulation of the peripheral cut ends of the descending oesophageal nerves causes a marked secretion of tracheal mucus; most of this response is cholinergically mediated since three-quarters of it is blocked by atropine (Phipps *et al.* 1977). Preliminary electron microscopic studies of gosling tracheal epithelium have shown that, unlike the cat, many intraepithelial nerve fibres of the goose contain an abundance of neurosecretory vesicles. In this regard, they resemble many of the nerve fibres found in the airway epithelium of the rat (Jeffery & Reid 1973). Clearly there is species variation in the nature and concentration of this epithelial innervation also.

ACKNOWLEDGEMENTS

I wish to acknowledge the technical assistance of Dr L. Al-Ugaily and Miss S. Barker and to thank Professor J. G. Widdicombe for the facilities made available to me.

The work presented here was funded in part by the Medical Research Council and by the Cystic Fibrosis Research Trust.

References

BASKERVILLE, A. (1970) Ultrastructure of the bronchial epithelium of the pig. *Zentralbl. Veterinärmed. A. 17*, 796–802

BREEZE, R. G., WHEELDON, E. B. & PIRIE, H. M. (1976) Cell structure and function in the mammalian lung: the trachea, bronchi and bronchioles. *Vet. Bull. 46*, 319–337

CHAKRIN, L. W. & SAUNDERS, L. Z. (1974) Experimental chronic bronchitis. Pathology in the dog. *Lab. Invest. 30*, 145–154

COVER, M. S. (1953) Gross and microscopic anatomy of the respiratory system of the turkey. II. The larynx, trachea, syrinx, bronchi and lungs. *Am. J. Res. 14*, 230–238

DAS, R. M., JEFFERY, P. K. & WIDDICOMBE, J. G. (1977*a*) The epithelial innervation of the lower respiratory tract of the cat. *J. Anat.*, in press

DAS, R. M., JEFFERY, P. K. & WIDDICOMBE, J. A. (1977*b*) Experimental degeneration of intra-epithelial nerve fibres in cat airways. *J. Anat.* in press.

FRASCA, J. M., AUERBACK, O., PARKS, V. R. & JAMIESON, J. D. (1968) Electron microscopic observations of the bronchial epithelium of dogs. I. Control dogs. *Exp. Mol. Pathol. 9*, 363–379

GALLAGHER, J. T., KENT, P. W., PASSATORE, M., PHIPPS, R. J. & RICHARDSON, P. S. (1975) The composition of tracheal mucus and the nervous control of its secretion in the cat. *Proc. R. Soc. Lond. B Biol. Sci. 192*, 49–76

JEFFERY, P. K. & DAS, R. M. (1977) Paper in preparation.

JEFFERY, P. K. & REID, L. (1973) Intra-epithelial nerves in normal rat airways: a quantitative electron microscopic study. *J. Anat. 114*, 35–45

JEFFERY, P. K. & REID, L. (1975) New observations of rat airway epithelium: a quantitative and electron microscopic study. *J. Anat. 120*, 295–320

JEFFERY, P. K. & REID, L. (1977) The respiratory mucous membrane, in *Respiratory Defense Mechanisms* (Brain, J. *et al.*, eds.) pp. 193–245, Dekker, New York

JONES, R., BOLDUC, P. & REID, L. (1973) Goblet cell glycoprotein and tracheal gland hypertrophy in rat airways: the effect of tobacco smoke with or without the anti-inflammatory agent phenylmethyloxadiazole. *Br. J. Exp. Pathol. 54*, 229–239

JONES, R., BASKERVILLE, A. & REID, L. (1975) Histochemical identification of glycoproteins in pig bronchial epithelium. (a) Normal (b) Hypertrophied from enzootic pneumonia. *J. Pathol. 116*, 1–11

MCCARTHY, C. & REID, L. (1964) Intracellular mucopolysaccharides in the normal human bronchial tree. *Q. J. Exp. Physiol. Cogn. Med. Sci. 49*, 85–94

PHIPPS, R. J., RICHARDSON, P. S., CORFIELD, A., GALLAGHER, J. T., JEFFERY, P. K., KENT, P. W. & PASSATORE, M. (1977) A physiological, biochemical and histological study of goose tracheal mucin and its secretion. *Proc. R. Soc. Lond. B Biol. Sci. 279*, 513–543

PURCELL, D. A. (1971) The ultrastructure of tracheal epithelium in the fowl. *Res. Vet. Sci. 12*, 327–329

REID, L. (1954) Pathology of chronic bronchitis. *Lancet 1*, 275–279

REID, L. (1960) Measurement of the bronchial mucous gland layer: a diagnostic yardstick in chronic bronchitis. *Thorax 15*, 132–141

REID, L. (1963) An experimental study of hypersecretion of mucus in the bronchial tree. *Br. J. Exp. Pathol. 44*, 437–445

RHODIN, J. (1966) Ultrastructure and function of the human tracheal mucosa. *Am. Rev. Respir. Dis. 93*, 1–15

RICHARDSON, P. S., PHIPPS, R. J., BALFRE, K. & HALL, R. L. (1978) The roles of mediators, irritants and allergens in causing mucin secretion from the trachea, in this volume, pp. 111–126

SPICER, S. S., CHAKRIN, L. W., WARDELL, J. R. Jr. & KENDRICK, W. (1971) Histochemistry of mucosubstances in the canine and human respiratory tract. *Lab. Invest. 25*, 483

Spicer, S. S., Chakrin, L. W. & Wardell, J. R. Jr. (1973) Respiratory mucous secretion, in *Sputum. Fundamentals and Clinical Pathology* (Dulfano, M. J., ed.), pp. 22–68, Thomas, Springfield, Ill.

Walsh, C. & McLelland, J. (1974) The ultrastructure of the avian extrapulmonary respiratory epithelium. *Acta Anat. 89*, 412–422

Discussion

Guz: What is the chemical basis for staining with substances like Alcian blue?

Jeffery: There is a lot of controversy about this dye but most will agree that Alcian blue stains acid glycoprotein and, in particular at pH 2.6, it stains weakly acidic groups. This is said to be by salt linkage to the acid groupings. It has been shown by a number of workers, e.g. Jones & Reid (1973*a*), that if one reduces the pH of the Alcian blue the staining becomes more specific for sulphated groups.

Guz: Are we talking about chemicals—in a test tube—or biological material?

R. Jones: We have looked at Alcian blue staining of epithelial glycoproteins in tissue. It is a very specific dye for these groups provided that the pH level of the staining solution is controlled (Jones & Reid 1973*a*, *b*). Quite a lot is known about the mechanism of its staining from the work of Dr John Scott and his colleagues (Scott *et al.* 1964, 1968; Quintarelli *et al.* 1964*a*, *b*). Their studies included *in vitro* work but they have also looked at the interaction of the dye and tissue groups. It is essentially a positive/negative charge attraction between polyanions in the tissue and cations in the dye.

Jeffery: One can compare the affinity of tissue for Alcian blue with two other techniques as well; for example, with the staining of cells with aldehyde fuchsin and especially with the uptake of radioactive sulphate by these same cells. There has been quite good correlation, but not 100% correlation, with the uptake of sulphate and the affinity for sulphate-specific stains of these cells.

R. Jones: But in fact very little is known about the way other dyes for sulphate groups, such as aldehyde fuchsin and high iron diamine, stain tissue—unlike Alcian blue, about which relatively speaking a good deal is known.

Silberberg: Could you indicate the nature of the electron-dense stain that was used in the electron micrographs? What does it indicate in terms of the chemistry?

Jeffery: It is glutaraldehyde and osmium tetroxide double fixation. It is the glutaraldehyde, coupled with uranyl acetate and lead citrate (which are the heavy metal stains used in these preparations), that imparts the electron-density to the serous cell granule. As the granules are not electron-dense after osmium alone, these results indicate a high protein content in the electron-dense areas and a lesser concentration of protein in those areas which are electron-lucent. But again this is empirical—little is known about the way in which these chemicals work.

Thurlbeck: Could you say something about the way in which cells in the epithelium can transform themselves from one to another, or the way a precursor cell differentiates in one particular way? Could you also comment on the work by Evans *et al.* (1976) which suggests that the non-ciliated (Clara) cell is the progenitor cell in the peripheral airways?

Jeffery: All I have are the results of recent experiments (Jeffery *et al.* 1976) on these airways using either tobacco smoke or sulphur dioxide, where one observes an increase in the number of goblet cells proximally or in the distal airways, respectively. When these animals are examined one finds, morphologically, transitional stages between the serous and the goblet cell and between the Clara and the goblet cell. The only trouble is that, as electron micrographs are 'still' pictures, one can arrange the sequence of cellular events involved in this transition in any order one chooses. What we are now trying to do is to put in tritiated thymidine to label the DNA and to follow this cell transformation sequentially to see which cell type is the stem cell in each case. I think there is already quite good evidence, from electron microscopy, that the serous cell can transform into a goblet cell and that a Clara cell can do so too (Jeffery 1973). It could well be that the Clara cell is a progenitor cell—indeed it is nice to think that the Clara cell may have another role than that of producing surfactant.

Richardson: I'd like to go back to the appearance of the granules in the serous and mucous cells on the electron micrographs. There seems to be quite a lot of difference in the kind of granules that you find even within one cell. In the serous cell, for instance, some are grey and some are almost black. Is this because the darker granules contain a lot of protein and little water and the lighter ones a lot of water and much less protein?

Jeffery: Possibly. Working on the hypothesis that it is the protein content that gives the electron density, I would say that the protein content does vary with the electron density of the granule. In some cells one finds, after irritation for example, that the granules change on their own and acquire an electron-lucent halo with a centrally located dense core, indicating that these granules can alter their morphology in respect to a given stimulus; enzyme systems may be adding extra end-groupings to the protein and altering the type of glycoprotein even at this late stage of synthesis.

Reid: Using density gradient ultracentrifugation one epithelial glycoprotein is recovered that is homogeneous but polydisperse, as one would expect for a molecule of such high molecular weight. Yet within the cell we found great variety in staining characteristics. This means that something is happening outside the cell to 'polymerize' the sort of material that we have been talking about.

There are two different types of cell—the serous and the mucous. In the serous cell the individual granule is surrounded by an intact membrane and secretes mucus continuously. In the mucous cell the granules 'fuse' and it may be that the contents of the granules in some way fuse even within the cell. In organ culture, using the radioactive precursors, and from histochemical methods, we find that serous cell and mucous cell granules have the same range of uptake of staining and precursors but the proportions are slightly different. Perhaps the most important difference we have found between serous and mucous cells is that, although the glycoprotein type is similar, the serous cells have a lower concentration of glycoproteins in the granules. This observation is based on the specific activity of our granules as judged electron microscopically by Dr Meyrick and carefully quantified (Meyrick & Reid 1975; Reid *et al.* 1976).

Nadel: Can you tell us something about the morphology of the microvilli? Are there any structures concentrated along them, and do they change physiologically when you manipulate them in various ways?

Jeffery: The microvilli on the ciliated cells are quite distinct. They are much longer than the microvilli on the goblet cells. The goblet cell—the secretory cell—has very few microvilli indeed and they are very short. On the ciliated cell they are about 2 μm long and about 0.2 μm wide, and they are very numerous. As to changes in function, the only thing I noticed was that their length increased after chronic exposure to tobacco smoke. I am not sure what one can conclude from this but it certainly seems that they are active structures. They are there for something, either to reabsorb fluid from the periciliary layer, or perhaps to provide a surface mucosubstance which may be a very real and important constituent of the epithelial surface.

J. G. Jones: A number of groups have reported on the differences in regional clearance of various labelled markers. You mentioned the distribution of goblet cells at different airway levels, Dr Jeffery. Could you say something more about regional differences in numbers of goblet cells, mucous cells and microvilli in airways of different sizes? Is there any anatomical reason why small airways should clear less rapidly than larger airways?

Jeffery: The specific pathogen-free rat has very few goblet cells and goblet cells are certainly absent from airways smaller than 0.4 mm in diameter. The submucosal gland is limited to the cranial aspect of the trachea. In the cat there is an abundance of goblet cells. Their number increases distally and they are very abundant in the small distal airways of 0.5 mm in diameter. It is also true to say that, as in the human, the gland is found in any airway where there is cartilage and in the cat the cartilage extends deep into the lung into very small airways. The cat seems to have an abundance of mucus-secreting tissue.

J. G. Jones: Is the upper part of the trachea a good place to get a representative sample of the whole airway?

Jeffery: We compared the numbers of goblet cells and the amount of gland in the upper and lower aspects of the trachea by using the Reid index (Reid 1960) and found that they were similar.

References

EVANS, M. J., JOHNSON, L. V., STEPHENS, R. J. & FREEMAN, G. (1976) Renewal of terminal bronchiolar epithelium in the rat following exposure to $NO_2 + O_3$. *Lab. Invest. 35*, 246–257

JEFFERY, P. K. (1973) Goblet cell increase in rat bronchial epithelium following irritation and drug administration: an experimental and electron microscopic study. Ph. D. Thesis, University of London

JEFFERY, P. K., REID, L. & WIDDICOMBE, J. G. (1976) Anatomical and physiological features of irritation of the bronchial tree, in *Air Pollution and the Lung* (Aharonson, E. F. *et al.*, eds.), pp. 253–267, Wiley, Chichester.

JONES, R. & REID, L. (1973*a*) The effect of pH on Alcian blue staining of epithelial acid glycoproteins. I. Sialomucins and sulphomucins (singly or in simple combinations). *Histochem. J. 5*, 9–18

JONES, R. & REID, L. (1973*b*) The effect of pH on Alcian blue staining of epithelial acid glycoproteins. II. Human bronchial submucosal gland. *Histochem. J. 5*, 19–27

MEYRICK, B. & REID, L. (1975) *In vitro* incorporation of H^3-threonine and H^3-glucose by the mucous and serous cells of the human bronchial submucosal gland; a quantitative electron microscopic study. *J. Cell Biol. 67*, 320–344

QUINTARELLI, G., SCOTT, J. E. & DELLOVO, M. C. (1964*a*) The chemical and histochemical properties of Alcian blue. II. Dye binding of tissue polyanions. *Histochemie 4*, 86–98

QUINTARELLI, G., SCOTT, J. E. & DELLOVO, M. C. (1964*b*) The chemical and histochemical properties of Alcian blue. III. Chemical blocking and unblocking. *Histochemie 4*, 99–112

REID, L. (1960) Measurement of the bronchial mucous gland layer: a diagnostic yardstick in chronic bronchitis. *Thorax 15*, 132–141

REID, L., MEYRICK, B. & COLES, S. (1976) Glycoprotein synthetic pathways in, and drug effects on, the human bronchial mucosa *in vitro*, in *Organ Culture in Biomedical Research* (Balls, M. & Monnickendam, M., eds.) *(Br. Soc. Cell Biol. Symp. 1)*, pp. 463–480, Cambridge University Press, London

SCOTT, J. E., QUINTARELLI, G. & DELLOVO, M. C. (1964) The chemical and histochemical properties of Alcian blue. I. The mechanism of Alcian blue staining. *Histochemie 4*, 73–85

SCOTT, J. E., DORLING, J. & STOCKWELL, R. A. (1968) Reversal of protein blocking of basophilia in salt solutions: implications on the localisation of polyanions using Alcian blue. *J. Histochem. Cytochem. 16*, 383–386

Site of synthesis, intracellular transport and secretion of glycoprotein in exocrine cells

M. F. KRAMER, J. J. GEUZE and G. J. A. M. STROUS

Department of Histology and Cell Biology, and Centre for Electron Microscopy, Medical School, University of Utrecht, The Netherlands

Abstract The site of attachment of the first sugar, *N*-acetylgalactosamine, to the seryl and threonyl residues of the protein chain is unknown in exocrine cells. The subsequent sugars of the carbohydrate side chains, galactose and *N*-acetylglucosamine alternately, and the end-group sugars, galactose, *N*-acetylgalactosamine and fucose, are attached in the Golgi complex. Sulphate too is attached in that structure. In the stomach, sulphate is probably transferred in the most mature cisterna of the Golgi stacks, galactose and fucose in other cisternae, suggesting a gradient in transferase activities along the stack. The possibilities of regulating the amount and relative sugar composition of the glycoproteins are discussed. The secretory product is stored in granules. Their polygonal, large and swollen appearance and complex formation by loss of bordering membranes, as observed in many kinds of glycoprotein-secreting cells ('mucous cells') might be caused by ineffective fixation techniques. Direct vascular perfusion results in a picture no different from what is found in non-mucous cells. Whether secretion is merely exocytotic, as in non-mucous cells, or whether it is accompanied by a loss of membrane and even cytoplasm needs thorough investigation, with the effects of various fixation techniques being compared.

SYNTHESIS, TRANSPORT AND COMPOSITION OF EPITHELIAL GLYCOPROTEINS

The site of synthesis of the protein moiety of secretory glycoproteins of epithelial cells is presumed to be no different from that of pure secretory proteins. In fact autoradiographic studies show that the area of the rough endoplasmic reticulum (RER) has the highest amount of radioactivity shortly after administration of radioactive amino acid to the glycoprotein-secreting cells of the Brunner gland (Rohr *et al.* 1967), bronchial mucous glands (Meyrick & Reid 1975), and the gastric surface of the rat (Kramer & Geuze 1977). The transport route of the protein moiety in these cells also does not differ from that described for the guinea-pig pancreas by Jamieson & Palade

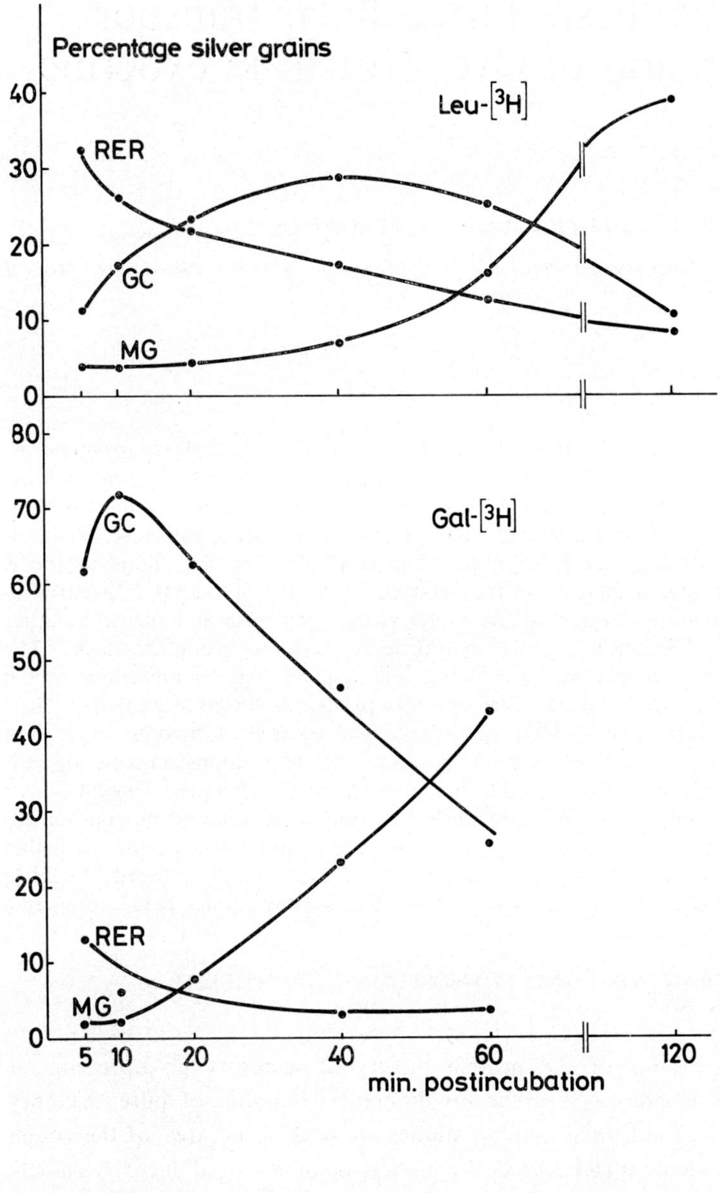

FIG. 1. Relative silver grain distribution over rough endoplasmic reticulum (RER), Golgi complex (GC) and mucous granules (MG) in electron microscope autoradiographs of surface mucous cells of the rat stomach, at various intervals after administration of [^{3}H]leucine or [^{3}H]galactose for 3 min *in vitro*.

(1967*a*, *b*), though the rate of transport appeared to be rather slow (Fig. 1).

Carbohydrates and sulphate are attached to the protein during its passage through the Golgi area, although it is believed that the first sugar of each carbohydrate side chain has already been attached to the seryl or threonyl residues of the protein main chain during its elongation and entrance into the cisternal space of the RER. However, there is no evidence for such an early attachment of the first sugar for secretory glycoproteins of epithelial origin. The evidence that the Golgi elements are the main site of sugar and sulphate attachment is based on autoradiographic demonstration of a high amount of radioactivity in the Golgi area shortly after administration of radioactive sugars or sulphate to glycoprotein-secreting cells (Neutra & Leblond 1966; Schmalbeck & Rohr 1967; Meyrick & Reid 1975; Kramer & Geuze 1977; Berg & Austin 1976). Moreover, the activities of glycosyltransferases are highest in subcellular fractions with characteristics of Golgi elements. These fractions consist of smooth microsomes with relatively low densities, lacking the enzyme activities characteristic of the plasma membrane. They show flat cisternae with swollen parts at their perimeter, sometimes still packed into stacks after special fractionation procedures.

In our study of the gastric surface cells, galactosyl and fucosyl transferase were found in a smooth microsomal fraction with density 1.11 g/ml, while sulphate transferase was found mainly in a fraction with a lower density (Fig. 2). Thiamine pyrophosphatase was also found in the lower density fraction. That enzyme is cytochemically demonstrated in the most mature *(trans)* cisterna of the Golgi stacks in the gastric surface cells (Fig. 3) and in many other cell types (Novikoff 1976). This suggests that the glycosyl transferases are located in elements of the immature *(cis)* side of the Golgi complex and the sulphate transferase, catalysing the last step in glycoprotein synthesis, in the most mature elements. Since transferase activity is found in the Golgi fractions even in the absence of exogenous acceptor molecules, endogenous substrate (probably the nascent glycoproteins) apparently passes along the membrane-bound transferases of the Golgi compartment. The presence of substrate and transferases in the immature elements confirms the results of cytochemical carbohydrate staining of ultrathin sections of Brunner gland and goblet cells, which show positive staining in the small vesicles of the Golgi periphery and in the first cisternae of the Golgi stacks (Thiéry 1969). In many cell types, the intensity of the carbohydrate staining increases from the first to the last cisternae (Fig. 4) (Rambourg *et al.* 1969; Wattel *et al.* 1977) as a result of either a continuous elongation of the carbohydrate chains, or a further concentration of the completed glycoproteins during their passage through the Golgi cisternae.

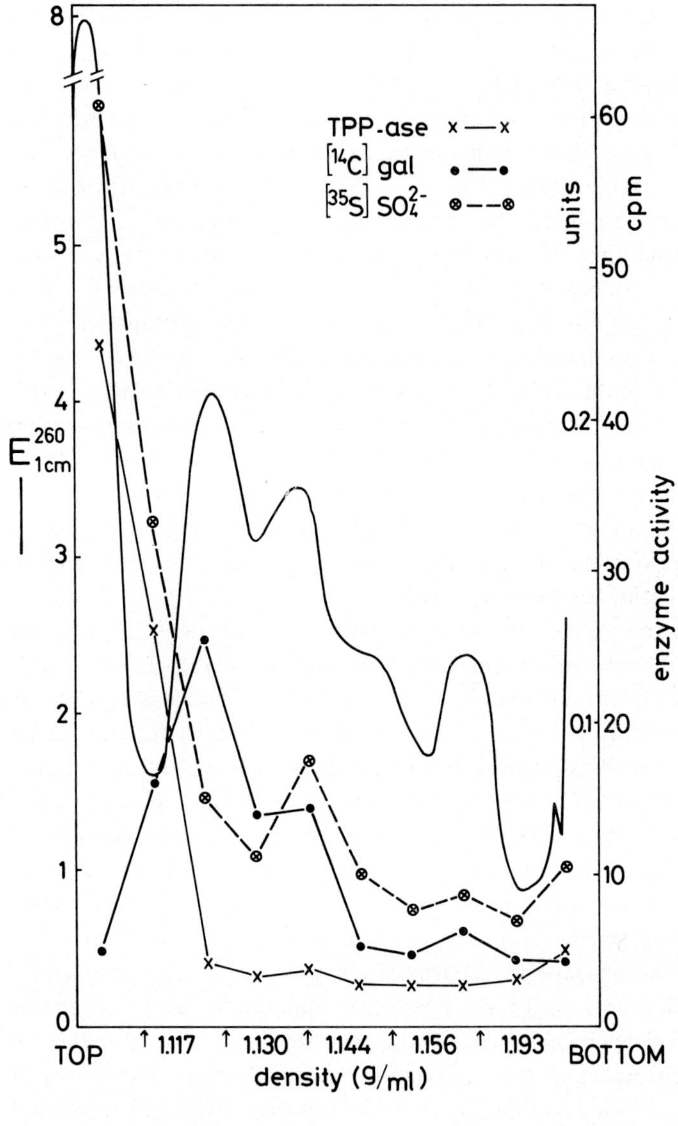

FIG. 2. Enzyme activities in smooth microsome fractions from rat gastric surface homogenate in a discontinuous sucrose gradient. E, extinction of the gradient at 260 nm; TPPase, thiamine pyrophosphatase activity in units; [^{14}C]gal, incorporation into exogenous acceptor from UDP-[^{14}C]galactose; [^{35}S]SO_4^{2-}, incorporation into endogenous acceptor from 3′-phosphoadenosine 5′-phosphosulphate-$^{35}SO_4$. The incorporation of [^{14}C]fucose parallels that of [^{14}C]galactose; inosine diphosphatase (IDPase) shows the same distribution as TPPase.

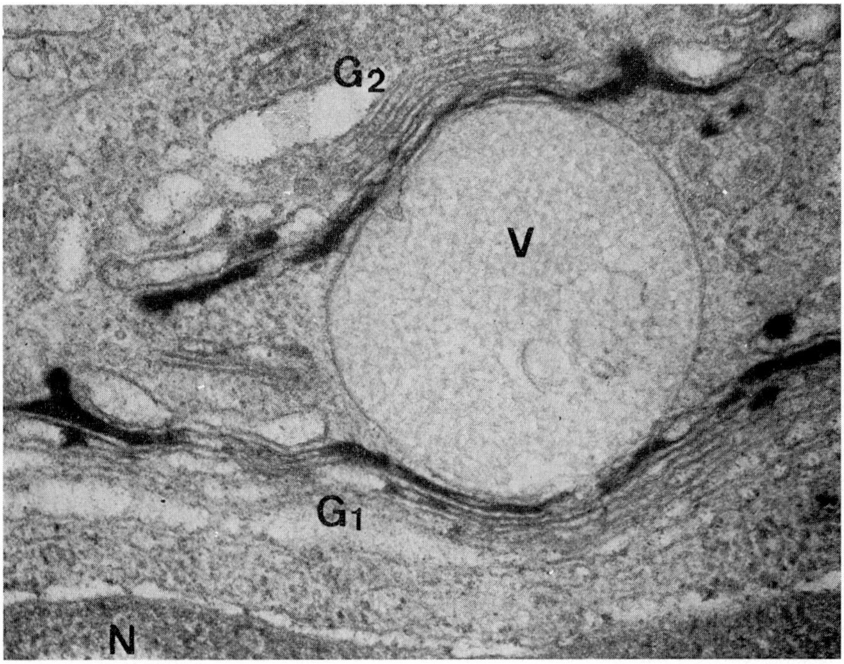

FIG. 3. Surface mucous cells, showing TPPase activity in the two most mature cisternae of the Golgi stacks (G_1, G_2). IDPase activity is found at the same sites. N, nucleus; V, condensing vacuole. Immersion fixation in glutaraldehyde (2%) and formaldehyde (2%) in 0.1 M-cacodylate buffer at pH 7.4. ×61 600

Once supplied with their sugar and sulphate moieties, the glycoproteins leave the Golgi stacks inside detaching vacuoles. The carbohydrate content of these vacuoles, and the secretory granules into which they transform, is shown cytochemically to be still increasing. Since these structures are not radioactive shortly after radioactive sugar administration, their increasing stainability reflects a further concentration of the glycoproteins at the onset of their rather long storage phase.

The secretory granules of glycoprotein-secreting cell types vary greatly in ultrastructure. Some glycoprotein-secreting cells show globular granules, limited by a continuous membrane surrounding a rather compact mass of secretory product, for example the surface cells of the stomach (Kramer & Geuze 1977; Wattel *et al.* 1977) (Fig. 5), the granular duct cells of the submandibular gland of rat and mouse (Cutler & Chaudhry 1973), and the acinar cells of the parotid gland (Castle *et al.* 1972). In many other cell types the granules have a quite different appearance. They are not globular but

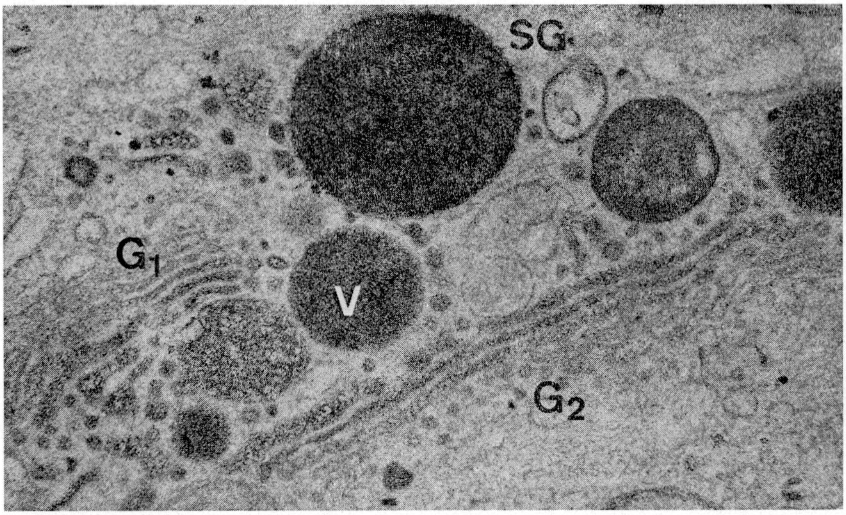

FIG. 4. Surface mucous cell, showing glycoproteins in the Golgi complexes (G_1, G_2). The staining intensity of the cisternae increases from the immature to the mature side of the stacks. Stained vesicles (or cross-sectioned tubules) are present at both sides of the stacks. Condensing vacuoles (V) and secretory granules (SG) show a further increase in stainability. Immersion fixation in glutaraldehyde (2%), formaldehyde (2%) in 0.1 M-phosphate buffer at pH 7.4, and postfixation in OsO_4 (1%) in Veronal acetate buffer of pH 6.9. Staining according to Thiéry (1967). × 24 000

polygonal, large and swollen structures, that contact and deform each other over large areas, leaving little space for the cytoplasmic matrix. The limiting membranes of neighbouring granules may even fuse and show discontinuities along the fusion sites, resulting in the formation of rather large complexes of granules. Their contents form a loose felt of fibrils or a flocculent mass. Often its density and stainability vary greatly, even between granules within one cell. Cells that show this kind of granule belong to what used, in light microscopy, to be called the mucous cell type. The mere presence of glycoproteins in the secretory granules is not a criterion for this cell type, because typical serous cells like those of the parotid and even the pancreatic gland may have glycoproteins in their granules, stainable by techniques for cytochemical detection of carbohydrates. Apart from the ultrastructure of their secretory granules, mucous cells have also a relatively small amount of rough endoplasmic reticulum, relatively low rates of protein synthesis, and a more or less flat nucleus near the basal plasma membrane. To this cell type belong human labial gland cells (Tandler *et al.* 1969), acinar cells of mammalian submandibular glands (Radley 1969; Dorey & Bhoola 1972; Bogart 1975;

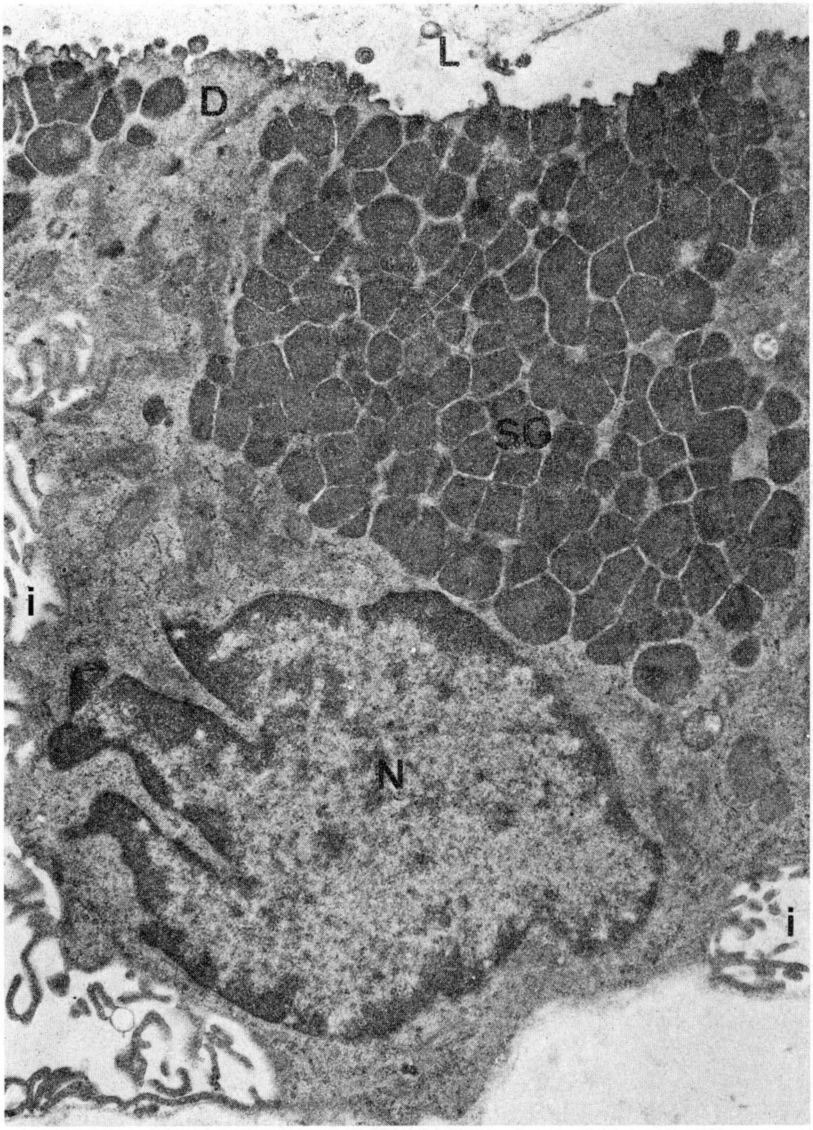

FIG. 5. Surface mucous cell, showing well-defined, darkly stained, individual secretory granules (SG) filling the apical part of the cell. N, nucleus; i, intercellular space with long slender microvilli; D, junctions between adjacent cells next to the gastric lumen (L). Immersion fixation in glutaraldehyde (1 %), formaldehyde (1 %), sucrose (1 %) in 0.1 M-phosphate buffer of pH 7.4, and postfixed as mentioned for Fig. 4. × 10 000

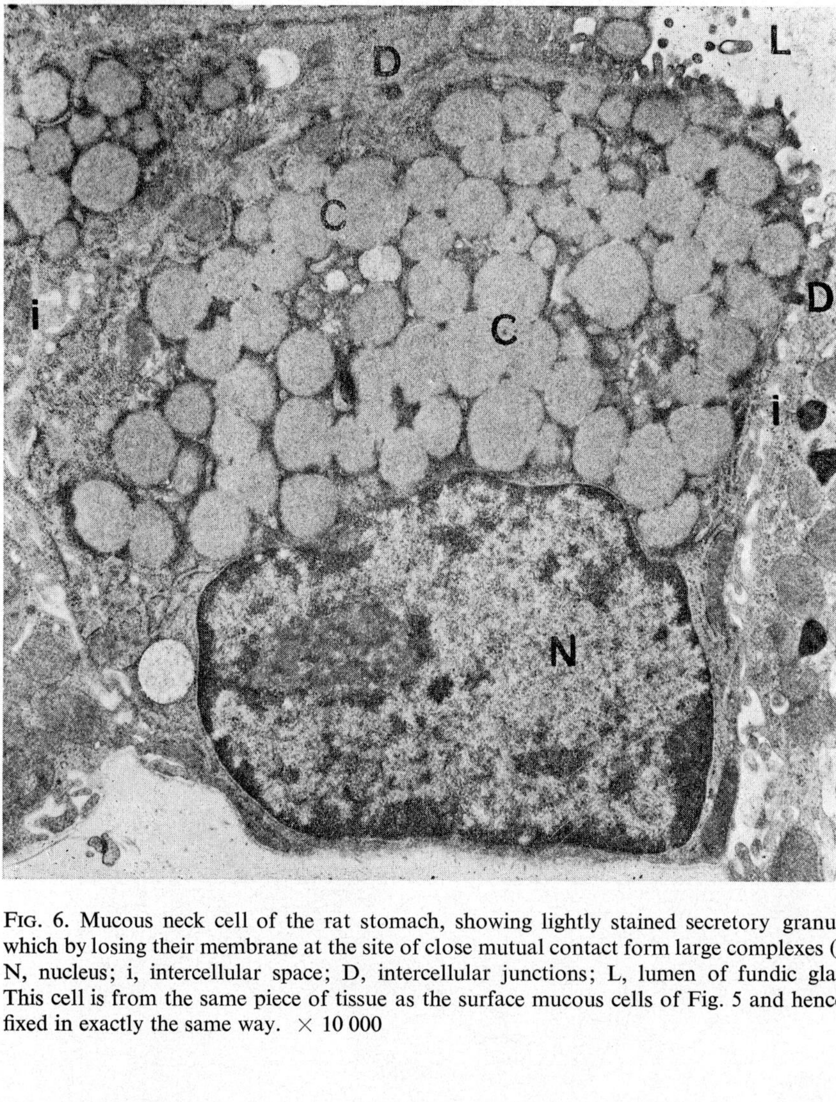

FIG. 6. Mucous neck cell of the rat stomach, showing lightly stained secretory granules, which by losing their membrane at the site of close mutual contact form large complexes (C). N, nucleus; i, intercellular space; D, intercellular junctions; L, lumen of fundic gland. This cell is from the same piece of tissue as the surface mucous cells of Fig. 5 and hence is fixed in exactly the same way. × 10 000

Tandler & Poulsen 1976), mucous cells of the rat sublingual gland (Kim *et al.* 1972), mucous neck cells of the rat stomach (Wattel *et al.* 1977) (Fig. 6), Brunner gland cells of the mouse (Rohr *et al.* 1967), goblet cells of the intestine (Neutra & Leblond 1966; Freeman 1966), mucous gland cells of the human bronchus (Meyrick & Reid 1975), epithelial cells of the human endocervix (Nilsson & Westman 1961), and bulbourethral gland cells of the rat (Geuze & Slot 1976) (Fig. 7).

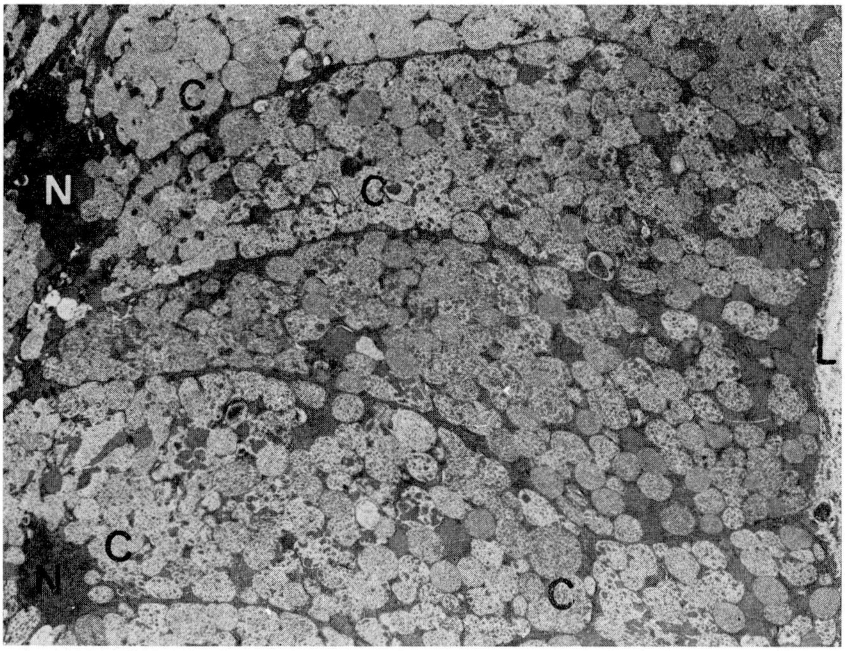

FIG. 7. Cells of the bulbourethral gland of the rat, showing dark nuclei (N) with irregular outline (shrunk by dehydration?) at their base, and numerous secretory granules filling the large apical part of the cell. The granules vary in stainability and form complexes (C). Complexing granules show a light and inhomogeneous content and are larger (swollen by hydration?). L, lumen of the gland. Immersion fixation as mentioned for Fig. 4. × 3900

The loose contents, the varying density and stainability, the large polygonal shape, the frequent membrane fusions, and the formation of complexes between the granules of mucous cells have often been said to be artifacts resulting from bad fixation. In labial mucous cells the granules had a darker and less swollen appearance after aldehyde and OsO_4 fixation than after OsO_4 fixation alone (Tandler *et al.* 1969). According to Martinez-Hernandez *et al.* (1972), fixation by direct (within 2 min) vascular perfusion alone prevents swelling and complex formation by the granules of the acinar cells of the mouse submandibular gland. However, Kim *et al.* (1972) found large polygonal granules and complexes in the same cells of the rat after vascular perfusion with aldehyde fixatives, while Tandler & Poulsen (1976) did not find complexes after fixation by immersion in aldehydes!

Our experience confirms the results of Martinez-Hernandez *et al.* (1972): after direct perfusion with aldehydes the cells of the bulbourethral gland

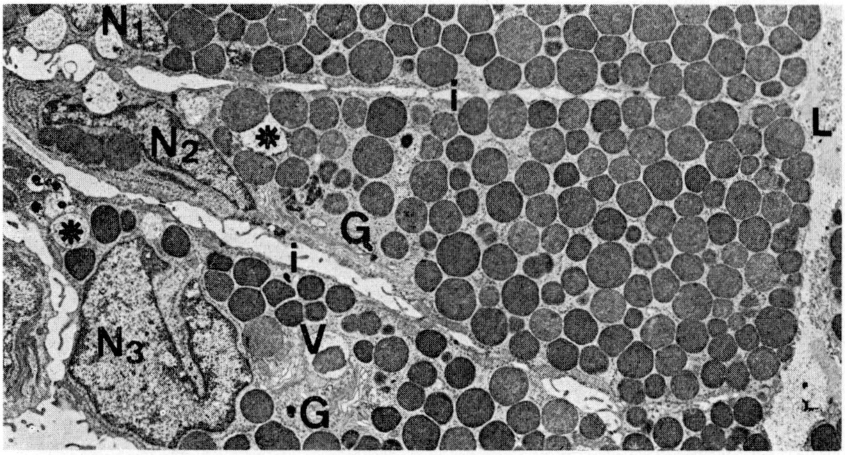

FIG. 8. Bulbourethral gland cells, fixed by direct vascular perfusion, showing normal nuclei (N), and secretory granules with darkly stained, homogeneous content that do not form complexes. Some granules (★) are inflated and have a lighter appearance (hydration during fixation?). G, Golgi complex; V, condensing vacuole; L, lumen of the gland; i, intercellular space with long, slender microvilli. Perfusion with glutaraldehyde (1%) and formaldehyde (1%) in 0.1 M-phosphate buffer of pH 7.4 through the aorta of the anaesthetized rat, breathing 95% O_2 and 5% CO_2. Postfixed as mentioned for Fig. 4. × 4000

show compact, globular, non-complexing granules (Fig. 8), while a vascular wash for some minutes with Tyrode solution to remove the mass of plasma proteins and the blood cells results in swollen granules with great variation in density and stainability and in the formation of many large complexes (Fig. 7). The great susceptibility of the mucous granules to even a short delay in fixation is clearly illustrated by Fig. 9, which shows badly fixed granules around a capillary plugged by erythrocytes, while the granules are well-preserved in cells near an empty capillary.

As to the cause of this high sensitivity we can only speculate. Radley (1969) suggests the presence of a membranolytic substance in the granule. Another explanation might be the membrane's great need of energy to prevent the net influx of ions and water. If, in the mucous granules, much water is bound to the glycoprotein molecules, the amount of free water is rather small and hence a small influx of ions is sufficient to increase the molality of these granules, resulting in swelling and even rupture of the granules. During the interval between the stopping of circulation and the arrival of the fixative in the cell, the amount of ATP might decrease below a value critical to ion transport in the granule membrane. A third possibility is that energy might be necessary to prevent membrane fusion and disintegration. The access of

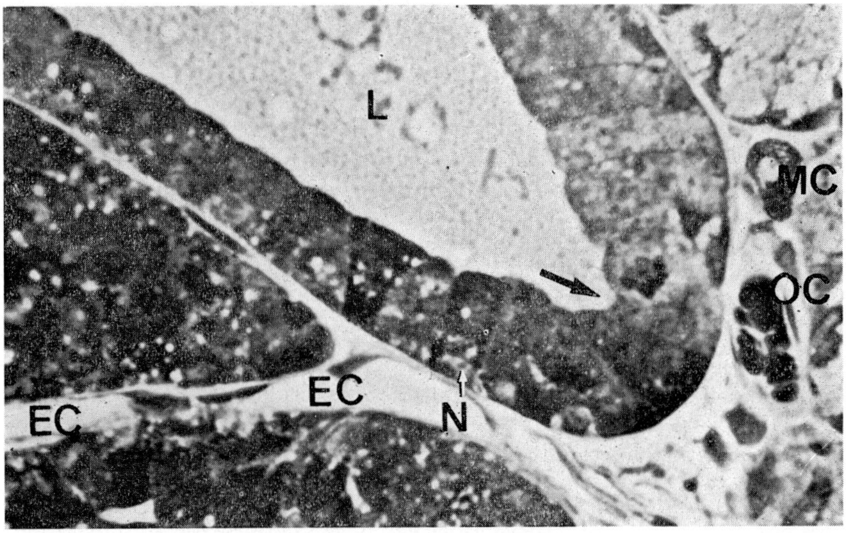

FIG. 9. Bulbourethral gland cells, showing empty capillaries (EC) and a capillary in which the passage is obstructed by erythrocytes (OC). The secretory granules are well-defined and stain deeply with methylene blue (1 %) in cells close to the empty capillaries, while around the obstructed vessel they have lost individuality and stainability. The black arrow indicates the boundary between the areas of good and bad preservation. N, nucleus of epithelial cell; L, lumen of the gland; MC, well-fixed mast cell. Perfusion fixation as described for Fig. 8. × 750

ATP along the narrow rims of cytoplasm to the membranes of the mucous granules might be more impeded than in serous cells where experimental lack of energy has been found to promote membrane fusion and exocytosis (Bauduin *et al.* 1969). Finally the drop in oxygen supply might lead to a disturbance in the Ca^{2+} movements in the cell, resulting in fusions of membranes or changes in membrane pump activities.

If the mucous granules are swollen and form complexes, the densities and stainabilities of the granule content may show great differences. This suggests that, as a result of membrane lysis, glycoproteins leave the granules and stream into the lumen through a series of intergranular openings (see Kim *et al.* 1972; Meyrick & Reid 1975) (Fig. 7). Since fixation of glycoproteins with many branched carbohydrate side chains might be rather ineffective, a loss of these molecules through the membrane discontinuities is conceivable even when the other structures of the cell are well fixed. Studies of glycoprotein transport with a radioactive pulse and a subsequent chase may lead to false conclusions for such cells, unless the loss of labelled glycoprotein by ineffective fixation can be excluded.

The final product of glycoprotein-secreting epithelial cells contains a relatively high amount of seryl and threonyl residues, a carbohydrate moiety with mainly *N*-acetylgalactosaminyl, *N*-acetylglucosaminyl, galactosyl, and fucosyl residues, a carbohydrate: protein ratio of 80:20 on a weight base, and only a small and varying amount of sialyl and sulphate groups. This composition has been found by analysis of a well-isolated secretory product of the surface of the stomach of man (Schrager & Oates 1974*a*), pig (Starkey *et al.* 1974), dog (Wousson-Colle *et al.* 1975), and rat.

The carbohydrate side chains start with a *N*-acetylgalactosaminyl residue *O*-glycosidically bound to the seryl and threonyl residues in the protein chain. Nearly all of these residues are occupied by the sugar. *N*-acetylgalactosamine is followed by a number of galactosyl and *N*-acetylglucosaminyl pairs. In man, the composition of the end group varies depending on the blood group genes active in the secretory cell. These genes (*A*, *B*, *H*, *Se*, Le^a, and Le^b) determine the glycosyltransferases present. Individuals with the *Se* gene secrete glycoproteins with the same antigenicity as the glycolipids on the surface of their erythrocytes. Galactose, *N*-acetylgalactosamine and fucose form the end groups (Schrager & Oates 1974*a*).

The epithelial glycoproteins can be isolated by centrifugation in CsCl. They equilibrate at rather high densities (1.56 for the pig [Starkey *et al.* 1974]; 1.45 for the rat), because of their large carbohydrate content. The glycosaminoglycans of the connective tissue have more carbohydrates and hence equilibrate at still higher densities, while pure proteins have lower densities. The glycoprotein of the pig gastric surface cells is a tetramer and can be separated into monomers by proteolytic digestion or breaking of disulphide bridges. Both treatments affect the carbohydrate-free N-terminal parts of the protein chains, which contain a number of cysteinyl residues interconnecting the monomers into a tetramer molecule (Starkey *et al.* 1974). Because of their large size, the glycoproteins, even in monomeric form, do not enter a normal acrylamide gel during SDS electrophoresis, but when the concentration of acrylamide is lowered from 10% to 2% and the solidity of the gel is increased by adding agarose (1.6%), the large molecules enter the gel and show up in well-defined bands, rich in periodic acid–Schiff-positive material and poor in proteins, as demonstrated by the Coomassie-blue stain. Column chromatography is also used to isolate gastric glycoproteins (Schrager & Oates 1974*a*, *b*; Starkey *et al.* 1974).

Components and structure of other epithelial glycoproteins such as saliva (Lombart & Winzler 1972; Schrager & Oates 1974*b*), trachea (Ellis & Stahl

1973; Gallagher *et al.* 1975), and intestinal goblet cells (Forstner *et al.* 1973; Jabbal *et al.* 1976; Marshall & Allen 1977) show close parallels with the glycoprotein from the gastric surface cells.

Apart from the genetic determination by blood group genes mentioned already, little is known about the regulation of glycoprotein synthesis. We may assume that the production of the protein moiety is regulated by the same factors as control the synthesis of pure secretory proteins and their movement into the cisternae of the endoplasmic reticulum (Campbell & Blobel 1976). But on the control of the attachment of sugars and sulphate we can only speculate. It is an open question whether such control exists at all, though some reports mention differences in the composition of the carbohydrates of the secretory product, released before and after stimulation of the secretion (Menguy 1969; Dische *et al.* 1969; André *et al.* 1971). Other explanations can be given: cells with different products can be stimulated to a different degree; different products from one cell may vary in solubility; the product may lose part of its attached sugar and sulphate groups after secretion. The studies cited did not rule out such possibilities. However, changes in composition are certainly conceivable. They may result from changes in precursor supply. Precursors are provided by various metabolic pathways, but their pool size is also affected by hydrolysing enzymes. Changes in composition may also result from variations in the insertion of transferases in the membranes of the transport route, which might turn over more rapidly when secretion is stimulated. And finally, variations in sugar composition may be caused by changes in the incidence of nascent glycoproteins running into the membrane-bound transferases, for example the incidence might decrease with increased synthesis or accelerated transport of the protein moiety along the transport route, after stimulation of the secretion.

We know from our own and from other autoradiographic studies (Lambert *et al.* 1968) that gastric surface cells, during their shift upwards from the deepest parts of the gastric pits, lose most of their capacity to incorporate sulphate groups. This may result from decreased production of PAPS transferase, decreased insertion of this enzyme into the Golgi membranes, a smaller amount of the enzyme that binds sulphate to 3′-phosphoadenosine 5′-phosphate (PAP), or a change in end-group composition of the glycoprotein to which the sulphate had to be attached.

Apart from the possibility, which is still theoretical, of qualitative or quantitative variations in the sugar and sulphate attachment to secretory glycoproteins, changes in the rate of production of the protein moiety and thus in the rate of sugar incorporation are less speculative; we found a substantial increase in leucine and galactose incorporation in the bulbourethral gland after stimulation of the secretion. But before we discuss this cellular reaction further, we have to describe the next step in the transport of secretory glycoprotein: its secretion.

SECRETION

The secretory granules in their various forms fill the apical part of the secretory cells. The number of granules and the part of the cell they fill vary greatly, but the number is large in mucous cells. The autoradiographic study of the goblet cell by Neutra & Leblond (1966) showed that the mucous granules filled with radioactive glycoprotein form a kind of layer in the mass of secretory granules that is gradually moved upwards by the new granules formed at the mature pole of the Golgi complex. Such a gradual and orderly shift of a layer or generation of secretory granules has been described also for the pancreatic (Kramer & Poort 1972) and the parotid exocrine cells (Williams & Cope 1973). It takes 4 h for the main part of a generation of glycoproteins in the goblet cells of the rat intestine to reach the site of secretion (Neutra & Leblond 1966). In mucous cells of the bronchial gland it takes more than 7 h (Meyrick & Reid 1975), and in gastric surface cells more than 2 h (Kramer & Geuze 1977).

Secretory proteins are released from the cell by a process called exocytosis, during which the membrane of the secretory granule fuses with the plasma membrane and the granular content moves through the fusion opening into the lumen. The process of membrane fusion, as deduced from electron microscopic observations of ultrathin sections and freeze-fracture preparations (Palade & Bruns 1968; Beisson *et al.* 1976; Chi *et al.* 1976), can be divided into a number of steps: contact between the secretory granule and the plasma membrane, the latter showing a ring of large intramembrane particles at that site; disappearance of intramembrane particles from the site of fusion; fusion of the two membranes into one five-layered septum between lumen and granule; transformation of the five-layered into a three-layered membrane by the disappearance of the central layer; conversion of the three-layered membrane into a diaphragm without any visible substructure; disruption of this diaphragm, giving rise to a continuity between lumen and granule through which the secretory product can flow into the lumen.

The membrane of the granule needs to reach a certain maturity before being able to fuse with the plasma membrane. The youngest granules, pinched off from the Golgi complex (frequently called condensing vacuoles), do not fuse even when the cell is strongly stimulated. This maturation is mirrored by changes in lipids and proteins resulting in a molecular composition of secretory granule membranes that has much in common with the plasma membrane, while Golgi membranes are very different (Geuze *et al.* 1976).

Fusion is not random. In exocrine cells the secretory granules fuse with the apical membrane and less often, or not at all, with the basal and lateral plasma membrane below the zone of tight junctions.

Since in exocrine secretory cells new (glyco)proteins are synthesized continuously and new secretory granules are added to those formed earlier, the cell has to remove granules from its store, even in the absence of a secretory stimulus. In endocrine cells crinophagy is supposed to be responsible for the control of the number of granules (Boudier & Picard 1976). In exocrine cells the redundant granules are secreted (Kramer & Poort 1972) and hence fusions between the granules and the plasma membrane are observed even in unstimulated cells.

Unstimulated secretion has also been reported in mucous epithelial cells but the process by which the glycoproteins can leave the granules differs from what has been described before. Neutra & Leblond (1966) and Kim *et al.* (1972) describe a disruption of the apical rim of the plasma membrane and underlying cytoplasm through which the membrane-bound granule slips into the lumen, where the membrane disintegrates and the contents become free. In the lumen sheets of membrane can be found. Tandler & Poulsen (1976) describe an avulsion of the plasma membrane as the only barrier between the granule and the lumen. Subsequent focal disintegrations of this three-layered membrane give rise to openings through which the mucus flows into the lumen. It is difficult to decide to what extent ineffective fixation contributes to the observed differences with pure merocrine secretion. In bulbourethral gland cells, well-preserved by direct vascular perfusion, the observed structures suggest a normal exocytotic process of unstimulated secretion, particularly towards the deep canaliculi present between neighbouring cells (Fig. 10). But even under these circumstances membrane is present in the lumen in the form of numerous small vesicles along the apical pole of the cells (Fig. 11). The presence of many membrane vesicles in the ejaculated semen of rabbits (Davies 1973) suggests that these luminal vesicles are not artifacts and one cannot exclude the possibility that secretion of mucous granules is accompanied by a shedding of cellular material, mainly of membrane origin.

The frequency of fusions between secretory granules and the apical plasma membrane can be increased by secretory stimuli (hormones, neurotransmitters or drugs). The chain of events from the interaction between the stimulating molecule and its receptor in the plasma membrane to the final secretory process is the subject of numerous studies, but is still not fully understood. To discuss

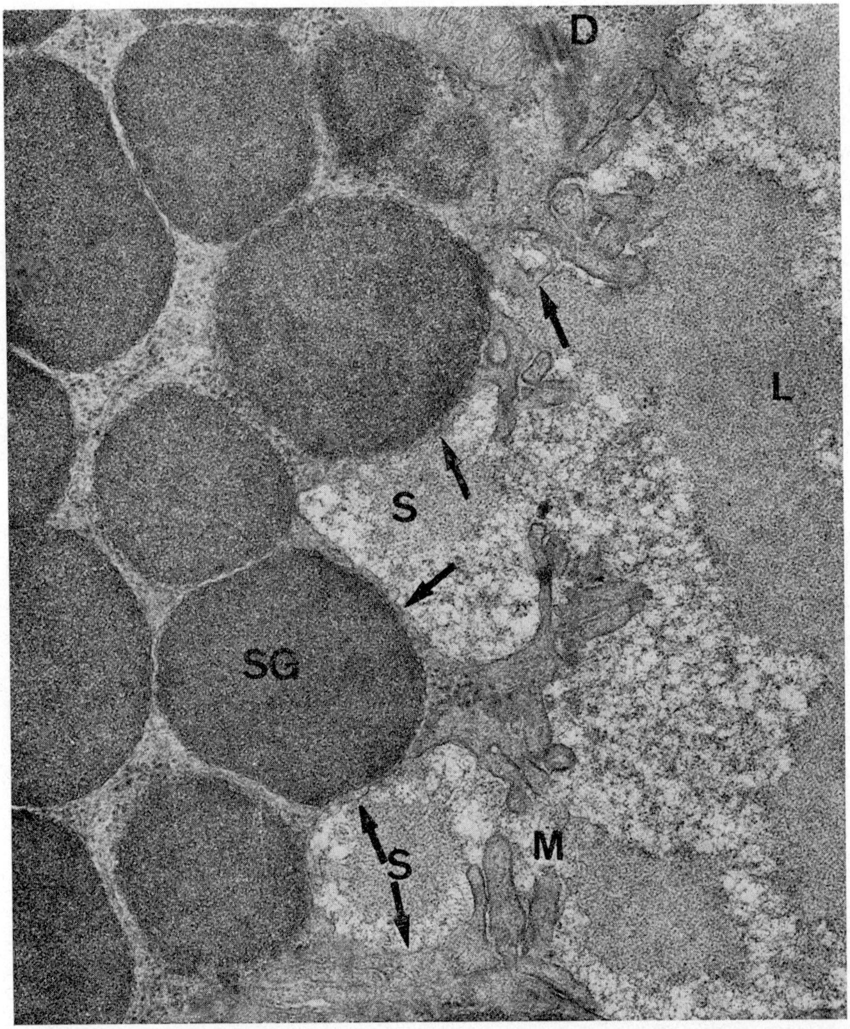

FIG. 10. Bulbourethral gland cell, lateral aspect, showing two caveolae (S) on the cell surface, clearly limited by membrane (arrows), strongly suggesting an exocytotic secretion of the granular content. SG, secretory granule; M, microvilli; D, intercellular junction; L, intercellular space filled by secretory product. Perfusion fixation as described for Fig. 8. × 50 000

it here would exceed the limits of this survey. We confine ourselves to a short list of the possible steps in the stimulus–secretion coupling: activation of purinylcyclases in the plasma membrane; increased amount of cyclic nucleotides; activation of protein kinases; increased amount of Ca^{2+} in the cytoplasm;

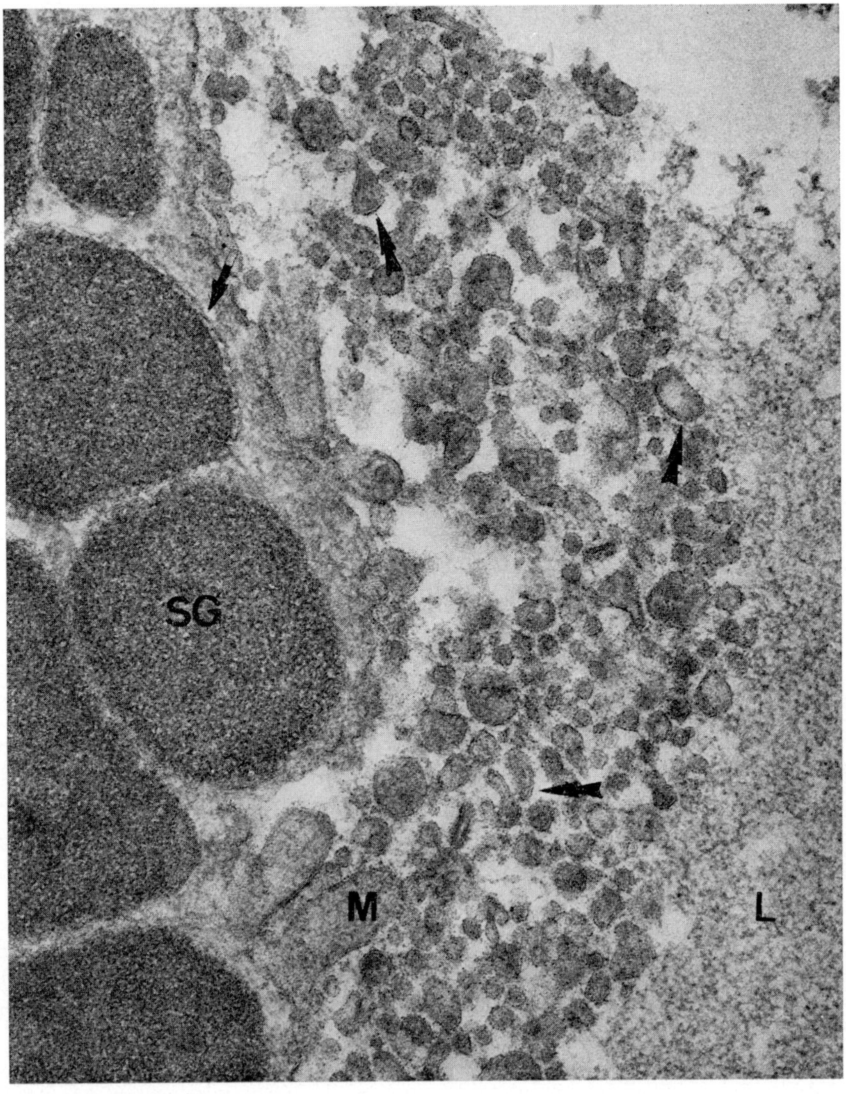

FIG. 11. Bulbourethral gland cell, apical aspect, showing secretory granules (SG), surrounded by a membrane (arrow). In the lumen (L) at the top of the cell a cluster of vesicles, formed by a triple-layered membrane (double arrows) and mostly dark contents. M, microvilli. Perfusion fixation as described for Fig. 8. × 69 600

a stronger cytoplasmic movement increasing the chance of contact between granule and plasma membrane; formation of pseudopodia by secretory granules; increased activities of microtubules and microfilaments guiding the transport of granules towards the membrane; loss of membrane charge at the cytoplasmic side of both plasma and granule membrane; formation of membranolytic lysophosphatidylserine. For all these possible steps indications exist, but which role they play in the final effect of stimulation is still unknown.

During stimulation the number of granules fusing with the plasma membrane per unit time increases compared with the number of new granules formed; the store of granules is therefore reduced or may even disappear altogether, while the plasma membrane increases in size through the addition of the membranes of the secretory granules. In the exocrine pancreas this increase may amount to 50%.

Among glycoprotein-secreting glands, stimulated secretion is reported for the salivary glands (Dische *et al.* 1969; Radley 1969; Kim *et al.* 1972; Cutler & Chaudhry 1973; Bogart 1975; Kuijper-Lenstra & Kramer 1975*a*), intestinal goblet cells (Freeman 1966), tracheal glands (Ellis & Stahl 1973; Gallagher *et al.* 1975), bronchial submucosal glands (Sturgess & Reid 1972), and the bulbourethral gland (Geuze & Slot 1976).

The high incidence of exocytotic fusion, though fundamentally a process of membrane interactions, may involve some loss of membrane and cytoplasm into the lumen, even in parotid (Harrop & Garrett 1974) and pancreatic exocrine cells. When the loss is absent or small, this type of secretion is called merocrine. A more dramatic loss of membrane and cytoplasm during stimulated secretion has been described for intestinal goblet cells (Freeman 1966) and sublingual gland cells (Kim *et al.* 1972). But Bogart (1975) found breaks in the outer rim of plasma membrane and cytoplasm of stimulated submandibular cells that cause such losses only after glutaraldehyde, not after trialdehyde fixation! This again illustrates the need for a thorough study of the effect of fixation before we try and describe the process of secretion in mucous cells.

At the end of stimulated secretion, the cells face the problem of an increased surface but a decreased cellular volume, because the granular membranes have been added to the plasma membrane. Redundant membrane is at least partly removed by endocytosis (Geuze *et al.* 1976). Whether the interiorized membrane is directly reutilized or broken down is still uncertain. Indirect evidence for reutilization is provided by the low rate of turnover of some membrane proteins of the secretory granules, indirect evidence for molecular breakdown being provided by the increased number of lysosomes.

After stimulated secretion the cell rebuilds the store of secretory granules, a process that takes many hours; but it is not known for certain whether the rate of synthesis of secretory protein is higher during that phase. Reports on the pancreas mention an absence of increase (Poort & Kramer 1969) but also a doubling of the rate of protein synthesis (Danielson *et al.* 1974). Salivary gland cells show no increase, except that the acinar cells of the parotid gland double their amino acid incorporation within 30 min of stimulation (Kuijper-Lenstra & Kramer 1975*b*). The bulbourethral cells increase their incorporation of radioactive leucine and galactose within 4 h of the start of stimulated secretion (Geuze & Slot 1976). The increased incorporation reaches its maximum between 6 and 13 h and lasts for about four days. By that time the cells have rebuilt a store of mucous granules nearly equal in size to the pre-stimulation phase. Whether the increased production of glycoprotein is determined by the rate of synthesis of the protein moiety only, or also by an increased amount or activity of transferase molecules, is now being studied, as is the question of whether the product shows changes in composition during the succeeding stages of the secretory cycle.

References

ANDRÉ, C., LAMBERT, R. & BÉRARD, A. (1971) Influence of prolonged stimulation on the composition of a salivary sulfated glycoprotein in man. *Digestion 4*, 257–263

BAUDUIN, H., COLIN, M. & DUMONT, J. E. (1969) Energy sources for protein synthesis and enzymatic secretion in rat pancreas in vitro. *Biochim. Biophys. Acta 174*, 722–733

BEISSON, J., LEFORT-TRAN, M., POUPHILE, M., ROSSIGNOL, M. & SATIR, B. (1976) Genetic analysis of membrane differentiation in Paramecium. *J. Cell Biol. 69*, 126–143

BERG, N. B. & AUSTIN, B. P. (1976) Intracellular transport of sulfated macromolecules in parotid acinar cells. *Cell Tiss. Res. 165*, 215–225

BOGART, B. I. (1975) Secretory dynamics of the rat submandibular gland. *J. Ultrastruct. Res. 52*, 139–155

BOUDIER, J.-A. & PICARD, D. (1976) Granulolysis in neurosecretory neurons of the rat supraoptico-posthypophyseal system. *Cell Tiss. Res. 172*, 39–58

CAMPBELL, P. N. & BLOBEL, G. (1976) The rôle of organelles in the chemical modification of the primary translational products of secretory proteins. *FEBS (Fed. Eur. Biochem. Soc.) Lett. 72*, 215–226

CASTLE, J. D., JAMIESON, J. D. & PALADE, G. E. (1972) Radioautographic analysis of the secretory process in the parotid acinar cell of the rabbit. *J. Cell Biol. 53*, 290–311

CHI, E. Y., LAGUNOFF, D. & KOEHLER, J. K. (1976) Freeze-fracture study of mast cell secretion. *Proc. Natl. Acad. Sci. U.S.A. 73*, 2824–2827

CUTLER, L. S. & CHAUDHRY, A. P. (1973) Release and restoration of the secretory granules in the convoluted granular tubules of the rat submandibular gland. *Anat. Rec. 176*, 405–420

DANIELSON, A., MARKLUND, S. & STIGBRAND, T. (1974) Effects of starvation and islet hormones on the synthesis of amylase in isolated exocrine pancreas of the mouse. *Acta Hepato-Gastroenterol. 21*, 289–299

DAVIES, B. K. (1973) Occurrence of vesicles in rabbit seminal plasma. *Experientia (Basel) 29*, 1484–1487

DISCHE, Z., BURGER, M. N., DANILCHENKO, A. & ROTHSCHILD, C. (1969) Variations in the composition of glycoproteins of the submaxillary and parotid saliva of the dog in relation to intensity of secretory stimulus. *Arch. Biochem. Biophys. 135*, 1–9

DOREY, G. & BHOOLA, K. D. (1972) Ultrastructure of acinar cell granules in mammalian submaxillary glands. I. *Z. Zellforsch. Mikrosk. Anat. 126*, 320–334

ELLIS, D. B. & STAHL, G. H. (1973) Biosynthesis of respiratory tract mucins. Incorporation of radioactive precursors into glycoproteins by canine tracheal explants *in vitro*. *Biochem. J. 136*, 837–844

FORSTNER, J., JABBAL, I. & FORSTNER, G. G. (1973) Goblet cell mucin of rat small intestine. Chemical and physical characterization. *Can. J. Biochem. 51*, 1154–1166

FREEMAN, J. A. (1966) Goblet cell fine structure, *Anat. Rec. 154*, 121–148

GALLAGHER, J. T., KENT, P. W., PASSATORE, M., PHIPPS, R. J. & RICHARDSON, P. S. (1975) The composition of tracheal mucus and the nervous control of its secretion in the cat. *Proc. R. Soc. Lond. B Biol. Sci. 192*, 49–76

GEUZE, J. J. & SLOT, J. W. (1976) Synthesis and secretion of glycoproteins in rat bulbourethral (Cowper's) gland. I. The effect of copulation on the glandular content and on the incorporation of galactose and leucine. *Biol. Reprod. 15*, 118–125

GEUZE, J. J., DE MAN, J. C. H. & KRAMER, M. F. (1976) Membranes of the endoplasmic reticulum and the secretory system and their rôle in plasma membrane regulation, in *Mammalian Cell Membranes*, vol. 2 (Jamieson, G. A. & Robinson, D. M., eds.), pp. 55–107, Butterworths, London

HARROP, T. J. & GARRETT, J. R. (1974) Effects of preganglionic sympathectomy on secretory changes in parotid acinar cells of rats on eating. *Cell Tiss. Res. 154*, 135–150

JABBAL, I., KELLS, D. I. C., FORSTNER, G. & FORSTNER, J. (1976) Human intestinal goblet cell mucin. *Can. J. Biochem. 54*, 707–716

JAMIESON, J. D. & PALADE, G. E. (1967*a*) Intracellular transport of secretory proteins in the pancreatic exocrine cell. I. Rôle of the peripheral elements of the Golgi complex. *J. Cell Biol. 34*, 577–596

JAMIESON, J. D. & PALADE, G. E. (1967*b*) Intracellular transport of secretory proteins in the pancreatic exocrine cell. II. Transport to condensing vacuoles and zymogen granules. *J. Cell Biol. 34*, 597–615

KIM, S. K., NASJLETI, L. E. & HAN, S. S. (1972) The secretion processes in mucous and serous secretory cells of the rat sublingual gland. *J. Ultrastruct. Res. 38*, 371–389

KRAMER, M. F. & GEUZE, J. J. (1977) Glycoprotein transport in the surface mucous cells of the rat stomach. *J. Cell Biol. 73*, 533–547

KRAMER, M. F. & POORT, C. (1972) Unstimulated secretion of protein from rat exocrine pancreas cells. *J. Cell Biol. 52*, 147–158

KUIJPER-LENSTRA, A. H. & KRAMER, M. F. (1975*a*) Rate of protein synthesis in rat salivary gland cells after pilocarpine or feeding. I. *Cell Tiss. Res. 164*, 435–446

KUIJPER-LENSTRA, A. H. & KRAMER, M. F. (1975*b*) Rate of protein synthesis in rat salivary gland cells after pilocarpine or feeding. III. *Cell Tiss. Res. 164*, 457–466

LAMBERT, R., MARTIN, F., ANDRÉ, C., DESCOS, L. & VOUILLON, G. (1968) Apical localization of glycoproteins in gastric mucous cells. *Am. J. Dig. Dis. 13*, 941–951

LOMBART, CHR. & WINZLER, R. J. (1972) Isolation and characterization of canine submaxillary mucin. *Biochem. J. 128*, 975–977

MARSHALL, TH. & ALLEN, A. (1977) The isolation of a high-molecular weight glycoprotein from pig colonic mucus. *Biochem. Soc. Trans 5*, 436–439

MARTINEZ-HERNANDEZ, A., NAKANE, P. K. & PIERCE, G. B. (1972) The secretory granules of the acinar cells of the mouse submaxillary gland. *Am. J. Anat. 133*, 259–268

MENGUY, R. (1969) Gastric mucus and the gastric mucous barrier. *Am. J. Surg. 117*, 806–812

MEYRICK, B. & REID, L. (1975) *In vitro* incorporation of [^{3}H]-threonine and [^{3}H]-glucose by the mucous and serous cells of the human bronchal submucosal gland. *J. Cell Biol. 67*, 320–344

NEUTRA, M. & LEBLOND, C. P. (1966) Synthesis of the carbohydrate of mucus in the Golgi complex as shown by electron microscope radioautography of goblet cells from rats injected with glucose-H^3. *J. Cell Biol. 30*, 119–136

NILSSON, O. & WESTMAN, A. (1961) The ultrastructure of the epithelial cells of the endocervix during the menstrual cycle. *Acta Obstet. Gynecol. Scand. 40*, 223–233

NOVIKOFF, A. B. (1976) The endoplasmic reticulum: a cytochemist's view. (A review). *Proc. Natl. Acad. Sci. U.S.A. 73*, 2781–2787

PALADE, G. E. & BRUNS, R. R. (1968) Structural modulations of plasmalemmal vesicles. *J. Cell Biol. 37*, 633–649

POORT, C. & KRAMER, M. F. (1969) Effect of feeding on the protein synthesis in mammalian pancreas. *Gastroenterology 57*, 689–696

RADLEY, J. M. (1969) Ultrastructural changes in the rat submaxillary gland following isoprenaline. *Z. Zellforsch. Mikrosk. Anat. 97*, 196–211

RAMBOURG, A., HERNANDEZ, W. & LEBLOND, C. P. (1969) Detection of complex carbohydrates in the Golgi apparatus of rat cells. *J. Cell Biol. 40*, 395–414

ROHR, H. P., SCHMALBECK, J. & FELDHAGE, A. (1967) Elektronenmikroskopisch-Autoradiographische Untersuchungen über die Eiweisz-Synthese in der Brunnerschen Drüse der Maus. *Z. Zellforsch. Mikrosk. Anat. 80*, 183–204

SCHMALBECK, J. & ROHR, H. P. (1967) Die Mukopolysaccharid-Synthese in ihrer Beziehung zur Eiweisz-Synthese in der Brunnerschen Drüse der Maus. *Z. Zellforsch. Mikrosk. Anat. 80*, 329–344

SCHRAGER, J. & OATES, M. D. G. (1974*a*) The isolation and partial characterization of a glycoprotein isolated from human aspirates and from extracts of gastric mucosae. *Biochim. Biophys. Acta 372*, 183–195

SCHRAGER, J. & OATES, M. D. G. (1974*b*) The chemical composition and some structural features of the principal salivary glycoprotein isolated from human mixed saliva. *Arch. Oral Biol. 19*, 1215–1220

STARKEY, B. J., SNARY, D. & ALLEN, A. (1974) Characterization of gastric mucoproteins isolated by equilibrium density-gradient centrifugation in caesium chloride. *Biochem. J. 141*, 633–639

STURGESS, J. & REID, L. (1972) An organ culture study of the effect of drugs on the secretory activity of the human bronchial submucosal gland. *Clin. Sci. (Oxf.) 43*, 533–543

TANDLER, B. & POULSEN, J. H. (1976) Fusion of the envelope of mucous droplets with the luminal plasma membrane in acinar cells of the cat submandibular gland. *J. Cell Biol. 68*, 775–781

TANDLER, B., DENNING, C. R., MANDELE, J. D. & KUTSCHER, A. H. (1969) Ultrastructure of human labial salivary glands. I. Acinar secretory cells. *J. Morphol. 127*, 383–408

THIÉRY, J. P. (1967) Mise en évidence des polysaccharides sur coupes fines en microscopie électronique. *J. Microsc. (Paris) 6*, 987–1018

THIÉRY, J. P. (1969) Rôle de l'appareil de Golgi dans la synthèse des mucopolysaccharides. Etude cytochimique. I. *J. Microsc. (Paris) 8*, 689–708

WATTEL, W., GEUZE, J. J. & DE ROOIJ, D. G. (1977) Ultrastructural and carbohydrate histochemical studies on the differentiation and renewal of mucous cells in the rat gastric fundus. *Cell Tiss. Res. 176*, 445–462

WILLIAMS, M. A. & COPE, G. H. (1973) A system for the study of zymogen granule genesis in rabbit parotid gland tissue in vitro. *J. Anat. 116*, 431–444

WOUSSON-COLLE, N. C., RASINSKI, C. & DE GRAEFF, J. (1975) Glycoprotéines du mucus gastrique du chien. *Biol. Gastro-Enterol. 8*, 275–289

Discussion

Silberberg: How does the glycoprotein that is synthesized enter the granules and how do the granules evolve? Is any synthesis still going on within the granules?

Kramer: No. The protein moiety is synthesized in the ribosomes attached to the endoplasmic reticulum. The signal peptide (for review, see Campbell & Blobel 1976) makes it possible for a protein to enter the membrane and to pierce through it to come into the cisterna. We don't know where the first sugar is attached to glycoproteins which are secreted by epithelial cells. The protein is transported in the cisternae towards the Golgi area, and there the other sugars are attached to it. Few if any sugars or sulphate are attached to the glycoproteins during their stay within the granules (Kramer & Geuze 1977). During transport and storage of glycoproteins within granules, the membrane continues to surround the secretory material. The granular contents are already out of the cell, within compartments.

Allison: Packaging starts with condensing vacuoles which are really quite small, and continues with large secretory granules, so presumably there is programmed fusion of the condensing vacuoles to form the secretory granules. Later there is again fusion of the membranes limiting the secretory granules with the cell membrane. There is also fusion when you fix the cells badly. So obviously the programming of membrane fusion is critical to the mechanism of secretion.

Kramer: Yes.

Phelps: One has to be careful not to confuse two sets of data. The evidence from subcellular fractionation would indicate activities found in certain fractions which are then putatively ascribed to either a mature or an immature Golgi system, but this would beg the question that there is no redistribution of activities during the time course of the making of that homogenate and the spinning of it. Your work would clearly put this in question.

Kramer: In the work I described, it was not a case of first labelling the cell and then fractionating it to localize the site of the transferases. The transferases studied in the gastric cells are membrane-bound proteins so there is little danger that they would have shifted during the fractionation procedure.

Phelps: I think there is clear evidence that some of the initial transferases can exist both in a soluble form and in a membrane-bound form. Perhaps the balance between the two is controlled by magnesium or calcium concentration which is not monitored in the extraction.

Kramer: We have never found galactosyl and fucosyl transferase activities in the cytosol fractions (Strous & Kramer 1976). Only when we use Triton do we find transferase activity in the cytosol. In these gastric cells transferase is absolutely a membrane-bound enzyme.

Allison: To put it simply, in the immature Golgi various sugars are added and in the mature Golgi there is sulphation. Do you object to that picture, Professor Phelps?

Phelps: No, I find it a very appealing picture but I think one ought to be quite clear what the evidence is and what the resulting construction is.

Reid: It may be a very good picture for the cell that Dr Kramer dealt with. It was interesting to see how uniform the granules were and I suspect therefore that what you have said may apply to that system. One of the interesting things about secretory cells that Dr Jeffery and Mrs Jones (Jones 1977; Reid 1977) have found in animal studies is that in the transforming cell, it is at the tip of the cell that acidification is first picked up; it is not found in the base near the Golgi. Therefore, in relation to airway cells, one of the things that we have to accept or that you will have to explain for us is how those granules are changing and why they change first of all close to the apical cell surface. I hope that Professor Phelps will tell us that here we still have membranes with their bound enzymes and that it may be just as easy to turn on an enzyme system when the membrane has migrated towards the surface of the cell as to turn it on when it is at the Golgi.

Allison: One of the current interests in cell biology is the phenomenon of so-called transglycosylation which is thought to happen at the cell membrane (Roth 1973) and which is now becoming scientifically respectable. This may be related to the formation of links between polypeptide chains in mucus.

Davis: Dr Kramer, you suggested that an ion pump system in the membrane surrounding the mucous granules might drive out the water and concentrate the mucin. Have you any evidence that ion pumps are present? Does an agent like ouabain, which inhibits sodium pumps, affect the formation of the granules?

Reid: We have done that. We can show interference with uptake, but we do not rinse the cells with Tyrode or anything else. So, to come back to this question of artifacts, Dr Kramer may have picked it up in his system but most of the work that we are now mentioning has been done with tissue that had not been washed. In organ culture medium we have added radioactive precursors, particularly threonine, glucose and glucosamine.

Depending on the radioactive pulse and when the drugs are added, one can watch the effect on uptake or on discharge. Ouabain and similar compounds have been used to study mucous and serous cells and we can block uptake of precursor (Coles 1976, 1978). What is interesting is that we can block uptake of precursor for an hour or two but, over a matter of several hours, we do not interfere with synthesis or discharge. Although, obviously, if synthesis in the cell is interfered with for a matter of hours, there will ultimately be nothing to be discharged.

Allison: The defined site of action of ouabain is on the plasma membrane, Na/K ATPase inhibiting transport of these ions across the membrane. An interesting possibility is that analogous pumps are present in the membranes limiting the granules.

Kramer: We can think in terms of a pump to understand why condensing vacuoles become secretory granules, but there is no reason to believe that these enzymes are shed from the membrane just after having finished their work: the concentration of the secretory granule content. So these enzymes —whether they are working or not—stay within the membrane when it moves upwards to the apical plasma membrane.

Jeffery: Perhaps the word artifact is being used in a rather unfortunate sense. I am fully prepared to accept that electron microscopy is the science of artifacts. An artifact may give some indication of a real chemical difference between the morphologically distinct granules of the different cell types.

Kramer: Of course. That is why I proposed fixation as a test for differences in glycoprotein content between the serous cells which do not attract, and mucous cells which apparently do attract, a lot of water the moment the anoxaemia starts.

Jeffery: So you still support the differentiation between serous and mucous cells?

Kramer: Yes, the gastric surface cells have different glycoprotein compared with the glycoprotein in bulbourethral cells and other cells with swelling granules. We don't yet know the chemical difference but there is a difference.

Phelps: Do you think that there is any post-synthetic modification going on inside these granules? It might be a case of losing something rather than adding something on.

Kramer: There might be. Allen suggests that monomers are organized into tetramers by cysteine bridges (Starkey *et al.* 1974). Perhaps that is one of the things that happen in some cell types but not in others. It can make a difference even to the molarity of the granule contents: if they are combined into tetramers, the molarity decreases.

Thurlbeck: We ought to be very careful in talking about good and bad fixation. If different fixation methods alter the appearance of a secretion, this may tell you a lot about the nature of the secretion. Have the microscopists looked at the effect of osmolarity of the fixative on the appearance of the granules?

Jeffery: It hasn't been looked at in the respiratory tract; it may have been elsewhere.

Kramer: I am not talking about good fixation, I am talking about shortening the period of anoxaemia. We didn't change our fixation fluids, we just started to perfuse them immediately without washing away the blood in animals breathing 95% oxygen. That is the whole difference. The idea was suggested by Martinez-Hernandez & Nakane (1972).

Douglas: Is there any evidence that you can get confluent granules if you inhibit the production of metabolic energy?

Kramer: We found the effect of different fixation procedures only recently and still have to do all the other experiments.

Douglas: I find it very difficult to imagine that perfusion with saline solution for a few minutes will substantially lower the energy substrates in the cell.

Allison: Wasn't perfusion designed to prevent that from happening, in the kidney for example?

Thurlbeck: Perfusion might add a lot of water to the tissue.

Reid: In almost all the work on the lung the blood should not be washed out. For electron microscopy it is best to perfuse immediately with glutaraldehyde or formaldehyde, either through the airways or the blood vessels or both, while the animal is still living and with the heart beating.

Allison: Yes, but nonetheless it would be interesting to try metabolic inhibitors just to see what happens to the granules.

Jeffery: Particularly in the airways, intratracheal inflation with fixative is better than vascular perfusion because in the airways the epithelium is not well supplied with vessels.

Allison: For the stomach do you fix from the surface or by vascular perfusion?

Kramer: By vascular perfusion, but after hours of perfusion with a fluorocarbon-containing mixture. Even during that experimental perfusion period something may go wrong with the granules. We still have to study this. Even anaesthesia might influence the oxygenation of cells.

Guz: You and Dr Jeffery have both suggested that the difference between serous and mucous cells might just be the concentration of glycoproteins.

Kramer: Not the concentration but the nature of the glycoproteins.

Jeffery: I think it is a mixture of both.

Guz: Then this is a vague area. But surely this sort of molecule will have the very alinear characteristics of the osmotic pressure/concentration relationship? Hyaluronic acid has been well studied for its osmotic properties. Up to a concentration of about 1 g/100 ml the osmosis/concentration relationship is pretty linear but above this concentration, the osmotic pressure really shoots up (Laurent 1970); so the osmotic forces that exist across the membrane (we know nothing about the reflection coefficients of this membrane, do we?) may be very dependent on the actual concentration of glycoproteins.

I just put this out because Dr Thurlbeck asked earlier about the effect of osmolarity; perhaps this could be studied by varying the osmolarity of the perfusing agents.

Phelps: Most of the osmotic pressure generated in hyaluronate systems is explainable in terms of excluded volume. This excluded volume comes about because of the vast volume occupancy of the polymer chains. In hyaluronate this can amount to 12 l/g polymer. Any other molecule is not free to occupy all the apparent liquid volume present and is therefore effectively more concentrated than simple volume considerations would predict. A large molecule will be denied sterically more volume than a small molecule—much as a large adult finds it more difficult to accommodate himself in a crowded tube train than does a small boy.

Nadel: Can you release electron-dense materials from some cells and electron-lucent materials from other cells, and are they selectively released either from the same cells or other cells?

Kramer: Most people think that all secretory granules have the same contents within one cell but different cells may have different contents. It is believed that one cell makes one type of secretory granule which has a population of different molecules within it, but that there are no differences between secretory granules within one cell. So if the membrane of the secretory granule in a cell fuses with the apical cell membrane all kinds of secretory enzymes —that is, all glycoproteins—that are packed within the cell then come out.

Nadel: Can you cause release of granules selectively from one cell type (i.e. serous or mucous cells)?

Reid: Yes, they have the same activity in terms of organ culture—the same response to drugs—so one can show, in organ culture, that both types of cell are susceptible to the same drugs and that whereas the mucous cell discharges intermittently, as it were, the serous cell, under basal conditions, discharges steadily. So there is a different pattern of basal discharge for the two cell types although each responds in the same way to the same stimuli.

Jeffery: We haven't done any experiments in the cat to answer Dr Nadel's question. With pilocarpine, for example, we know that the glycoprotein is virtually exhausted from all the cells of the submucosal glands. In other words, a simple maximal stimulation involves a response of both the serous and the mucous cells, although we know that, in the cat, the ratio of cells is about 60:40, serous:mucous; but both cell types seem to be affected. Innervation hasn't really been examined fully although, in the cat, both serous and mucous cells appear to be innervated (unpublished data).

Godfrey: What causes the granules to move away from the Golgi apparatus to the cell membrane?

Kramer: Many factors can cause the granules to move. There is pushing by granules formed later (Kramer & Poort 1972). Maybe microtubules and microfilaments are the guiding apparatus. There could be a stream of cytoplasm from the Golgi towards the apical cell membrane—but this is just speculation.

Allison: Nowhere are membranes more densely stacked together than they are in the Golgi, and presumably there is just more space elsewhere. There are also questions of curvature and so on.

Silberberg: Could some of the difference in staining of the granules be due to a difference in the permeability of their membranes, so that the stain does not actually enter all the granules?

Kramer: No. The granules are stained after the sections have been made, and the sections are so thin (50 to 100 nm) that all the membranes are cut.

References

CAMPBELL, P. N. & BLOBEL, G. (1976) The role of organelles in the chemical modification of the primary translational products of secretory proteins. *FEBS (Fed. Eur. Biochem. Soc.) Lett. 72*, 215–226

COLES, S. J. (1976) *The Nature and Control of Glycoprotein Secretion by Human Bronchial Glands*, Ph. D. Thesis, University of London

COLES, S. J. (1978) An organ culture study of mucous glycoprotein secretion by human airway. (Submitted for publication)

JONES, R. (1977) Modification of mucus in animal models of disease, in *Mucus in Health and Disease* (Elstein, M. & Parke, D. K., eds.), Plenum Press, London

KRAMER, M. F. & GEUZE, J. J. (1977) Glycoprotein transport in the surface mucous cells of the rat stomach. *J. Cell Biol. 73*, 533–547

KRAMER, M. F. & POORT, C. (1972) Unstimulated secretion of protein from rat exocrine pancreas cells. *J. Cell Biol. 52*, 147–158

LAURENT, T. C. (1970) Chemistry of hyaluronic acid, in *Chemistry and Molecular Biology of the Intercellular Matrix* (Balazs, E. A., ed.), vol. 2, Academic Press, London

MARTINEZ-HERNANDEZ, A. & NAKANE, P. K. (1972) The secretory granules of the acinar cells of the mouse submaxillary gland. *Am. J. Anat. 133*, 259–268

REID, L. (1977) Secretory cells., *Fed. Proc. 36* (Abstr.)

ROTH, S. (1973) A molecular model for cell interactions. *Q. Rev. Biol. 48*, 541–563

STARKEY, B. J., SNARY, D. & ALLEN, A. (1974) Characterization of gastric mucoproteins isolated by equilibrium density-gradient centrifugation in caesium chloride. *Biochem. J. 141*, 633–639

STROUS, G. J. A. M. & KRAMER, M. F. (1976) Glycoprotein synthesis in gastric epithelial cells of the rat. Properties of microsomal glycoprotein glycosyltransferases. *Biochim. Biophys. Acta 451*, 201–211

General discussion I

Proctor: One question of importance is, what factors influence the ability of a particle containing a virus to move through the surface of airway secretions to establish contact with a cell wall? This has to be done before it can penetrate the cell and start an infection. And, if a glycoprotein is secreted which coats the cilia in addition to materials which are in the supernatant above periciliary fluid, this might be another factor impeding the capacity of the virus to penetrate the cell.

Jeffery: We expected, when we put in tritiated glucose, that it would be taken up most actively by the goblet cells, but the goblet cells seemed to shut it out, though it was taken up avidly by 'other cells'. I suggest that the 'other cells' are in fact ciliated cells. So there is a high turnover of glucose by ciliated cells and it seems that the ciliated cells were in fact secreting something onto their surface. It suggests there is a very active secretory process by ciliated cells.

Proctor: Dr Nadel (p. 22) asked whether the microvilli change when manipulated. Dr Spicer (personal communication, 1977) believes that the microvilli of ciliated cells may secrete a glycoprotein which coats the cilia and that this is of some importance in the functioning of the ciliated cell. Has anyone else noted this?

Richardson: We are coming round to the same conclusion. As Dr Jeffery showed, the microvillous border of the ciliated cells takes up some labels, including tritiated glucose and to some extent [^{35}S]sulphate, very avidly, and this suggests to us that it is a very actively synthesizing microvillous border. I shall be showing later (p. 125) that a lot of the glycoprotein, which has become labelled with ^{3}H from the glucose, is released from the microvillous border even in the absence of any irritant stimulus, so we have two sets of evidence that there is a physiological release of glycoprotein from ciliated cells. I don't know whether this constitutes a true secretion or whether it is just little bits of the cell dropping off. In either case ammonia vapour, given directly into the tracheal segment, greatly increases the rate at which this glycoprotein appears in tracheal washings.

Widdicombe: This high concentration of ammonia—500 p.p.m.—is extremely unpleasant to inhale and I wonder if it does any damage to the surface. Do electron microscopic pictures taken after ammonia has been given show that the microvilli and cilia are still intact and, physiologically speaking, are the cilia still beating after that concentration of ammonia? Are there more physiological stimuli that produce secretion of the surface substance?

Jeffery: We haven't done electron microscopy to see whether the microvilli are damaged; light microscopy shows that the epithelium is still intact in most cases—not all—and the cilia are still there. I don't know whether the cilia are still motile. We have yet to try other irritants.

Richardson: After some of the experiments in which we gave ammonia, we opened the trachea and sprinkled carbon dust onto the epithelium. In three out of four experiments the dust moved, so the cilia were working. Dalhamn (1956) found that when he gave ammonia into the rat trachea there was first stasis of mucus, which lasted for some time, but later the cilia recovered their function. This may well have happened in the tracheas we used.

Guz: I share Professor Widdicombe's fear about the concentration of ammonia. Isn't there an inflammatory reaction and doesn't the epithelium look red compared with untreated epithelium?

Richardson: Yes. There is some reddening.

Guz: Therefore, on light microscopy presumably you would see a cellular infiltrate as well. What do you see that explains the redness?

Allison: The redness is vasodilatation.

Guz: Have red cells come out of the capillaries?

Jeffery: No, definitely not. They may be dilated, they are often congested, but there is no cellular infiltration.

Guz: But there is a definite vascular effect from this concentration of ammonia?

Richardson: Yes.

Reid: It is interesting to compare the uptake of the radioactive precursor given from tracheal lumen with its uptake from the blood. Our experience, again, has been with organ culture, and we find that the secretory cells take up glucose and incorporate it into the macromolecule. Have you any evidence whether that glucose is taken up into a glycoprotein or into something else?

Richardson: We have never given [^{3}H] or [^{14}C]glucose into the bloodstream. We did try with [^{3}H]glucosamine but tracheal mucous cells failed to incorporate it. Other tissues, such as the liver, seemed to remove it all. [^{35}S]Sulphate given intravenously is not taken up so avidly by all the organs of the body so enough is left for the trachea to have a share. The tracheal glands again take up a lot of labelled sulphate and our impression is that, though the ciliated cells incorporate some of the isotope given by this route (see appendix, in Gallagher *et al.* 1975), their labelling is less than when [^{35}S]sulphate is given directly into the lumen of the trachea, as you would expect.

Nadel: Can you define what you would 'expect'? Because of the non-specificity of glucose uptake, the amount of glycogen and its location might not be quite so predictable. However, the observation that sodium sulphate is taken up from the luminal surface appears to have more specific implications. Normally, mucoproteins are secreted *into* the lumen. Does the fact that sulphate is avidly taken up from the luminal surface imply 'recycling' of these materials?

Jeffery: They need not necessarily be taken up from the luminal aspect of the cell; they could still be coming in from the base of the cell after passing through 'leaky junctions' (shall we say) between the cells.

Richardson: When we give labelled sulphate, very little—probably about 1% or less—of the total dose actually gets taken up in the wrong way, that is from the lumen to the cells. The other 99% just gets washed away.

Silberberg: Have you any evidence that the glucose is in fact chemically part of these glycoprotein structures, that it is not simply attached to the surface by some physical interaction?

Richardson: Yes. The first step in our analysis is to dialyse the tracheal washings for a week with five changes of distilled water, and we find that the macromolecules retain their radioactivity. Moreover, when we mix secretions with radioactively labelled glucose *in vitro* and then dialyse, all the labelled glucose is dispersed in the dialysis water and the glycoproteins do not become radioactive. So I don't think this is a passive labelling but depends on a living cell taking up the glucose, putting it through some synthetic pathway, and attaching it to the molecule.

Kramer: If you put glucose into the lumen of the trachea, do you find incorporation only in the goblet cells?

Jeffery: No, we find it mainly in the 'surface mucosubstance'.

Kramer: When we put galactose, serine, or leucine in the medium in the lumen of the stomach, we see incorporation only in the superficial layer of cells and never in the deeper layer, but when we administer them through the bloodstream, we see incorporation of serine, leucine, and even galactose in deep-lying cells too. One has to be careful in interpreting the effect of a luminal administration of a precursor because the superficial layers can cause a steep gradient by taking away the radioactive precursor.

Jeffery: That is a good point. However, the precursor is left for about an hour within the tracheal lumen, and since the submucosal glands have ducts, parts of which are quite dilated, I imagine that the glucose could easily come down the duct and into the gland that way.

Kramer: Perhaps in the duct the flow is in the opposite direction and could counteract the diffusion.

Guz: Can we get away from giving radioactive precursors via the lumen? That is not the way precursors reach the lumen in real life. Is it technically possible to isolate the segment of trachea under study so as to determine the uptake in a single pass of sulphate? And how avid is the trachea when the sulphate is given through the arterial system?

Richardson: It would be difficult to isolate it vascularly because several arteries supply the trachea and several veins drain its blood supply. Probably the best way to work out the dynamics of it would be to do the experiment *in vitro*, as Professor Nadel has done (Olver *et al.* 1975).

Reid: We studied it in rat, both in the living animal and in organ culture. We did not isolate trachea but if just one injection of sulphate is given to the living animal it is taken up avidly.

Nadel: But you don't know which surface of the cells in organ culture is taking it up.

Reid: It comes in via the base of the cell. We can show that glucose is incorporated into the epithelial glycoprotein. We haven't done that particular experiment with the sulphate. An interesting thing about sulphate is that in some cells it is added early, but in many of the airway cells no sulphate is seen at the base. It is when the granules are near the apex that one can first identify sulphate. We know from Glyn Roberts' purification studies (Roberts 1974, 1976) that it is the longer oligosaccharide side chains that have the most sulphate. The membranes around the packaged secretion may add this extra sulphate towards the apex of the cell. We have always wondered what is the role of this acidification, and particularly of sulphation, in the behaviour of the membrane and in the mechanism of discharge. One area of conflict between chemists and histochemists is that chemists find relatively little sulphate in the purified glycoprotein while histochemists see a heavy uptake of radioactive sulphate into the secretory cells, but, 20 years ago, chemists weren't prepared to accept that we were really dealing with a sulphated epithelial glycoprotein.

Allison: Isn't it possible that there are two components: you are dealing with one but most of the sulphate is on what may be a relatively small molecule?

Reid: No; because when we obtain the purified glycoprotein by density gradient ultracentrifugation it is sialylated and sulphated so that in the end there is mixing of these various types of building blocks. But I would like to know whether there is any way in which hydration is more effective once there is a sulphated molecule with a sulphate in a terminal position. Is this a packaged granule which, when it bursts, is going to open up more easily because of charge, or something like that?

Nadel: So far we have been talking about the granules inside the cells. Can you tell us what happens immediately after the granule is secreted into the lumen, Dr Jeffery?

Jeffery: All I can say is that one doesn't see the granules in the lumen. The granular nature of the secretion is lost once it leaves the cell.

Allison: So presumably the plasma membrane fuses with the granule membrane?

Jeffery: I imagine that it is an exocytotic process.

Silberberg: I have recently seen an electron micrograph of a cell caught in the process of secretion—it looks like a volcanic eruption.

Jeffery: I think it depends on whether the cell type we are talking about secretes in an apocrine or merocrine way. We have to make a distinction.

Allison: I want to come back to the question of the microvilli. They are prominent in the cells in the respiratory system but we know very little about them. As a cell biologist I think of microvilli as occurring in the intestine, in the renal tubules and so on. I don't think that Spicer would believe that microvilli by themselves could synthesize protein, as there are no ribosomes associated with them. So protein must be synthesized somewhere else but the microvilli could very well modify secretions. In other situations we know that microvilli extend the surface area of plasma membranes which are chiefly associated with absorptive capacity, so that the kind of absorption seen with sulphates and so on from the airways may take place through this enormously increased surface area of plasma membrane.

Microvilli also have a microfilament core but no microtubules. They can be isolated, for example, from the intestine and their properties analysed. So I think it might be possible to isolate microvilli from the respiratory system and to find out what they do—whether they have membrane-associated hydrolytic enzymes and concentrations of transport systems.

Silberberg: Dr Jeffery, you said earlier that all mucus produced by the lung is swallowed. Could there not also exist some mechanism by which mucus, or rather the mucin, is reabsorbed by the epithelium? Mucus, as we have shown, is undergoing a kind of spontaneous degradation. Hence, in resting epithelia (no mucus flow) the mucus may be in some sort of cycle which, in the respiratory tract, does not necessarily involve the need for each mucin molecule to come all the way up and then be swallowed. You did suggest that there might be a reabsorbing mechanism which would restore material back to the cell.

Jeffery: It could well be that much of it is absorbed.

Nadel: Have electron probes been used to see whether specific cations or anions are concentrated on the surfaces of microvilli?

Allison: The technical problem is that in the preparation of materials for electron microscopy a lot of these evanescent associations are lost. Moreover, unless one has increased concentrations of calcium or other material of high atomic number the method is inapplicable.

Jeffery: Yes, that is right, and as far as I know no such studies have been done, but it might be worth trying.

Douglas: My comment relates to the question of the 'right' side and the 'wrong' side for uptake of substances by the mucous cells. I am impressed by the fact that they are almost certainly secreting by exocytosis. We know this involves a massive addition of granule membrane to the cell surface, and we know from other cells that this is accompanied by some restorative process—recapture by pinocytic activity. Surely there must be a lot of reincorporation of luminal materials by pinocytic activity. What is known about such activity in these cells?

Reid: Dr Hogg's work (Simani *et al.* 1974) gets closest to endocytosis. He used peroxidase as a label. Admittedly he was mainly interested in what got through between the cells, but certainly that is one of the few occasions when material taken up into goblet cells has been identified.

Jeffery: Garrett has shown that secretory cells in the salivary gland of the rabbit actively take up horseradish peroxidase (Garrett & Parsons 1976). One has also to explain somehow the pinocytic vesicles that are often present in ciliated cells.

Douglas: If the peroxidase is put in the lumen does it get into the cell?

Jeffery: Yes.

Douglas: At the apex or along the side?

Reid: It looks as though it is in the apex of the goblets, although it does get down between the cells as well. The point of the experiment was that one was able to convert a tight junction to a leaky junction by either tobacco smoke or an antigen to which the animal was sensitive.

Thurlbeck: With that particular technique, how much is really endogenous peroxidase rather than the exogenous horseradish peroxidase? As you know, there is a lot of endogenous peroxidase activity in cells of the epithelium.

Jeffery: Not in the rabbit.

Reid: This is a crude method, but it is about the only one available.

Douglas: It is important to bear in mind when studying specific uptake mechanisms that pinocytic activity complicates the picture.

Reid: The serous cells in the human submucosal gland have intracellular canaliculi that open into the intracellular spaces and penetrate deep within the cell. Also, certainly in the human the collecting duct can be quite a long structure (up to 1 mm or so) lined with cells stuffed with mitochondria maybe up to about 70 μm high. This collecting duct with its collecting duct cell is very like the striated duct of the salivary gland, except that it doesn't have basal striations. So in thinking of total activity of the gland and of relating structure to function, we must take into account that collecting duct cell —and also a so-called 'clear' cell (Meyrick & Reid 1970; Meyrick *et al.* 1969). We also have to bear in mind the way the cells are arranged within the gland: the serous cells are always distal—upstream as it were to the mucous cells. The secretions of the serous cell must flow over the mucous cell and then over the duct cell. From some of the recent freeze-dried material that has been studied it is possible to see that the really sticky stuff coming out from the gland does tend to lie centrally as it comes out, but then what was a more liquid layer on top of the cells may have been lost. This cellular arrangement must say something about the way the various secretions are going to be related to each other spatially.

References

DALHAMN, T. (1956) Mucous flow and ciliary activity in the trachea of healthy rats and rats exposed to respiratory irritant gases. *Acta Physiol. Scand. 36*, 1–161

GALLAGHER, J. T., KENT, P. W., PASSATORE, M., PHIPPS, R. J. & RICHARDSON, P. S. (1975) The composition of tracheal mucus and the nervous control of its secretion in the cat. *Proc. R. Soc. Lond. B Biol. Sci. 192*, 49–76

GARRETT, J. R. & PARSONS, P. A. (1976) Movement of horseradish peroxidase in rabbit submandibular glands after ductal injection. *Histochem. J. 8*, 177–189

MEYRICK, B. & REID, L. (1970) Ultrastructure of cell in the human bronchial submucosal glands. *J. Anat. 107*, 281–299

MEYRICK, B., STURGESS, J. M. & REID, L. (1969) A reconstruction of the duct system and secretory tubules of the human bronchial submucosal gland. *Thorax 24*, 729–736

OLVER, R. E., DAVIS, B., MARIN, M. G. & NADEL, J. A. (1975) Active transport of Na^+ and Cl^- across the canine tracheal epithelium *in vitro*. *Am. Rev. Respir. Dis. 112*, 811–815

ROBERTS, G. P. (1974) Isolation and characterisation of glycoproteins from sputum. *Eur. J. Biochem. 50*, 265–280

ROBERTS, G. P. (1976) The role of disulfide bonds in maintaining the gel structure of bronchial mucus. *Arch. Biochem. Biophys. 173*, 528–537

SIMANI, A. S., INOUÉ, S. & HOGG, J. (1974) Penetration of the respiratory epithelium of guinea pigs following exposure to cigarette smoke. *Lab. Invest. 31*, 75–81

Stimulus-secretion coupling: variations on the theme of calcium-activated exocytosis involving cellular and extracellular sources of calcium

W. W. DOUGLAS

Department of Pharmacology, Yale University School of Medicine, New Haven, Connecticut

Abstract The term stimulus–secretion coupling refers to all those events occurring in the cell on exposure to an appropriate stimulus that lead to discharge of secretory product. In cells whose secretory product is sequestered in membrane-limited secretory granules a common secretory mechanism seems to operate whose principal features are: (1) An action of the stimulus on the plasma membrane that leads, in one way or another, to a rise in the concentration of free calcium ions at some critical site within the cell, probably the inner aspect of the plasma membrane. (2) The activation, by this calcium, of some energy-dependent step which results in: (3) Merging of the membranes of secretory granules with the limiting membrane of the cell with subsequent rupture and expulsion of the secretory granule core to the exterior (exocytosis). The mechanisms whereby secretory stimuli raise the intracellular concentration of free calcium ions fall into two broad classes: those promoting calcium influx and those mobilizing cellular calcium. In the former category are cells whose plasma membranes possess potential (voltage)-dependent calcium channels (which open on depolarization and are associated with sodium-spiking or calcium-spiking), and other cells where the secretagogue opens calcium channels insensitive to membrane potential. The presence of potential-dependent calcium channels may reflect developmental origin in neuroectodermal tissue: cells with this mechanism include neurons, neurosecretory fibres, and various endocrine cells of the APUD series. Different stimuli applied to the same cell (e.g. mast cells or exocrine salivary cells) may preferentially activate calcium influx or mobilization. Various stratagems that allow calcium to flow into the cell from without or otherwise cause free calcium to accumulate within the cell will initiate exocytosis. The calcium-activated process seemingly involves ATP: calcium fails to induce exocytosis in cells exposed to various inhibitors of energy production. Whether ATP is consumed during exocytosis (fusion–fission) is uncertain. Model systems using isolated granules, with or without membranes, indicate that calcium can cause fusion–fission. The occurrence, in intact cells, of 'compound exocytosis' (wherein granules fuse with one another) probably offers important clues to the nature of the fusion–fission reaction.

Of the various aspects of secretory function that capture the experimenter's interest many are unique to individual secretory systems and relate to particular syntheses and secretory products or particular secretory stimuli or secretagogues. But it is possible to discern certain features that are shared by secretory cells of widely different form and function whose product is stored in and expelled from membrane-limited secretory granules. These include the cellular machinery for the synthesis, packaging and transport of the secretory product and a common mechanism for extrusion of the secretory product, exocytosis, in which the membranes of the secretory granule and the limiting membrane of the cell fuse and rupture to transfer the secretory product from the cellular to the extracellular domain (Palade 1975). Exocytosis and its control by calcium are the subjects with which this paper will be concerned. There is now considerable evidence that exocytosis, however induced, may result from a rise in the concentration of free calcium ions at some intracellular site during stimulation. Ten years ago (Douglas 1968) I advanced the general hypothesis that calcium-activated exocytosis might be a common link in stimulus–secretion coupling and my colleagues and I had toyed with this idea for several years before that as a result of our work with several different types of secretory cells which we had selected as possible models of the three main classes of secretory system: endocrine, neuroendocrine and exocrine, namely, adrenal medulla, posterior pituitary and salivary glands. I shall discuss here some aspects of the involvement of calcium in stimulus–secretion coupling, this term being 'intended to embrace all the events occurring in the cell exposed to its immediate stimulus that lead, finally, to the appearance of the characteristic secretory product in the extracellular environment' (Douglas 1968). Most experiments have been performed on cells other than those specifically associated with mucus secretion, but there are good reasons for supposing that mucus-secreting cells probably conform to the same general pattern; certainly this is true of submaxillary salivary glands and mucus-secreting cells of invertebrates.

According to one view exocytosis is the universal calcium-sensitive mechanism for release of packaged, preformed, secretory product. When this argument was being developed (see Douglas 1966, 1967, 1968) convincing evidence of exocytosis had been obtained from only a small group of cells and alternative conjectures were abundant. The view that exocytosis probably operated in systems where it had not been detected (even when deliberately and vigorously sought) was based on argument by analogy. The widespread involvement of calcium in secretory activity, the remarkable parallelism of ionic influences and the general requirement for metabolic energy all seemed to indicate a common secretory process. Exocytosis had been clearly demonstrated in some cells and similar packaging of secretory product in membrane-limited secretory granules would clearly allow for the operation of the mechanism in the other secretory cells. Moreover exocytosis, which involves the interaction of membranes presumably more uniform than the diverse secretory products, would, I argued, neatly explain the common ionic influences and energy dependence. Now, a decade or more later, the literature is replete with illustrations and documentation of exocytosis in all sorts of secretory systems, not only in exocrine and endocrine glands of the familiar classes, but in all manner of cells with secretory function including unicellular organisms; and exocytosis may be viewed as a 'probably general mechanism for the discharge of macromolecular secretory products' (Palade 1975). Some very interesting electron micrographs of exocytosis have been obtained from mucus-secreting systems, for example the mucocysts of *Tetrahymena* (Satir *et al.* 1973). Even in neurons and neurosecretory fibres, where the existence of exocytosis has been so long and heatedly debated, and where alternative *ad hoc* hypotheses have flourished for so long, evidence for exocytosis is becoming more impressive. My colleagues and I (Douglas *et al.* 1971), and others since, have obtained electron micrographs of exocytosis in the neurosecretory fibres of the posterior pituitary gland. Moreover, biochemical evidence shows that protein stored along with the peptide hormones in the neurosecretory granules escapes *pari passu* with the hormone without any loss of cytoplasmic molecules of corresponding size. The only known secretory mechanism that would permit this is exocytosis (see reviews by Douglas 1973, 1974*a*, *b*). It was combined morphological and biochemical evidence of this sort that established beyond doubt that secretion occurred by exocytosis in the adrenal medullary chromaffin cells, the system that originally provided evidence of the involvement of calcium in stimulus–secretion coupling (see reviews by Douglas 1975*a* and Viveros 1975). In ordinary nerves, such as those secreting acetylcholine or noradrenaline, both morphological and chemical evidence for exocytosis has been more difficult to obtain (there are forbidding technical difficulties) but there is now some chemical evidence in favour of the process (see for example Smith 1971; De Potter 1976), and morphological evidence indicative of exocytosis has been obtained with a variety of methods including transmission electron microscopy (see for example Couteaux 1974) and freeze–fracture methods (Heuser & Reese 1974). Moreover studies on dynamic changes induced by nerve impulses in the membrane in the secretory granules and nerve terminal which are accompanied by uptake of tracer substances seem consistent only with the view that exocytosis provides the mechanism for release of transmitter substances (Ceccarelli *et al.* 1973; Heuser & Reese 1973). It may seem odd to devote space here to the question of exocytosis in nerves and neurosecretory terminals, which are a far cry indeed from mucus-secreting cells, but the problem is most relevant to my topic; such preparations have provided some of the clearest and most direct evidence on the involvement of calcium in stimulus–secretion coupling, particularly with regard to calcium fluxes and the intracellular free calcium ion concentration (see reviews by Katz 1969; Douglas 1974*a*, *b*; Baker 1972; Llinas *et al.* 1976).

What then of calcium and the suggestion that it serves as a mediator or messenger in stimulus–secretion coupling? The evidence that led us to propose such a scheme was obtained from adrenal chromaffin cells more than a decade ago (Douglas & Rubin 1961, 1963; Douglas & Poisner 1962; Douglas *et al.* 1967*a*, *b*) and is familiar to many working in the field. But inasmuch as the chromaffin cell can now be recognized as a valid paradigm of calcium-mediated exocytosis it is worth reviewing the findings briefly (for a more extensive review see Douglas 1975*a*). The medullary chromaffin cells are innervated by cholinergic nerves and release their product when exposed to the neurotransmitter, acetylcholine (ACh). Such nerve-evoked release of secretory product is, of course, a pattern familiar to those working with mucus-secreting cells. My colleagues and I found:

1. That calcium was essential for ACh-induced secretion.
2. That calcium was also a sufficient ionic condition for secretion.
3. That calcium influx, as gauged by isotope accumulation or electrophysiological measurement, was increased by ACh.
4. That substances blocking calcium influx (Mg or local anaesthetic) blocked secretion.
5. That barium, which penetrates membranes more readily than calcium, elicited secretion in the absence of ACh or other secretagogue; and, most critical:
6. That calcium itself was capable of eliciting secretion provided that the plasma membrane had been rendered leaky to it (by prolonged exposure to a calcium-free medium).

These results pointed clearly to a mediator role for calcium ions (Fig. 1). Intracellular recording revealed to us that acetylcholine depolarized the chromaffin cells and provided evidence that some of the depolarizing current was carried by calcium ions, in line with the postulated mediator role of this ion (Douglas *et al.* 1967*a*, *b*). But most of the depolarization was clearly attributable to inward sodium current. To account for this we suggested that depolarization might help to open calcium channels: in other words that the chromaffin cell possessed calcium channels sensitive to transmembrane potential which opened as this potential fell. The fact that we were able to demonstrate a calcium-dependent secretory response when extracellular potassium was raised to depolarizing levels supported this interpretation. We recognized

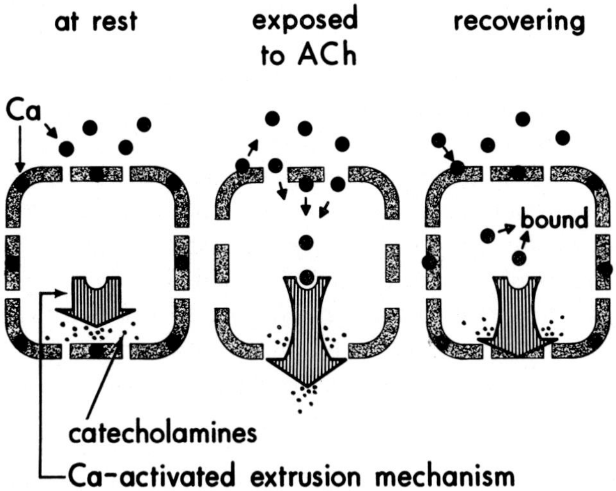

FIG. 1. Calcium as a mediator of stimulus–secretion coupling in the chromaffin cell.
The black circles represent calcium ions or calcium bound to the cell membrane. The secretagogue acting on the membrane causes a rise in the concentration of free intracellular calcium ion which then initiates secretion (exocytosis). The action on the membrane is depicted as increasing permeability to calcium ions, allowing them to enter passively down their electrochemical gradient. Displacement of membrane calcium may also contribute to the secretory response. Secretion is supposed to cease, on withdrawing the stimulus, as free calcium is bound. (From Douglas 1966.)

that this endocrine cell, the chromaffin cell, was behaving much like the cholinergic nerve terminal (see Katz 1969) where depolarization accompanying the arrival of the propagated nerve impulse also appeared to set in motion a calcium-dependent secretory process. The fact that chromaffin cells shared a common developmental origin with neurons led us to study the developmentally related neurosecretory system, the hypothalamo-neurohypophysial tract that secretes posterior pituitary hormones. Our evidence showed that release of these hormones was also calcium-dependent and was accompanied by calcium uptake, and we concluded that the appearance of free calcium ions somewhere in the cell was sufficient to initiate the secretory response (Douglas 1963*a*; Douglas & Poisner 1964*a*, *b*; and review by Douglas 1974*b*). Meanwhile a long line of evidence, involving some exquisite electrophysiological methods, was being developed by B. Katz and R. Miledi from studies of the cholinergic neuromuscular junction which was to lead them, in 1967, to a specific hypothesis for the quantal release of chemical transmitter by calcium influx (see Katz 1969, p. 39). Studies of nerve endings, particularly large presynaptic terminals of squid giant synapses, have now provided some of the most striking evidence for inward calcium current during excitation and for its relation to the release of neurotransmitter (see for example Katz 1969; Llinas *et al.* 1976).

As all this evidence was coming together, a certain unity of events in stimulus–secretion coupling became obvious in these three developmentally related cells. In each instance the stimulus to the cell involved depolarization and calcium influx and the action potential in the cells with long secretory processes (axons) clearly served simply to telegraph this primitive 'go' signal to the distant secretory poles of the neuron and neurosecretory fibres (see Douglas 1966, 1973, 1974*a*, *b*, 1975*a*). Recent experiments have shown that the parallelism is even closer than was suspected; for example Biales *et al.* (1976) and Brandt *et al.* (1976) have discovered that chromaffin cells, like neurons and neurosecretory fibres, generate action potentials attributable to regenerative sodium influx. In the light of the evidence I have cited, indicating that depolarization is an adequate stimulus for calcium influx in the chromaffin cells (see also Baker & Rink 1975), such action potentials, appearing in response to acetylcholine, must obviously play a part in stimulus–secretion coupling.

In the three systems mentioned it would thus appear that the sodium spikes mediate, or contribute importantly to, stimulus–secretion coupling by depolarizing and opening potential-dependent calcium channels which allow calcium to run passively down its electrochemical gradient and enter the cells to initiate exocytosis. How many other secretory cells conform to this pattern remains to be seen. Some exocrine cells of invertebrates, including mucus-secreting cells, have recently been shown to generate sodium spikes and to require calcium for their secretory responses (Mackie 1976; Kater 1977), but many other secretory cells, including mammalian exocrine systems, do not use this mechanism of stimulus–secretion coupling, but rather some variation of it.

CALCIUM SPIKING SYSTEMS

The first of these variations is not far removed from the theme just described, inasmuch as one can recognize, as a central feature, potential-dependent calcium influx and a critical dependence on extracellular calcium to effect the exocytotic response. Among the most familiar cells in this category are those of the endocrine pancreas and the anterior pituitary. On the rather tenuous grounds of morphological similarity with chromaffin cells we early suspected that the lessons learned from the chromaffin cell might apply to these also (Douglas & Poisner 1963), and when these cells were subsequently exposed to the ionic manipulations used in the analysis of chromaffin cell function similarities at once became apparent (see reviews by Geschwind 1971; Malaisse 1972; Randle & Hales 1972). As in the chromaffin cell, secretion showed critical dependence on extracellular calcium and the response to the physiological secretagogue—an increase in blood sugar or hypophysiotropic hormone—could be mimicked by an increase in extracellular potassium to presumably depolarizing levels. Likewise secretion could be elicited by calcium provided the cells were rendered permeable to that ion by a calcium ionophore (see reviews by Labrie *et al.* 1976 and by Gerich *et al.* 1976). But on closer inspection the behaviour of these cells clearly differs from that of the chromaffin cell. This has become apparent from a series of elegant electrophysiological experiments initiated and pursued by E. K. Matthews and his colleagues at Cambridge and others who have adopted the electrophysiological approach (see Dean *et al.* 1975; Meissner 1976). This work has shown that the pancreatic beta cell generates electrical impulses in response to an increase in extracellular glucose, which is the physiological stimulus for insulin secretion. Moreover, the impulses appear to be generated and sustained by influx of calcium ions rather than sodium ions: in the electrophysiological idiom the cells show calcium spikes. These calcium spikes, unlike the sodium spikes characteristic of nerve, are unaffected by tetrodotoxin, the classic blocker of most potential-dependent sodium channels, but are inhibited by substances such as Mn and the verapamil derivative D600 which are known to block potential-dependent calcium channels (see Baker 1972). Experiments recently conducted by Kidokoro (1975) on a clonal line of transformed (adenomatous) anterior pituitary cells (GH3) have revealed the presence there also of spikes blocked by Mn but not by tetrodotoxin. This raises the possibility that calcium spiking activity may also participate in stimulus–secretion coupling in normal anterior pituitary cells. Dr P. S. Taraskevich and I have subsequently shown the existence of spiking in another clonal cell line (GH4) and demonstrated its calcium-dependence directly by showing that spike amplitude increases as the extracellular concentration of calcium is increased. We have extended the study to *normal* anterior pituitary cells and discovered that spiking is present in these too, and moreover that spikes may be induced, or their frequency increased, by the stimulant hypophysiotropic hormone (hypothalamic 'releasing factor') TRH. The impulses in the normal cells are resistant to tetrodotoxin, persist in the absence of sodium, and are blocked by D600. They are thus probably calcium spikes. Dr Taraskevich and I believe that stimulation or inhibition of action potentials involving calcium influx may be a key element in the hypothalamic control of normal adenohypophysial cells (Taraskevich & Douglas 1977; Douglas & Taraskevich 1977).

There are thus at least two categories of secretory cell (sodium spiking and calcium spiking) in which potential-dependent calcium influx figures in stimulus-secretion coupling. As I shall point out shortly, such potential-dependence is by no means universal in secretory cells and some important exocrine cells such as those of salivary glands and exocrine pancreas do not possess it, as shown by their failure to secrete in response to an increase in extracellular potassium. A possibility which I have raised before (Douglas 1974*a*) is that the presence of potential-dependent calcium channels in certain secretory cells, which we have seen is associated with spike-generating capacity, may reflect developmental origins in neural crest or related neuroectodermal tissues. Pearse has long argued that endocrine pancreatic and adenohypophysial, as well as many other endocrine cells which he refers to as the APUD series, have such an origin (see Pearse & Takor Takor 1976). The discovery of electrical activity in cancerous C cells (thyroid adenomata) is consistent with this interpretation, as pointed out by Tischler *et al.* (1976). If this view is correct then we may expect to find electrical activity, potential-dependent calcium channels, and perhaps calcium spiking in a large number of endocrine cells, including, for example, those secreting gastrointestinal peptide hormones of various sorts (Pearse & Polack 1971; Johnson 1977). Scratcherd *et al.* (1976) have provided evidence that potential-dependent calcium channels exist by showing that pancreozymin-cholecystokinin can be released from a site of storage by an increase in extracellular potassium and that this response is calcium-dependent. The converse may also be true: that if a cell shows a calcium-dependent exocytotic secretory response to excess potassium, this may be taken as evidence, at least suggestive, of origin in neuroectodermal tissue. Here I am referring only to vertebrate material: the potential-dependent secretory activity in some exocrine cells in invertebrates indicates the possible limitations of this argument, but I repeat the suggestion (Douglas 1974*a*) that a comparative approach may be helpful not only to broaden our understanding of secretion but also to provide clues to the embryological origins of secretory cells and their influence on the pattern of stimulus–secretion coupling.

CELLS WITHOUT POTENTIAL-DEPENDENT CALCIUM INFLUX

What now of cells that seem to possess no potential-dependent calcium influx mechanism? The most familiar examples are the exocrine cells of the pancreas and salivary glands, but free-floating cells of less conventional, but nevertheless real, secretory activity such as basophils, mast cells, and platelets, also fall into this class. None of these cells secrete when challenged with depolarizing concentrations of potassium. Yet calcium seems to be intimately involved in secretion and, in some instances at least, secretion seems attributable to calcium influx in response to stimulation. The mast cell provides a good illustration of this. As far as is known, the normal stimulus for mast cell secretion (the discharge of histamine and other substances) is the acute hypersensitivity reaction, a reaction of specific antigen with antibodies (IgE) bound on the cell surface which may be regarded as receptors that have been grafted onto the cells. Some 15 years ago, Mongar & Schild (1962) observed that the acute hypersensitivity reaction that leads to histamine release has a unique requirement for calcium. Confronted with our evidence identifying the role of calcium in the chromaffin cell, Rubin and I proposed that 'anaphylactic' secretion of histamine and other amines from various cellular sites of storage might be due to calcium influx (Douglas & Rubin 1961). Later, reviewing the general problem of stimulus–secretion coupling in the light of more extensive evidence, I pointed out that antigen, acting on sensitized cells such as the mast cell, might be regarded as simply another secretagogue acting on its membrane receptors to increase membrane permeability to calcium, thereby promoting calcium influx and activating exocytosis (Douglas 1968, 1970, 1975*b*). There is now compelling chemical and morphological evidence that secretion in mast cells in response to antigen is by exocytosis (see Goth & Johnson 1975; Anderson *et al.* 1973) and is mediated by calcium influx. Much of the evidence on the role of calcium has been provided by Foreman *et al.* (1976), who have shown that histamine secretion from sensitized mast cells on exposure to specific antigen is profoundly inhibited by withdrawal of calcium from the extracellular medium and varies with the extracellular calcium concentration over a wide range. Furthermore they found that mast cells exposed to antigen accumulate ^{45}Ca even when the secretory response is inhibited by the cells being deprived of energy; they thereby showed that calcium accumulation is not secondary to the secretory response but is probably an antecedent event. And in a pioneering experiment with the calcium ionophore A23187 they showed that calcium could stimulate histamine release (Foreman *et al.* 1973). Shortly thereafter my colleagues and I demonstrated by light and electron microscopy that this secretory response to calcium involves the classic 'degranulating response' by exocytosis (Cochrane & Douglas 1974; Kagayama & Douglas 1974). The mast cell response, readily seen under the light microscope, provides a vivid illustration of the operation of calcium-activated exocytosis (Fig. 2). A similar exocytotic response can be elicited by introducing calcium to calcium-deprived mast cells (Fig. 3), about which I shall say more later.

The mast cell, unlike others I have discussed, does not secrete in response to an increase in extracellular potassium: even isosmotic KCl (150 mM) in

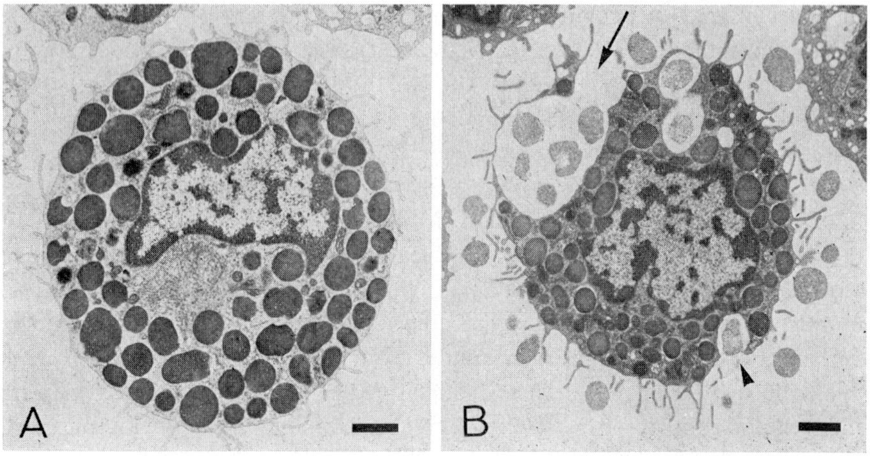

FIG. 2. Exocytosis induced by calcium in mast cells treated with a calcium ionophore (A 23187).

A. Control. A mast cell suspended 10 min in Ca-free Locke solution containing 0.1 mM-EDTA with the addition of A23187 (2.5 μg/ml). The cell appears normal. Secretory granules are dense and membrane-limited.

B. Response to calcium. Another mast cell treated as above but with the further addition of Ca (1.0 mM) 60 s before fixing. The long arrow indicates a site of compound exocytosis: note the large exocytotic pit containing several granule cores which are swollen, less dense, and devoid of membrane. Two other altered granules to the right of this pit (at 12 o'clock) are probably lying in an exocytotic pit whose opening to the cell surface is out of the plane of section. At another site (arrowhead) exocytosis appears to involve only a single granule. Extruded granules surround the cell. Scale 1 μm. (Experiment by Kagayama & Douglas from Douglas 1974*c*; see also Kagayama & Douglas 1974.)

the presence of Ca fails to elicit secretory responses. But excess potassium does not impede responses to the calcium ionophore (Cochrane & Douglas 1974, 1976). It seems clear that mast cells lack any potential-dependent calcium channels (Douglas 1974*a*). Calcium channels in this cell seem to be opened directly by the interaction of the antigenic stimulus with the membrane-fixed antibody (IgE) 'receptors' and not by any mechanism dependent on fall in transmembrane potential.

Other cells that show no secretory response to an increase in potassium and seem to lack potential-dependent calcium channels are those present in mammalian exocrine glands such as salivary glands and exocrine pancreas. But these cells, unlike mast cells responding to antigen, seem to rely relatively little on extracellular calcium for their moment-to-moment secretory activity; rather, the physiological stimuli appear able to induce exocytosis by 'mobilizing' calcium from some cellular source.

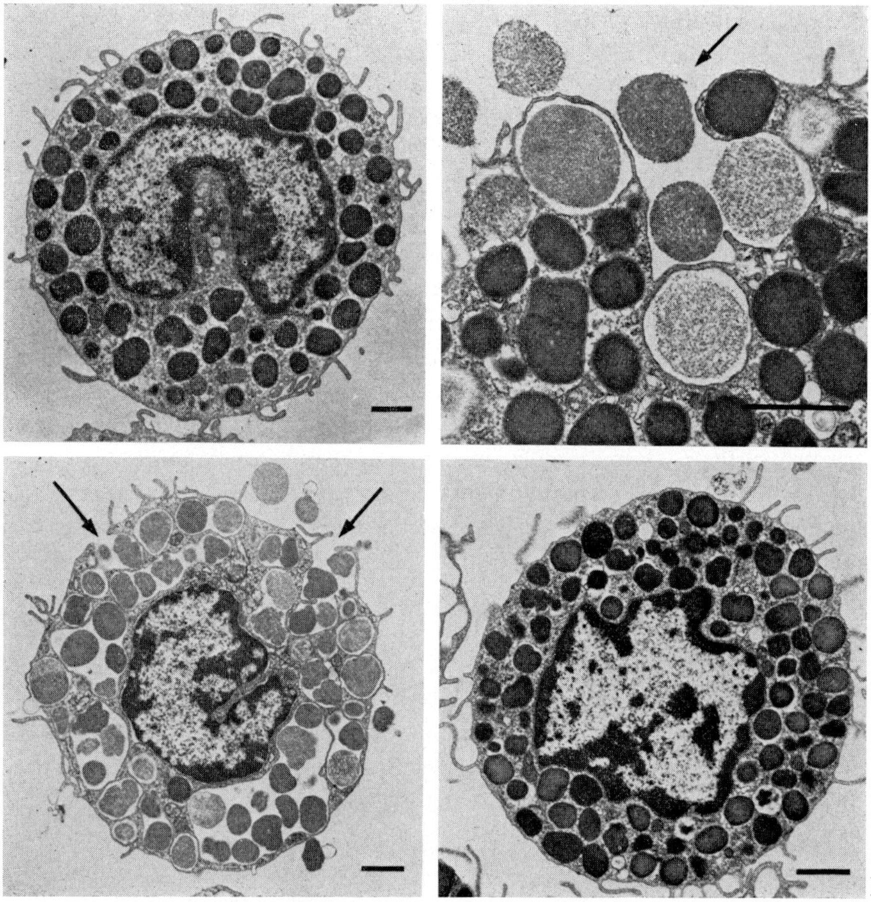

A B C D

FIG. 3. Exocytosis induced in mast cells by calcium after calcium deprivation to increase membrane permeability.

A. Control mast cell in Ca-free Locke solution after 2 h incubation in Ca-free Locke containing 1 mM-EDTA. The appearance is normal.

B. A mast cell treated as in A and then exposed to high Ca (110 mM) Locke solution for 10 min. A site of compound exocytosis is indicated by the arrow.

C. Another EDTA-treated mast cell exposed to high Ca for 30 min, showing a more extensive compound exocytotic reaction. All but one of the granules (lying just below the nucleus) have been altered and lie in pits, two of whose openings are evident in the section (arrows).

D. Another EDTA-treated mast cell exposed to high Mg (110 mM) Locke solution for 30 min. There is no response. (From experiments by Douglas & Kagayama 1977.)

CALCIUM MOBILIZATION

The experiments that initially revealed an involvement of calcium in stimulus–secretion coupling in an exocrine system were done on cat submaxillary salivary glands (Douglas & Poisner 1963), whose secretion is rich in mucoproteins (Burgen & Emmelin 1961). We applied to these glands the same procedures as had revealed the involvement of calcium in the adrenal medulla. The results, in the main, paralleled those obtained from the adrenal gland and led us to conclude that calcium might act in stimulus–secretion coupling in exocrine as well as endocrine systems. Thus, secretion to acetylcholine could be reversibly inhibited by perfusion with calcium-free medium, and an increase in the extracellular calcium concentration augmented secretory responses. At the same time, we were impressed by certain differences between the two systems. For example, to inhibit the secretory response we had to deprive the exocrine preparation of calcium for a much longer period than the endocrine preparation. The effects, on the evoked secretion, of varying the extracellular calcium concentration were smaller; magnesium was a feeble inhibitor; and reintroduction of calcium into the calcium-deprived gland was not an adequate stimulus for secretion (Douglas & Poisner 1963). Eventually the pieces of the puzzle began to fall into place, largely as a consequence of work carried out on the exocrine pancreas (see Case 1973; Argent *et al.* 1976). This work confirmed that extracellular calcium had a role (see Hokin 1966 and below) but suggested that cellular sources of calcium could be mobilized in sufficient amounts to sustain secretory responses, provided that the cell had not been deprived of calcium for a prolonged period. These conclusions were based on two main observations: that secretion could be elicited for a considerable time after extracellular calcium had been removed and chelating agent added, and that the stimulus evoked discharge of cellular ^{45}Ca even when there was no calcium in the extracellular medium. The relative importance of cellular and extracellular calcium for stimulus–secretion coupling in different exocrine glands, including the pancreas, is still debated (see for example Chandler & Williams 1974; Schulz & Kondo 1976). There is little doubt, however, that in some circumstances extracellular calcium makes an important contribution, for example in the submaxillary glands as Poisner and I studied them (Douglas & Poisner 1963) and in the parotid stimulated through α-adrenergic or cholinergic receptors (Schramm & Selinger 1976; Petersen 1976), and also in the rat pancreas either perfused (Kanno & Nishimura 1976) or *in vitro* (Argent *et al.* 1977). Moreover, the exocrine cells clearly become increasingly dependent on extracellular calcium as stimulation is prolonged; and an influx of extracellular calcium can certainly provide an intense stimulus for secretion, as shown by the vigorous responses to calcium in pancreas treated with the calcium ionophore A23187 (see Poulsen & Williams 1977). But the point to be stressed here is that some cells may call on cellular stores of calcium to effect the exocytotic response and this may be especially significant for responses to particular stimuli, for example catecholamines acting through β-receptors of the parotid gland (Schramm & Selinger 1976).

Another example of this sort of behaviour involving calcium mobilization is provided by the mast cell (Douglas 1975*b*). If, instead of antigen, we use a stimulus such as the polyamine 48/80 or some other basic polymeric histamine releaser, the response is reduced relatively little by the omission of extracellular calcium. This long-known fact had suggested that the secretory response to 48/80, which is known to be exocytosis (see Röhlich *et al.* 1971), might be an exception to the rule of calcium dependence. Mrs Ueda and I have found, however, that when mast cells are incubated with chelating agents such as EDTA or EGTA for an hour or so the response to 48/80 can be completely abolished and may be regained by incubating the cells for a few minutes in a calcium-containing medium (Douglas & Ueda 1973; see also Kagayama & Douglas 1974; Cochrane & Douglas 1974). We have noted a similar phenomenon with polymyxin B (W. W. Douglas and Y. Ueda, unpublished results). We take this behaviour to mean that the mast cells can draw on some cellular source of calcium to sustain the response to these polyamines. Both substances are known to act on receptors on the cell membrane and it is possible that this action causes the membrane to release calcium to the cytoplasm (see Cochrane & Douglas 1976; Douglas 1976). A similar suggestion has been made by Petersen (1976) for the action of acetylcholine on exocrine cells; indeed, this was long ago indicated as a possible adjuvant factor in the chromaffin cell response to acetylcholine (Douglas 1963*b*, 1966) (see Fig. 1).

I am not suggesting that one kind of stimulus to the cell acts exclusively by one mechanism and relies solely on calcium influx or on calcium mobilization to effect the secretory response. On the contrary, the response of mast cells to 48/80 is somewhat reduced in the absence of extracellular calcium; and in Ca-depleted mast cells (EDTA-treated) 48/80 'primes' the cell in much the same way as does a calcium ionophore (possibly by increasing membrane permeability); as a result, the reintroduction of calcium to the extracellular medium gives an immediate exocytotic response (Cochrane & Douglas 1974; Kagayama & Douglas 1974). Moreover, the response of sensitized mast cells to antigen is not completely lost when extracellular calcium is absent and, by analogy with 48/80 and other stimuli, we have proposed that this residual response to antigen is not a calcium-independent process but reflects mobilization of cellular calcium (Cochrane & Douglas 1976; see also

Foreman *et al.* 1976). The old model illustrated in Fig. 1 suggests that stimuli acting primarily to open calcium channels may act by some mechanism involving removal of membrane calcium (Douglas, 1963*a*, 1966) so that mobilized calcium then appears as a by-product contributing to the calcium-sensitive secretory mechanism; likewise, stimuli acting primarily to mobilize calcium might incidentally increase membrane permeability, allowing passive calcium influx. Perhaps such complexity is common in exocrine and endocrine secretory systems and may explain the many discrepant observations and opinions on the precise nature of the sources of calcium contributing to the secretory response. In multicellular animals where the extracellular environment is body fluid containing calcium, the use of cellular calcium to effect exocytosis is certainly not dictated by lack of calcium in the extracellular fluid. Some cells, however, have to use cellular calcium because little is present in the extracellular environment. Thus exocytotic discharge of secretory vesicles (mucocysts and trichocysts) from freshwater organisms such as *Tetrahymena* and *Paramecium* probably results from mobilization of cellular calcium (Wissig & Satir 1976; Plattner 1974), as does the exocytotic discharge of cortical granules from eggs, including those of freshwater species (see Vacquier 1976; Ridgway *et al.* 1977).

In summary, stimulus–secretion coupling can be effected by several different mechanisms which draw on cellular or extracellular calcium in different ways, although all seem directed to the same end: the increase in the intracellular concentration of free calcium ions at some critical site, presumably just under the limiting membrane of the cell. The calcium hypothesis of stimulus–secretion coupling (Douglas 1968) therefore needs updating to take this diversity into account and Table 1 is an attempt to classify discernible mechanisms of stimulus–secretion coupling that may have some heuristic value. Like most classifications it tends to give the impression that particular examples fall neatly into one category or another but, as I have already said, the same cell may use different mechanisms, and I have indicated this by certain double entries in the table. Even where alternative mechanisms are not indicated (I, a, i, ii), they are not necessarily excluded. On the contrary, there is abundant evidence that calcium mobilization by various treatments involving drugs, toxins and ions (see below) will elicit secretion in all the cell types I have listed as characteristically operating through the calcium influx mechanism; moreover for endocrine cells of the APUD series there are indications of secretion attributable to calcium mobilization in response to physiological secretagogues (see Gerich *et al.* 1976; Labrie *et al.* 1976).

This variety of mechanisms for raising the intracellular concentration of free calcium ions in secretory cells is similar to what takes place in muscles,

TABLE 1

Mechanisms of stimulus-secretion coupling: ways in which stimuli raise intracellular Ca^{2+}

	Extracellular Ca^{2+} essential	*Depolarization (excess K^+) elicits secretion*
1. CALCIUM INFLUX		
a) Potential-dependent Ca channels	YES	YES
(i) *Na spiking cells*		
Neurons		
Neurosecretory fibres		
Chromaffin cells		
Invertebrate exocrine cells		
(ii) *Ca spiking cells*		
Endocrine pancreas B cell		
Adenohypophysial cells		
? all other APUD cells		
b) Potential-independent Ca channels	YES	NO
Mast cell (antigen)		
Basophil (antigen)		
Platelet (antigen)		
Salivary glands (ACh and α agonists)		
2. CALCIUM MOBILIZATION	NO	NO
Exocrine pancreas		
Salivary glands (β agonists)		
Mast cell (48/80)		
Platelet (thrombin)		
Unicellular organisms: Tetrahymena		
Egg cortical granules		

where a rise in the concentration of free calcium ions is the universal trigger for contraction, yet where the means by which this is achieved are equally diverse. In some smooth and cardiac muscles calcium influx contributes importantly and calcium spikes are demonstrable in preparations of such muscles, whereas in skeletal striated muscle the required calcium is mobilized from cellular stores (sarcoplasmic reticulum). From the time of the experiments on the adrenal that led to the concept of stimulus–secretion coupling, my colleagues and I have repeatedly drawn attention to the parallels between contraction and secretion, and to the great many ionic and other manipulations that affect both systems similarly. Indeed, it was the initial indications of parallelism that led us to coin the term 'stimulus–secretion coupling' (Douglas &

Rubin 1961; see also Douglas 1968). And I long ago suggested that those of us working in the field of stimulus–secretion coupling might profitably view our endeavours on the involvement of calcium in the broader perspective of 'stimulus–response coupling' (Douglas 1966). This is all the more evident today.

One question that emerges from such a comparative approach is whether those secretory cells that use cellular sources of calcium possess a special calcium-sequestering and releasing apparatus analogous to the sarcoplasmic reticulum that serves such a function in striated muscle. There is as yet no convincing evidence for this but it may be rewarding to seek such a system in large 'polarized' secretory cells where the receptors for the stimulus are far removed from the site of exocytosis, and where there is no evidence of a propagated disturbance of the plasma membrane (depolarization with or without spike generation) that could be implicated as a calcium-mobilizing factor. The relatively large exocrine cells in the pancreas and salivary glands might fall into this category. Certainly, if a rise in free calcium ions is critical for the membrane fusion–fission process occurring in exocytosis, there must be some means of providing calcium at the exocytotic site. It seems unlikely that a stimulus restricted to one part of a large cell will cause a rise in the concentration of free calcium ions throughout the cell even if it has this effect locally, and Rose & Loewenstein (1975) have demonstrated that calcium injected into a large secretory cell at one point does not spread unless the calcium-sequestering capacity of the cell has been inhibited. However, although by analogy we might be tempted to seek a specialized calcium-sequestering and releasing organelle in secretory cells we need to keep in mind the different functional considerations in striated muscle cells and exocytotic secretory mechanisms. In the striated muscle fibre the functional response—actin–myosin interaction—occurs *throughout the cytoplasm*, including sites far removed from the surface; free Ca^{2+} ions must therefore be delivered instantly throughout the cell. By contrast, exocytosis involves only the surface of the cell and presumably free calcium ions need appear only at the *cytoplasmic aspect of the cell surface membrane* or nearby.

COMPOUND EXOCYTOSIS

There is one characteristic of exocytosis that is not widely appreciated but which, as I have argued (Douglas 1974*a*), must be recognized if we are to understand that process and the role of calcium. Exocytosis always involves an interaction between the membrane of the secretory granule and that forming the cell surface. This is usually interpreted to mean that the reaction always involves two *distinct* entities—granule membrane and plasmalemma; and this, in turn, has suggested an interplay between complementary constituents of two different membranes: perhaps enzyme and substrate (see reviews by Douglas 1974*b*, 1975*a*, *b*) or something comparable to hormone receptor interaction (Palade 1975). But the fact remains that in many secretory cells interaction between functionally distinct membranes can account for only a fraction of the exocytotic events since, once exocytosis begins in these cells, granules may fuse and rupture among themselves in serial fashion. When this occurs each reaction still involves granule membrane and cell surface membrane, but this cell surface membrane is now composed of granule membrane incorporated by a previous exocytotic event. This process has been detected repeatedly in various exocrine and endocrine cells and in the mast cell is rapidly produced in exuberant form by any number of 'degranulating agents' such as antigen (in sensitized cells) or 48/80. The enormous exocytotic pits thus formed may contain many secretory granule cores (see Anderson *et al.* 1973; Röhlich *et al.* 1971; Lagunoff 1972) which have undergone exocytosis in the strict sense of transfer from cellular to extracellular medium but which are retained within the 'territorial limits' of the cell in deep fjords of extracellular medium (see Figs. 2 & 3). To distinguish this kind of reaction from 'simple' exocytosis (where 'virgin' plasmalemma and secretory granule membrane interact), I have proposed the term 'compound exocytosis' (Douglas 1974*a*). The essential features of the process are evident in Fig. 4. As I pointed out in 1974, compound exocytosis has important functional implications, perhaps the most obvious of which is that the essential ingredients for the fusion–fission reaction are present in secretory granules themselves. It follows that studies on isolated secretory granules (see later) may well be relevant to the problem of exocytosis.

Compound exocytosis also suggests that granules may themselves provide the source of calcium required for exocytosis. Granules and granule membranes have been shown, in the exocrine pancreas, to be rich in calcium (Meldolesi 1975); and Vacquier (1975) has obtained evidence suggesting that the propagated wave of granule–granule fusion in secretory (cortical) granules of sea urchin eggs might be explained in this way (see also Ridgway *et al.* 1977).

In seeking factors that allow compound exocytosis to occur, and with it the possible release of calcium from granules or their membranes, we should have in mind that whenever the membrane of a secretory granule is incorporated in the cell surface by an exocytotic event, its environment is abruptly altered. The former inside of the granule membrane is now confronted with the extracellular milieu and its very different ionic composition, and, as noted earlier (Douglas 1974*a*), the granule membrane now has the huge electrical

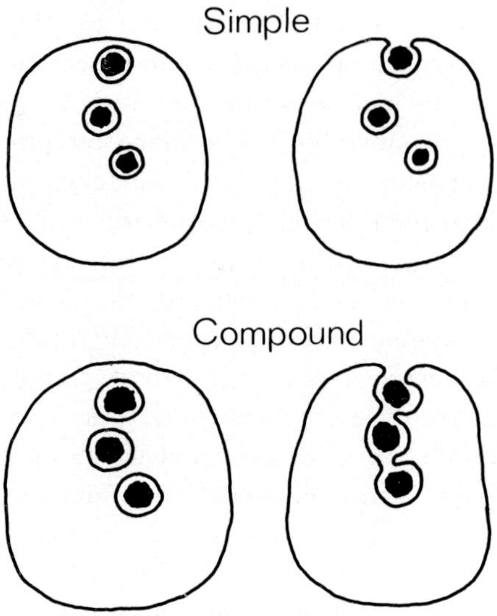

FIG. 4. The two forms of exocytosis: simple and compound.

In simple exocytosis a single granule approaches the plasma membrane, merges with it and, after rupture of the fused plasma and granule membranes, voids its contents into the extracellular space. The essential fusion–fission reaction involves two functionally and chemically distinct membranes: plasmalemma and granule membrane. In compound exocytosis the initial event is as above but thereafter other granules merge with the first and undergo the fusion–fission reaction. In these subsequent events the membranes involved are thus similar: the interaction is between granule membranes. The functional implications of the two forms of exocytosis are discussed in the text. (From Douglas 1974*a*.)

field—say 10 000 V/cm—imposed across it as it is subjected to the transmembrane potential; and granule contents, which could, conceivably, contribute to the normal characteristics of the granule membrane within the cytoplasmic domain have been lost. Alone, or in concert, these or other factors could alter the membrane of the exocytosed granule in such a way that an adjacent granule would now recognize it as 'surface membrane' with which fusion–fission can take place. But perhaps granules can undergo this reaction without one of them first opening to the extracellular environment, and the preferential peripheral locus of fusion that is the basis of compound exocytosis may simply reflect the steepness of the gradient of the free calcium ion concentration from the cell surface inwards. These are interesting and little-explored points.

FURTHER COMMENTS ON CALCIUM AS A SECRETAGOGUE

The ability of calcium to elicit secretion is the lynchpin of the calcium hypothesis of stimulus–secretion coupling. I have so far mentioned two procedures that indicate that calcium possesses the essential property of a mediator: introduction of calcium to cells whose membranes have been rendered permeable to it by (1) calcium deprivation or depolarization (in cells that possess potential-dependent calcium channels) or by (2) exposure to a calcium ionophore such as A23187. Further, and more direct, evidence has been obtained from experiments in which calcium has been injected into cells iontophoretically through micropipettes. The efficacy of this procedure was demonstrated independently by Miledi (1973), who elicited release of chemical transmitter from the squid giant synapse by such means; and by my colleagues and I (Kanno *et al.* 1973) who injected calcium into rat mast cells and observed extrusion of secretory granules.

Besides the above, several manipulations known to raise the concentration of free calcium ions intracellularly have been found to evoke exocytotic secretion. These manipulations all involve disruptions of the normal mechanism that maintains the concentration of free calcium ions within the cell at its typically low level (about 10^{-7} M). The active extrusion of calcium from the cytoplasm to the extracellular environment is driven, at least in part, by the energy derived from the inwardly directed sodium gradient (Baker 1972, 1976; Blaustein 1976) and calcium accumulates intracellularly when this gradient is diminished either by lowering extracellular sodium or by causing sodium to accumulate intracellularly as, for instance, when the sodium pump is inhibited by cardiac glycosides. Both these procedures elicit exocytosis in various cell types (see for example Baker 1972; Douglas 1974*a*, *b*, 1975*a*). Likewise secretion ensues when the calcium-sequestering activity of mitochondria is reduced by metabolic inhibitors and other agents (see Alnaes & Rahamimoff 1975). The converse of this is seen in experiments by Rotshenker *et al.* (1976) who demonstrated a *fall* in spontaneous secretory activity in cholinergic nerves under conditions permitting calcium *efflux* (depolarization while the extracellular concentration of free calcium ions was held at a value lower than the intracellular concentration).

THE ENERGY REQUIREMENT OF THE CALCIUM-SENSITIVE MECHANISM

Secretory responses to different secretagogues in many cell types can be blocked by inhibitors of energy production, but most experiments do not tell where or when the energy is needed. It is obviously important to know whether energy is required before or after calcium influx or mobilization. We first tested this on the neurohypophysis (Douglas *et al.* 1965) by depolarizing the neurosecretory terminals with potassium (thereby short-circuiting the initial membrane events in stimulus-secretion coupling) and thereafter eliciting secretion with pulses of calcium. The secretory responses were abolished by various inhibitors of energy production and we concluded that ATP was needed for the calcium-activated step. The same conclusion has been arrived at by experiments on mast cells stimulated with calcium after different treatments (Foreman *et al.* 1973; Diamant & Patkar 1975; Douglas & Kagayama 1977). The conventional explanation is that the fusion–fission event is energy-consuming; an alternative, suggested in the initial study (Douglas *et al.* 1965), is that ATP might be required to prime the calcium receptive mechanism, for example by binding to some molecular complex to yield the appropriate conformation for calcium triggering. There have been repeated indications, in other contexts, that ATP can subserve 'structural' or conformational roles. Certain observations on mast cells could be interpreted in this way. Thus Diamant & Patkar (1975) have reported that restoring an energy source to energy-deprived mast cells exposed to a calcium ionophore does not elicit secretion, whereas restoring the energy source for a brief period before exposure to ionophore allows secretion to occur. This could mean that the sequence *ATP followed by Ca* allows exocytosis while the opposite sequence *Ca followed by ATP* does not. Clearly this deserves a closer look, for the experiments are complicated and subject to other interpretations. Nevertheless, it may be relevant that in a model system using isolated secretory granule and plasma membranes (Davis & Lazarus 1976) an adjuvant effect of ATP on escape of secretory product was mimicked by non-metabolizable ATP congeners. Here, however, we must recognize that in this system there is, as yet, no proof that exocytosis occurs. The findings taken together with the observations in the whole cell are certainly provocative.

CONTRACTILE HYPOTHESES

The repeated emphasis in the literature on parallels between stimulus–secretion coupling and excitation–contraction coupling have prompted much speculation on the involvement of contraction-like processes in exocytosis and there has been a particular focus on microtubules and microfilaments (see Douglas 1968, 1974*a*). The fact that drugs such as colchicine and cytochalasin B, which can disrupt microtubules and microfilaments respectively, affect secretion has been advanced in support of the idea (see, for example, Allison & Davies 1974; Poisner & Cooke 1975). Our own experience with these drugs suggests that some inhibitory actions at least can be attributed to quite different pharmacological properties of the drugs and, moreover, do not directly address the question of exocytosis. In the adrenal medulla, for example, although colchicine strongly inhibited the secretion due to acetylcholine, it had little effect on secretion evoked by potassium, although this too involves calcium-dependent exocytosis (Douglas & Sorimachi 1972); and in mast cells Mrs Ueda and I saw no obvious inhibitory effect of cytochalasin B such as was reported by Orr *et al.* (1972) unless the cells had been exhausted of endogenous substrates for energy production. In our experiments, cytochalasin B proved to be a very potent inhibitor of secretory responses to 48/80 when cells were poisoned with dinitrophenol and thereby rendered dependent on glycolysis; but it did not inhibit, even in 100-fold higher concentration, when mast cells were respiring normally (Douglas & Ueda 1973; also Fig. 6 in Douglas 1974*c*). The demonstrated capacity of cytochalasin B to inhibit glucose transport seems to be the factor responsible for inhibiting mast cell secretion. Analysis of the effects of cytochalasin on transmitter secretion from neurons also led to a similar conclusion (Nakazato & Douglas 1973). The problem is complex, but I wish here to make two points. Firstly, that in cells showing compound exocytosis granules do not move to the surface (and hence need no propulsion by any contractile machinery); on the contrary the cell surface moves inwards to meet the more deeply located granules (see Fig. 4). Secondly, recent demonstrations that isolated granules can undergo fusion–fission on exposure to calcium (see below) indicate that other cellular components are not needed. Perhaps microfilaments, microtubules and other such cellular elements have a supportive role in exocytosis, inasmuch as they may help move granules towards sites of release but are not involved in the exocytotic event proper. Conceivably they could also participate in granule expulsion after the critical fusion–fission event. Thus my colleagues and I have noted that in the presence of a large excess of calcium (110 mM) compound exocytosis in mast cells occurs without the usual vigorous expulsion of granules from the depths of the exocytotic pits (Douglas 1975*b*; Douglas & Kagayama 1977). The observation of exocytosis in 110 mM-Ca calls into question the view (Poste & Allison 1973) that depletion of membrane calcium is an important preliminary to the fusion–fission reaction.

MODEL IN VITRO SYSTEMS USING ISOLATED GRANULES AND MEMBRANES

I have already pointed out that granules may undergo fusion and fission among themselves during compound exocytosis and that this indicates the relevance of model systems using isolated secretory granules. In one such study Dahl & Gratzl (1976) have obtained electron microscopic evidence that calcium (10^{-6} M) can induce granule–granule fusion–fission (so that two granule cores come to lie in a single investing membrane). And Davis & Lazarus (1976) have shown Ca-dependent escape of insulin from such granules incubated with islet cell membrane. These are most promising developments and it will be interesting to see whether they accommodate the evidence that the response to calcium in the intact cell seems to require ATP. It could be that ATP is present in the components studied: ATP has been detected in secretory granules as well as in cell membrane (see for example Reporter 1972). Moreover Davis & Lazarus (1976) have noted a potentiating effect of ATP in their granule–cell membrane system, and because of mimicry by AMP-PNP, a non-phosphorylating analogue of ATP, they suspect an allosteric effect (see above, p. 80). However, they have offered no morphological or other evidence that release of insulin in their model system involves the fusion and fission of membranes characteristic of exocytosis. Vacquier (1976), working with isolated cortical granules and membranes from sea urchin eggs has, however, obtained electron microscopic evidence for calcium-induced fusion–fission. Whether ATP is involved in this reaction remains to be tested.

In conclusion, there is now much evidence that calcium derived from extracellular or cellular sources acts as a mediating agent in stimulus–secretion coupling whose role is to initiate exocytosis, and recent studies on isolated granules and granule–cell membrane systems promise fresh insights into the function of calcium.

ACKNOWLEDGEMENT

The work by myself and my colleagues cited in this paper was supported by grants from the United States Public Health Service.

References

ALLISON, A. C. & DAVIES, P. (1974) Interaction of membranes, microfilaments, and microtubules in endocytosis and exocytosis, in *Cytopharmacology of Secretion* (Ceccarelli, B. *et al.*, eds.) *(Adv. Cytopharmacol. Ser.)* vol. 2, pp. 237–256, Raven Press, New York

ALNAES, E. & RAHAMIMOFF, R. (1975) On the role of mitochondria in transmitter release from motor nerve terminals. *J. Physiol. (Lond.) 248*, 285–306

ANDERSON, P., SLORACH, S. A. & UVNÄS, B. (1973) Sequential exocytosis of storage granules during antigen induced histamine release from sensitized rat mast cells *in vitro*. An electron microscopic study. *Acta Physiol. Scand. 88*, 359–372

ARGENT, B. E., SMITH, R. K. & CASE, R. M. (1976) The role of calcium in pancreatic enzyme and electrolyte secretion, in *Stimulus-Secretion Coupling in the Gastrointestinal Tract* (Case, R. M. & Goebell, H., eds.), pp. 237–250, Medical and Technical Publishing, Lancaster

ARGENT, B. E., CASE, R. M. & HIRST, F. C. (1977) Effects of manganese on amylase secretion and calcium efflux in the rat pancreas. *J. Physiol. (Lond.) 269*, 70–71P

BAKER, P. F. (1972) Transport and metabolism of calcium ions in nerve. *Prog. Biophys. Mol. Biol. 24*, 177–223

BAKER, P. F. (1976) Regulation of intracellular Ca and Mg in squid axons. *Fed. Proc. 35*, 2589–2595

BAKER, P. F. & RINK, T. J. (1975) Catecholamine release from bovine adrenal medulla in response to maintained depolarization. *J. Physiol. (Lond.) 253*, 593–620

BIALES, B., DICHTER, M. & TISCHLER, A. (1976) Electrical excitability of cultured chromaffin cells. *J. Physiol. (Lond.) 262*, 743–754

BLAUSTEIN, M. P. (1976) The ins and outs of calcium transport in squid axons: internal and external ion activation of calcium efflux. *Fed. Proc. 35*, 2574–2579

BRANDT, B. L., HAGIWARA, S., KIDOKORO, Y. & MIYAZAKI, S. (1976) Action potentials in the rat chromaffin cell and effects of acetylcholine. *J. Physiol. (Lond.) 262*, 417–440

BURGEN, A. S. V. & EMMELIN, N. G. (1961) *Physiology of the Salivary Glands*, Williams & Wilkins, Baltimore

CASE, R. M. (1973) Calcium and gastrointestinal secretion. *Digestion 8*, 269–288

CECCARELLI, B., HURLBUT, W. P. & MAURO, A. (1973) Turnover of transmitter and synaptic vesicles at the frog neuromuscular junction. *J. Cell Biol. 57*, 499–524

CHANDLER, D. E. & WILLIAMS, J. A. (1974) Pancreatic acinar cells: effects of lanthanum ions on amylase release and calcium ion fluxes. *J. Physiol. (Lond.) 243*, 831–846

COCHRANE, D. E. & DOUGLAS, W. W. (1974) Calcium-induced extrusion of secretory granules (exocytosis) in mast cells exposed to 48/80 or the ionophores A-23187 and X-537A. *Proc. Natl. Acad. Sci. U.S.A. 71*, 408–412

COCHRANE, D. E. & DOUGLAS, W. W. (1976) Histamine release by exocytosis from rat mast cells on reduction of extracellular sodium: a secretory response inhibited by calcium, strontium, barium, or magnesium. *J. Physiol. (Lond.) 257*, 433–448

COUTEAUX, R. (1974) Remarks on the organization of axon terminals in relation to secretory processes at synapses, in *Cytopharmacology of Secretion* (Ceccarelli, B. *et al.*, eds.) *(Adv. Cytopharmacol. Ser.)* vol. 2, pp. 369–379, Raven Press, New York

DAHL, G. & GRATZL, M. (1976) Calcium-induced fusion of isolated secretory vesicles from the islet of Langerhans. *Cytobiologie 12*, 344–355

DAVIS, B. & LAZARUS, N. R. (1976) An *in vitro* system for studying insulin release caused by secretory granules – plasma membrane interaction: a definition of the system. *J. Physiol. (Lond.) 256*, 709–730

DEAN, P. M., MATTHEWS, E. K. & SAKAMOTO, Y. (1975) Pancreatic islet cells: effects of monosaccharides, glycolytic intermediates and metabolic inhibitors on membrane potential and electrical activity. *J. Physiol. (Lond.) 246*, 459–478

DE POTTER, W. P. (1976) *Peripheral Sympathetic Neurotransmission,* Arscia, Brussels

DIAMANT, B. & PATKAR, S. A. (1975) Stimulation and inhibition of histamine release from isolated rat mast cells. *Int. Arch. Allergy Appl. Immunol. 49*, 183–207

DOUGLAS, W. W. (1963*a*) A possible mechanism of neurosecretion: release of vasopressin by depolarization and its dependence on calcium. *Nature (Lond.) 197*, 81–82

DOUGLAS, W. W. (1963*b*) Acetylcholine as a secretagogue: calcium-dependent links in 'stimulus-secretion coupling' at the adrenal medulla and submaxillary gland, in *Pharmacology of Cholinergic and Adrenergic Transmission*, vol. 3 (Carlsson, A. *et al.*, eds.) *(Proc. 2nd Int. Pharmacol. Meet. Prague 1963)*, pp. 95–111, Pergamon, New York

DOUGLAS, W. W. (1966) Calcium-dependent links in stimulus-secretion coupling in the adrenal medulla and neurohypophysis, in *Mechanisms of Release of Biogenic Amines* (von Euler, U. S. *et al.*, eds.), pp. 267–290, Pergamon, New York

DOUGLAS, W. W. (1967) Stimulus-secretion coupling in the adrenal medulla and the neurohypophysis: cellular mechanisms of release of catecholamines and posterior pituitary hormones, in *Neurosecretion* (Stutinsky, F., ed.), pp. 178–190, Springer, Heidelberg

DOUGLAS, W. W. (1968) Stimulus-secretion coupling: the concept and clues from chromaffin and other cells (The First Gaddum Memorial Lecture, Cambridge 1967). *Br. J. Pharmacol. 34*, 451–474

DOUGLAS, W. W. (1970) Histamine and antihistamines; 5-hydroxytryptamine and antagonists, in *The Pharmacological Basis of Therapeutics*, 4th edn. (Goodman, L. & Gilman, A., eds.), pp. 628–629, Macmillan, New York

DOUGLAS, W. W. (1973) How do neurones secrete peptides? Exocytosis and its consequences, including 'synaptic vesicle' formation, in the hypothalamoneurohypophyseal system. *Prog. Brain Res. 31*, 21–39

DOUGLAS, W. W. (1974*a*) Involvement of calcium in exocytosis and the exocytosis-vesiculation sequence, in *Calcium and Cell Regulation* (Smellie, R. M. S., ed.) *(Biochem. Soc. Symp. 39)*, pp. 1–28, Academic Press, New York

DOUGLAS, W. W. (1974*b*) Mechanism of release of neurohypophyseal hormones: stimulus-secretion coupling, in *Handb. Physiol.* Sect. 7: *Endocrinology*, vol. 4: *The Pituitary Gland and its Neuroendocrine Control* (Knobil, E. & Sawyer, eds.), pp. 191–224, American Physiological Society, Washington D.C.

DOUGLAS, W. W. (1974*c*) Exocytosis and the exocytosis-vesiculation sequence: with special reference to neurohypophysis, chromaffin and mast cells, calcium and calcium ionophores, in *Secretory Mechanisms of Exocrine Glands* (Thorn, N. A. & Peterson, O. H., eds.) *(Alfred Benzon Symp. 7, Copenhagen 1973)*, pp. 116–129, Munksgaard, Copenhagen

DOUGLAS, W. W. (1975*a*) Secretomotor control of adrenal medullary secretion: synaptic, membrane, and ionic events in stimulus-secretion coupling, in *Handb. Physiol.* Sect. 7: *Endocrinology*, vol. 6: *Adrenal Gland* (Blaschko, H., Sayers, A. & Smith, A. D., eds.), pp. 367–388, American Physiological Society, Washington D.C.

DOUGLAS, W. W. (1975*b*) Stimulus-secretion coupling in mast cells: regulation of exocytosis by cellular and extracellular calcium, in *Calcium Transport in Contraction and Secretion* (Carafoli, E. *et al.*, eds.), pp. 167–174, North-Holland, Amsterdam

DOUGLAS, W. W. (1976) The role of calcium in stimulus-secretion coupling, in *Stimulus-Secretion Coupling in the Gastrointestinal Tract* (Case, M. & Goebell, H., eds.), pp. 17–29, Medical and Technical Publishing, Lancaster

DOUGLAS, W. W. & KAGAYAMA, M. (1977) Calcium and stimulus-secretion coupling in the mast cell: stimulant and inhibitory effects of calcium rich media on exocytosis. *J. Physiol. (Lond.) 270*, 691–705

DOUGLAS, W. W. & POISNER, A. M. (1962) On the mode of action of acetylcholine in evoking adrenal medullary secretion: increased uptake of calcium during the secretory response. *J. Physiol. (Lond.) 162*, 385–392

DOUGLAS, W. W. & POISNER, A. M. (1963) The influence of calcium on the secretory response of the submaxillary gland to acetylcholine or to noradrenaline. *J. Physiol. (Lond.) 165*, 528–541

DOUGLAS, W. W. & POISNER, A. M. (1964*a*) Stimulus-secretion coupling in a neurosecretory organ: the role of calcium in the release of vasopressin from the neurohypophysis. *J. Physiol. (Lond.) 172*, 1–18

DOUGLAS, W. W. & POISNER, A. M. (1964*b*) Calcium movement in the neurohypophysis of the rat and its relation to the release of vasopressin. *J. Physiol. (Lond.) 172*, 19–30

DOUGLAS, W. W. & RUBIN, R. P. (1961) The role of calcium in the secretory response of the adrenal medulla to acetylcholine. *J. Physiol. (Lond.) 159*, 40–57

DOUGLAS, W. W. & RUBIN, R. P. (1963) The mechanism of catecholamine release from the adrenal medulla and the role of calcium in stimulus-secretion coupling. *J. Physiol. (Lond.) 167*, 288–310

DOUGLAS, W. W. & SORIMACHI, M. (1972) Colchicine inhibits adrenal medullary secretion evoked by acetylcholine without affecting that evoked by potassium. *Br. J. Pharmacol. 45*, 129–132

DOUGLAS, W. W. & TARASKEVICH, P. S. (1977) Action potentials (probably calcium spikes) in normal and adenomatous cells of the anterior pituitary and the stimulant effect of thyrotropin-releasing hormone, TRH. *J. Physiol. (Lond.)*, in press

DOUGLAS, W. W. & UEDA, Y. (1973) Mast cell secretion (histamine release) induced by 48/80: calcium-dependent exocytosis inhibited strongly by cytochalasin only when glycolysis is rate-limiting. *J. Physiol. (Lond.) 234*, 97–98P

DOUGLAS, W. W., ISHIDA, A. & POISNER, A. M. (1965) The effect of metabolic inhibitors on the release of vasopressin from the isolated neurohypophysis. *J. Physiol. (Lond.) 181*, 753–759

DOUGLAS, W. W., KANNO, T. & SAMPSON, S. R. (1967*a*) Effects of acetylcholine and other medullary secretagogues and antagonists on the membrane potential of adrenal chromaffin cells: an analysis employing techniques of tissue culture. *J. Physiol. (Lond.) 188*, 107–120

DOUGLAS, W. W., KANNO, T. & SAMPSON, S. R. (1967*b*) Influence of the ionic environment on the membrane potential of adrenal chromaffin cells and on the depolarizing effect of acetylcholine. *J. Physiol. (Lond.) 191*, 107–121

DOUGLAS, W. W., NAGASAWA, J. & SCHULZ, R. A. (1971) Electron microscopic studies on the mechanism of secretion of posterior pituitary hormones and significance of microvesicles ('synaptic vesicles'): evidence of secretion by exocytosis and formation of microvesicles as a by-product of this process. *Mem. Soc. Endocrinol. 19*, 353–378

FOREMAN, J. C., MONGAR, J. L. & GOMPERTS, B. D. (1973) Calcium ionophores and movement of calcium ions following the physiological stimulus to a secretory process. *Nature (Lond.) 245*, 249–251

FOREMAN, J. C., GARLAND, L. E. & MONGAR, J. L. (1976) The role of calcium in secretory processes: model studies in mast cells. *Symp. Soc. Exp. Biol. 30*, 193–218

GERICH, J. E., CHARLES, M. A. & GRODSKY, G. M. (1976) Regulation of pancreatic insulin and glucagon secretion. *Annu. Rev. Physiol. 38*, 353–388

GESCHWIND, I. I. (1971) Mechanisms of release of anterior pituitary hormones: studies *in vitro*. *Mem. Soc. Endocrinol. 19*, 221–229

GOTH, A. & JOHNSON, A. R. (1975) Current concepts on the secretory function of mast cells. *Life Sci. 16*, 1201–1214

HEUSER, J. E. & REESE, T. S. (1973) Evidence for recycling of synaptic vesicle membrane during transmitter release at the frog neuromuscular junction. *J. Cell Biol. 57*, 315–344

HEUSER, J. E. & REESE, T. S. (1974) Morphology of synaptic vesicle discharge and reformation at the frog neuromuscular junction, in *Synaptic Transmission and Neuronal Interaction* (Bennet, M. V. L., ed.), pp. 59–77, Raven Press, New York

HOKIN, L. E. (1966) Effects of calcium omission on acetylcholine-stimulated amylase secretion and physiological synthesis in pigeon pancreas slices. *Biochim. Biophys. Acta 115*, 219–221

JOHNSON, L. R. (1977) Gastrointestinal hormones and their functions. *Annu. Rev. Physiol. 39*, 135–158

KAGAYAMA, M. & DOUGLAS, W. W. (1974) Electron microscopic evidence of calcium-induced exocytosis in mast cells treated with 48/80 or the ionophores A-23187 and X-537A. *J. Cell Biol. 62*, 519–526

KANNO, T. & NISHIMURA, O. (1976) Stimulus-secretion coupling in pancreatic acinar cells: inhibitory effects of calcium removal and manganese addition on pancreozymin-induced amylase release. *J. Physiol. (Lond.) 257*, 309–324

KANNO, T., COCHRANE, D. E. & DOUGLAS, W. W. (1973) Exocytosis (secretory granule extrusion) induced by injection of calcium into mast cells. *Can. J. Physiol. Pharmacol. 51*, 1001–1004

KATER, S. B. (1977) Calcium electroresponsiveness and its relationship to secretion in molluscan exocrine gland cells, in *Approaches to the Cell Biology of Neurons* (Cohen, W. M. & Ferrendelli, J. A., eds.) *(Soc. Neurosci. Symp. 2)*, pp. 195–214, Society for Neurosciences, Bethesda, Md.

KATZ, B. (1969) *The Release of Neural Transmitter Substances (The Sherrington Lectures)*, Thomas, Springfield, Ill.

KIDOKORO, Y. (1975) Spontaneous calcium action potentials in a clonal pituitary cell line and their relationship to prolactin secretion. *Nature (Lond.) 258*, 741–742

LABRIE, F., BORGEAT, P., BARDEN, N., BEAULIEU, M., FERLAND, L., DROUIN, J., DE LEAN, A. & MORIN, O. (1976) Role of cyclic AMP in neuroendocrine control, in *Subcellular Mechan-*

isms in Reproductive Neuroendocrinology (Naftolin, F. *et al.*, eds.), pp. 391–406, Elsevier, Amsterdam

LAGUNOFF, D. (1972) The mechanism of histamine release from mast cells. *Biochem. Pharmacol. 21*, 1889–1896

LLINAS, R., STEINBERG, I. Z. & WALTON, K. (1976) Presynaptic calcium currents and their relation to synaptic transmission: voltage-clamp study in squid giant synapse and theoretical model for the calcium gate. *Proc. Natl. Acad. Sci. U.S.A. 73*, 2918–2922

MACKIE, G. O. (1976) Propagated spikes and secretion in a coelenterate glandular epithelium. *J. Gen. Physiol. 68*, 313–325

MALAISSE, W. J. (1972) Hormonal and environmental modification of islet activity, in *Handb. Physiol.* Sect. 7: *Endocrinology*, vol. 1: *Endocrine Pancreas* (Steiner, D. F. & Freinkel, N., eds.), pp. 237–260, American Physiological Society, Washington D.C.

MEISSNER, H. P. (1976) Electrophysiological evidence of coupling between B cells of pancreatic islets. *Nature (Lond.) 262*, 502–504

MELDOLESI, J. (1975) Calcium and pancreatic secretion. 1. Subcellular distribution of calcium and magnesium in the exocrine pancreas of the guinea pig. *J. Cell Biol. 65*, 88–102

MILEDI, R. (1973) Transmitter release induced by injection of calcium ions into nerve terminals. *Proc. R. Soc. Lond. B Biol. Sci. 183*, 421–425

MONGAR, J. L. & SCHILD, H. O. (1962) Cellular mechanisms in anaphylaxis. *Physiol. Rev. 42*, 226–270

NAKAZATO, Y. & DOUGLAS, W. W. (1973) Cytochalasin blocks sympathetic ganglionic transmission: a presynaptic effect antagonized by pyruvate. *Proc. Natl. Acad. Sci. U.S.A. 70*, 1730–1733

ORR, T. S. C., HALL, D. E. & ALLISON, A. C. (1972) Role of contractile microfilaments in the release of histamine from mast cells. *Nature (Lond.) 236*, 350–351

PALADE, G. E. (1975) Intracellular aspects of the process of protein synthesis. *Science (Wash. D.C.) 189*, 347–358

PEARSE, A. G. E. & POLACK, J. M. (1971) Neural crest origin of the endocrine polypeptde (APUD) cells of the gastrointestinal tract and pancreas. *Gut 12*, 783–788

PEARSE, A. G. E. & TAKOR TAKOR, T. (1976) Neuroendocrine embryology and the APUD concept. *Clin. Endocrinol. Suppl. 5*, 229S–244S

PETERSEN, O. H. (1976) Stimulus-secretion coupling of salivary acinar cells: the role of membrane permeability change, Ca^{2+} and cyclic AMP, in *Stimulus-Secretion Coupling in the Gastrointestinal Tract* (Case, R. M. & Goebell, H., eds.), pp. 281–291, Medical and Technical Publishing, Lancaster

PLATTNER, H. (1974) Intramembraneous changes on cationophore-triggered exocytosis in *Paramecium*. *Nature (Lond.) 252*, 722–724

POISNER, A. M. & COOKE, P. (1975) Microtubules and the adrenal medulla. *Ann. N.Y. Acad. Sci. 253*, 653–669

POSTE, G. & ALLISON, A. C. (1973) Membrane fusion. *Biochim. Biophys. Acta 300*, 421–465

POULSEN, J. H. & WILLIAMS, J. A. (1977) Effect of the calcium ionophore A23187 on pancreatic acinar cell membrane potentials and amylase release. *J. Physiol. (Lond.) 264*, 323–340

RANDLE, P. F. & HALES, C. N. (1972) Insulin release mechanism, in *Handb. Physiol.* Sect. 7: *Endocrinology*, vol. 1: *Endocrine Pancreas* (Steiner, D. F. & Freinkel, N., eds.), pp. 219–236, American Physiological Society, Washington D.C.

REPORTER, M. (1972) An ATP pool with rapid turnover within the cell membrane. *Biochem. Biophys. Res. Commun. 48*, 598–604

RIDGWAY, E. B., GILKEY, J. C. & JAFFE, L. F. (1977) Free calcium increases explosively in activating medaka eggs. *Proc. Natl. Acad. Sci. U.S.A. 74*, 623–627

RÖHLICH, P., ANDERSON, P. & UVNÄS, B. (1971) Electron microscope observations on compound 48/80-induced degranulation in rat mast cells. Evidence for sequential exocytosis of storage granules. *J. Cell Biol. 51*, 465–483

ROSE, B. & LOEWENSTEIN, W. R. (1975) Calcium ion distribution in cytoplasm visualized by aequorin: diffusion in cytosol restricted by energized sequestering. *Science (Wash. D.C.) 190*, 1204–1206

ROTSHENKER, S., ERULKAR, S. D. & RAHAMIMOFF, R. (1976) Reduction in the frequency of miniature end-plate potentials by nerve stimulation in low calcium solutions. *Brain Res. 101*, 362–365

SATIR, B., SCHOOLEY, C. & SATIR, P. (1973) Membrane fusion in a model system. Mucocyst secretion in *Tetrahymena. J. Cell Biol. 56*, 153–176

SCHRAMM, M. & SELINGER, Z. (1976) Neurotransmitter receptors, second messengers and responses in parotid gland and pancreas, in *Stimulus-Secretion Coupling in the Gastrointestinal Tract* (Case, R. M. & Goebell, H., eds.), pp. 49–60, Medical and Technical Publishing, Lancaster

SCHULZ, I. & KONDO, S. (1976) Discussion paper on the role of extracellular calcium in the mechanism of pancreatic enzyme secretion, in *Stimulus-Secretion Coupling in the Gastrointestinal Tract* (Case, R. M. & Goebell, H., eds.), pp. 269–271, Medical and Technical Publishing, Lancaster

SCRATCHERD, T., SYME, G. M. & WYNNE, R.D. A. (1976) The release of cholecystokinin-pancreozymin from the isolated jejunum of the ferret, in *Stimulus-Secretion Coupling in the Gastrointestinal Tract* (Case, M. & Goebell, H., eds.), pp. 341–353, Medical and Technical Publishing, Lancaster

SMITH, A. D. (1971) Secretion of proteins (chromogranin A and dopamine B-hydroxylase) from a sympathetic neuron. *Phil. Trans. R. Soc. Lond. B Biol. Sci. 261*, 363–370

TARASKEVICH, P. S. & DOUGLAS, W. W. (1977) Action potentials occur in cells of the normal anterior pituitary gland and are stimulated by the hypophysiotropic peptide thyrotropin-releasing hormone. *Proc. Natl. Acad. Sci. U.S.A.* in press

TISCHLER, A., DICHTER, M., BIALES, B., DELELLIS, R. & WOLFE, H. (1976) Neural properties of cultured human endocrine tumors of proposed neural crest origin. *Science (Wash. D.C.) 192*, 902–904

VACQUIER, V. D. (1975) The isolation of intact cortical granules from sea urchin eggs: calcium ions trigger granule discharge. *Dev. Biol. 43*, 62–74

VIVEROS, O. H. (1975) Mechanism of secretion of catecholamines from the adrenal medulla, in *Handb. Physiol.* Sect. 7: *Endocrinology*, vol. 6: *Adrenal Gland* (Blaschko, H. *et al.*, eds.), pp. 389–426, American Physiological Society, Washington D.C.

WISSIG, S. L. & SATIR, B. (1976) Ionophore-induced secretion in *Tetrahymena. J. Cell Biol. 70*, 172*a* (abstract No. 514, International Congress on Cell Biology)

Discussion

Allison: Professor Schramm's group in Israel have evidence that some types of fusion are associated with an increase in the level of cyclic AMP rather than with calcium (Schramm & Selinger 1976). Do you accept that?

Douglas: I find it extremely difficult to develop a unifying theme out of all the *ad hoc* hypotheses on the involvement of cyclic nucleotides in secretion. The field is so littered with arrows that it looks like the battle of Agincourt. Sometimes the nucleotide levels rise: sometimes they fall. Sometimes the nucleotides stimulate; sometimes they inhibit. For example, in the mast cell cyclic AMP inhibits exocytotic secretion (see Foreman *et al.* 1976) whereas in the endocrine pancreas it stimulates. In the latter system cyclic AMP was proposed as the second messenger many years ago, but with time this suggested role has been relegated to smaller print and removed to the further recesses of the cell; and we find diagrams with arrows leading directly from calcium to secretion (see Gerich *et al.* 1976). I don't want to diminish the significance of observations on the cyclic nucleotides but it is very difficult for me to fit them into a coherent scheme. I should point out, however, that in parotid cells, for example, where adrenaline appears to stimulate in the absence of extracellular calcium, there is a massive efflux of calcium which, Schramm & Selinger (1976) have recently argued, is due to mobilization of calcium through cyclic AMP. But then the muscle people tell us that cyclic AMP facilitates sequestering of calcium. It is all very complicated.

Richardson: In my laboratory Kim Balfre has been working on a possible role of calcium in the secretion of mucin from hen trachea. She suspends a hen trachea in an organ bath and puts in some radioactive glucose which is taken up by the mucous cells and incorporated into the mucins. She has measured the rate of secretion of radio-labelled mucins and has simultaneously recorded potential difference (p.d.) across the tracheal wall. When she increases the calcium concentration in the organ bath fluid both mucin secretion and the p.d. across the trachea increase. That seems to fit in with what you have been saying; but now she has a puzzling observation that when she removes all the calcium from the organ bath fluid there is quite a big increase in the amount of mucin secreted and in the tracheal potential (see Fig. 1). She has done this experiment twice. Have you any explanation for this?

Douglas: It is delightful to be confronted with puzzles such as this. In nerves—and nerves are the only example I know of—one can get repetitive electrical activity when one withdraws calcium and sometimes this can produce a little blip of secretion. In the invertebrate world there is evidence that mucus-secreting glands develop action potentials, so something of the same sort could operate there: but we have no evidence of spiking in vertebrate mucus cells.

Allison: You could explain it like this. If you have, say, a sialoglycoprotein it will have a negative charge which will be partially neutralized by having calcium ions or magnesium ions associated with it. If you remove the calcium or magnesium ions you will increase the charge difference across the membrane.

Kramer: It is not a part of the membrane; I think it is the whole epithelium.

Allison: Yes, but even then the same would apply.

Richardson: What you are suggesting is that the p.d. is a Gibbs–Donnan potential but I don't think that is right because one can abolish the potential if one replaces O_2 in the organ bath with N_2, although we haven't actually

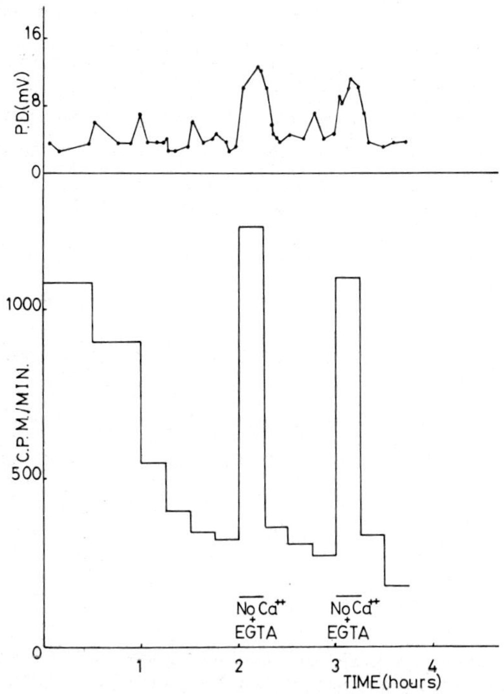

FIG. 1. (Richardson). Graphs showing the effect on hen trachea of withdrawal of Ca^{2+} from organ bath and the simultaneous addition of the chelating agent EGTA.

Upper: Potential difference across tracheal wall (submucosa positive with regard to lumen) against time.

Lower: rate of output of mucin-bound radioactivity against time.

done this in the presence of low calcium. The protein would not be reabsorbed during anoxia!

Allison: But that is another story, because active transport processes will be stopped.

Richardson: But the protein won't be reabsorbed so it can't just be a Gibbs–Donnan potential.

Allison: There must be two components. Part of the potential follows from active transport across the membrane, but part of it is due to fixed charges.

Richardson: Yes, we find that when we make the tissue anoxic there is still a tiny potential left, about 0.25 millivolt. I think that is the Gibbs–Donnan part of the potential and the major part is probably caused by ion pumps.

Phelps: Would you try and repeat the effect by using calcium in EGTA buffers? This would be a way of modulating the free calcium levels. Alternatively this system could be used as a means of finding out the triggering level of calcium at which mucus secretion is elicited.

Richardson: Yes, we should do that. It looks as though there is a U-shaped effect; when calcium concentration in the organ bath is increased from zero there is first a reduction of secretion to a minimum and then, when calcium is increased further, secretion increases again.

Douglas: How sure are you that this is an orthodox secretory response? Is it abolished by metabolic inhibitors?

Richardson: We haven't tried that.

Douglas: From what we have already heard these cells may be rather fragile. Certainly they seem to be for the electron microscopists. One may be seeing something which is not exocytotic secretion. If so, one would want to know about the escape of lactic dehydrogenase and other markers from the cell and also something about the energetics.

References

FOREMAN, J. C., GARLAND, L. E. & MONGARD, J. L. (1976) The role of calcium in secretory processes: model studies in mast cells, in *Calcium in Biological Systems* (Dundan, C. J., ed.) *(Symp. Soc. Exp. Biol. 30)*, pp. 193–218, Cambridge University Press, London

GERICH, J. E., CHARLES, M. A. & GRODSKY, G. M. (1976) Regulation of pancreatic insulin and glucagon secretion. *Annu. Rev. Physiol. 38*, 353–388

SCHRAMM, M. & SELINGER, Z. (1976) Neurotransmitter receptors, second messengers and responses in parotid gland and pancreas, in *Stimulus-Secretion Coupling in the Gastrointestinal Tract* (Case, R. M. & Goebell, H., eds.), pp. 49–60, Medical and Technical Publishing, Lancaster

Studies on the control of mucin production

CHARLES F. PHELPS and AILEEN M. STEVENS

Department of Biological Sciences, University of Lancaster

Abstract The process of synthesizing a mucin molecule is discussed, primarily from the standpoint of glycoconjugate biosynthesis. The control of the activation steps in the making of nucleotide sugars is detailed, stressing the molecular mechanisms operating. These include: supply of glycolytic intermediates; the pyridine nucleotide redox potential; the energy state as expressed in nucleotide potential; and feedback modifiers. Next, the glycosyl transferases are discussed, as are suggestions of control at the first commitment step and the subjects of specificity of donor and acceptor molecules and the associational state of the glycosyl transferases.

The second part of the paper describes a model system *in vivo*. The paired cat submandibular glands are exposed and, in one, blood supply and salivary duct are cannulated and the parasympathetic and sympathetic nerve exposed. This preparation uses the contralateral gland as control and enables certain questions to be asked:

1. Does the cell produce incomplete mucins when the biosynthetic rate is high?
2. Does the energy state of the cell 'keep up with' the high rates of synthesis?
3. What is the extent of post-synthetic modifications?
4. What cell types are involved in mucin elicited by different chemical or electrical stimuli?
5. What is the time involved in synthesis and storage?

> *Ah! don't say that you agree with me.*
> *When people agree with me I always feel*
> *that I must be wrong.*
> OSCAR WILDE *(The Critic as Artist,* 1891*)*

The following account falls into two parts. The first is an attempt to describe, synoptically, the complex molecular mechanisms, at present imperfectly understood, which condition the biosynthesis of mucins. The second is an account of a physiological system *in vivo* which we have exploited biochemically so that we could ask certain questions generated by the first part.

THE THEORETICAL EXEGESIS

The cellular processes whereby a mucin molecule is created are extraordinarily complex, and a rigorous timetable has to be adhered to so that the many contributory components can be assembled. These components are diverse and the translational machinery for production of the correct messenger RNA is needed to effect synthesis of the protein core of the mucin. This in turn requires the activation of amino acids and the charging of relevant transfer RNA molecules. This process occurs on membrane-bound ribosomes and it has been argued (Winterburn & Phelps 1972) that the nascent peptide chain traverses the endoplasmic reticulum into the cisternal space by a process as yet undescribed.

The protein core presumably contains sequences which can act as binding sites for the glycosyl transferases as well as for chemically reactive groupings capable of accepting a glycosyl donor group. These glycosyl transferases are membrane-bound and disclose an almost breathtaking specificity in their enzyme requirements. The sugar substrates are supplied primarily in the form of activated nucleoside diphosphate sugars, though their transference across the cisternal membrane from the cytosol where they are formed from sugar phosphates and nucleotide triphosphates is still unexplained. Membranes are notoriously impermeable to nucleotides and there has been no evidence whatever of lipid-bound intermediates in mucin biosynthesis such as have been reported for *N*-aspartamido-linked glycoconjugates (for a comprehensive review see Hemming 1974).

The biosynthesis and interconversions of nucleotide sugars represent a complex metabolic pathway where conjugation reactions at the pyrophosphorylase level are few in number whereas interconversion reactions are legion. The chemistry of these processes is exceedingly complicated and can include oxidation, reduction, inversion and decarboxylation. As an example of the subtleties employed, consider the interconversion of GDP-D-mannose to GDP-L-fucose. This requires an internal oxidation on $C_{(4)}$, reduction of the primary alcohol on $C_{(6)}$ to a methyl group, inversion of configuration on $C_{(3)}$ and $C_{(5)}$ and finally reduction on $C_{(4)}$ to restore the hydroxyl moiety. All of these operations appear to be performed by a single enzyme.

The nucleotide sugars also represent a considerable investment of the cellular economy in nucleotide triphosphate potential, and it is no surprise to observe in the interconversion some of the most elegant examples of feedback inhibition designed to conserve that potential. It is indeed usual to find that the end-product of one pathway influences the flux of substrates through the first enzyme in the scheme. One example of this working is seen in the control of the first enzyme in the hexosamine pathway which transfers an amino group from glutamine to fructose-6-phosphate to create glucosamine-6-phosphate. This enzyme responds in a remarkable way to the end-product of the hexosamine pathway—UDP–*N*-acetylglucosamine. The enzyme is inhibited by this product with a $K_i = 10$ μM. However, the cellular levels of this nucleotide sugar in tissues synthesizing mucus glycoproteins can range from 200–800 μM. It is clear that the enzyme is almost completely inhibited and that steady-state fluxes through this pathway will be only a few per cent of maximal. In times of need, then, how is this flow to be increased? It is found that the inhibition by the nucleotide sugar can be modulated by a series of secondary effectors, so that UTP relieves the inhibition, thereby raising fluxes through the pathway, whereas AMP and glucose-6-phosphate increase the inhibition (Winterburn & Phelps 1973). Thus the energy state of the cell in the form of mixed nucleotide ratio AMP/UTP controls the flux through this pathway. Analogously, the hexose monophosphate pool constituents can also modulate the capabilities of the enzyme. Table 1 lists examples of agents capable of exercising discretion over enzymes in the nucleotide sugar pathway, where in addition to the factors mentioned above it can be observed that the redox state of the cell may also play an important part. This attracts attention as the mechanisms of sugar interconversion often involve an initial oxidation to the $C_{(4)}$-keto semichair structure in a reaction requiring NAD,

TABLE 1

Control mechanisms operating on nucleotide sugar biosynthesis

A. Supply of glycolytic intermediates	UDP galactose interconversions Glucosamine synthetase UDP glucose pyrophosphorylase GDP mannose biosynthesis
B. Nucleotide potential	Glucosamine synthetase UDP glucose pyrophosphorylase
C. Pyridine nucleotide redox state	UDP glucose dehydrogenase Epimerases: UDP galactose UDP *N*-acetylgalactosamine GDP mannose – GDP fucose interconversions
D. Feedback inhibition	UDP *N*-acetylglucosamine on glucosamine synthetase CMP sialate on *N*-acetylmannosamine formation GDP mannose pyrophosphorylase by GDP fucose UDP xylose on UDP glucose dehydrogenase

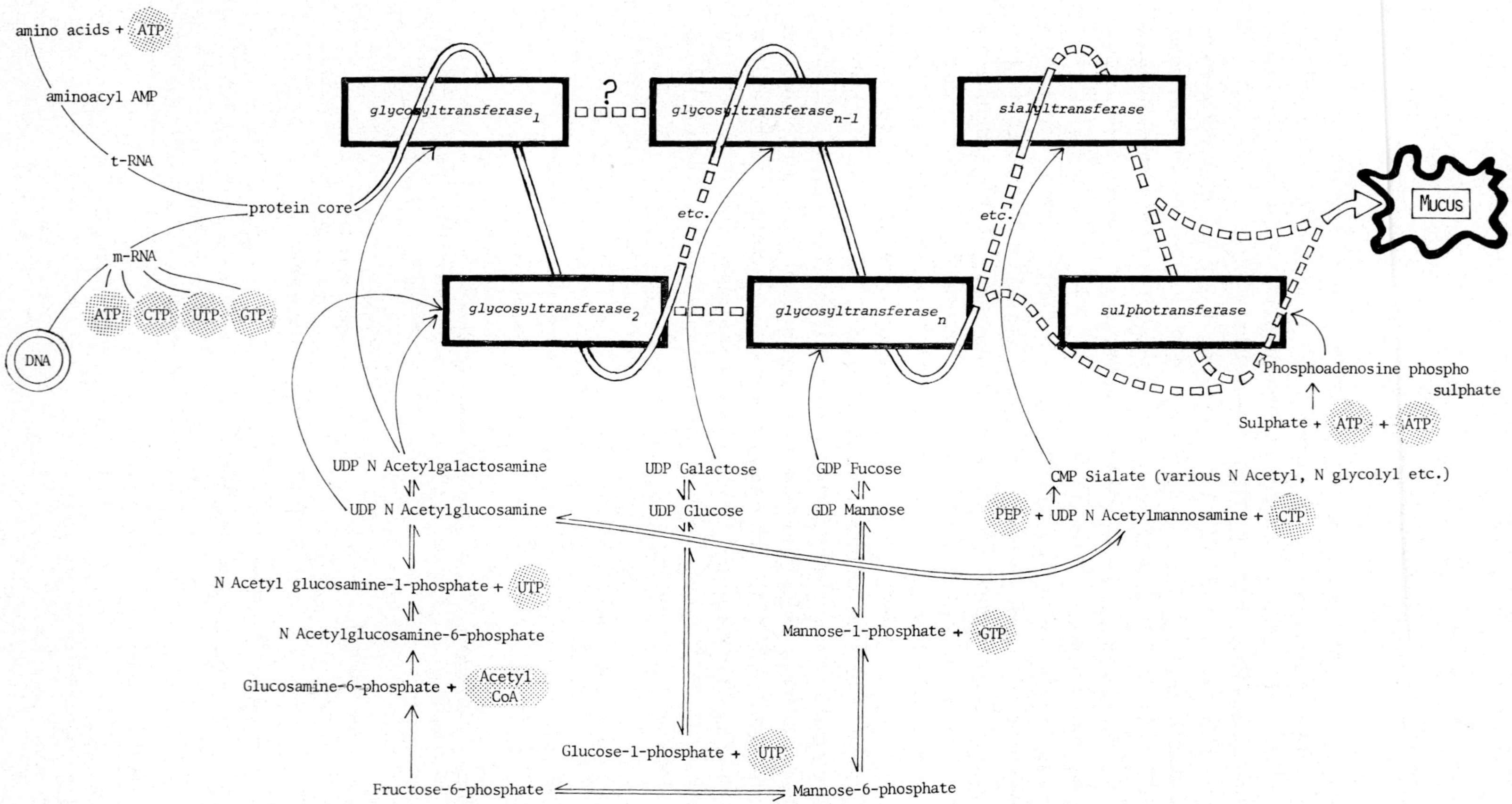

FIG. 1. Schematic diagram of mucus biosynthesis.

The Ciba Foundation

for the Promotion of International Cooperation
in Medical and Chemical Research

ORDER FORM | 1977

Current and forthcoming publications

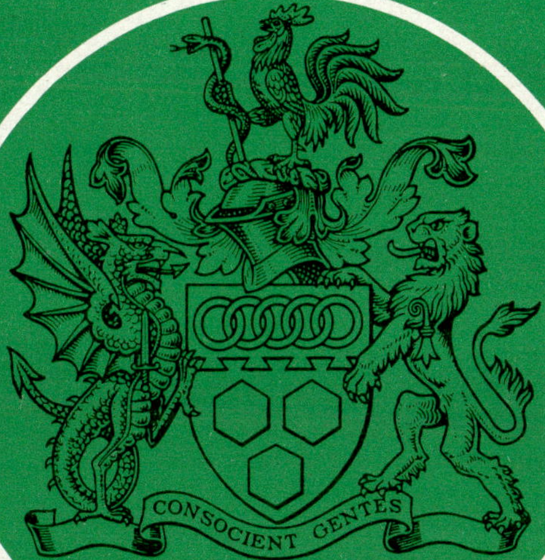

ELSEVIER
EXCERPTA MEDICA
NORTH-HOLLAND

ASSOCIATED SCIENTIFIC PUBLISHERS

the ciba foundation - what it is, what it does

The Ciba Foundation is a scientific and educational charity, well known for its interdisciplinary and international symposia and for the hospitality it offers to scientists on working visits to London. The Foundation was established in 1947 by CIBA (now CIBA-GEIGY) Ltd, the Swiss chemical and pharmaceutical company, with the aim of encouraging communication between scientists from different countries and disciplines. Although supported financially by CIBA-GEIGY Ltd, the Foundation operates under English trust law independently of the company. Its activities are controlled, through its Director, by five Trustees and by the members of the Executive Council, all of whom are leading figures in science or public life.

The Foundation's house in Portland Place, London, has ten bedrooms available for those attending meetings in the house and for others in London on short working visits. People from other countries working in medical or allied fields may apply to stay for 1 to 14 days when the rooms are not occupied by symposium members, and no charge is made for bed and breakfast - though donations are now welcomed. Many scientific friendships have begun in the breakfast-room and this part of the Foundation's work is perhaps as valuable as the symposia themselves.

As well as the bedrooms and handsome reception rooms, the Foundation has a library which is open to visiting scientists and to postgraduate research workers and medical and scientific undergraduates in London. The conference room and other rooms are used for meetings of many kinds, in addition to the Foundation's symposia.

The Foundation does not itself undertake research or give grants for research or travel, except through an exchange scheme with France and in certain other minor ways. Its chief contribution to research is made through the eight to ten symposia which the staff organize and edit for publication every year. These symposia, whose membership is limited to about 25, bring together people from different disciplines who are interested in various aspects of the same subject. The meetings cover a wide range of topics, as can be seen from the titles listed in this order form. Since 1950, when the first symposium was published, some 210 titles have appeared and over 700000 books have been sold. The earlier series of colloquia on Endocrinology and Ageing, together with the shorter study groups (all published by J. & A. Churchill, London - now Churchill Livingstone, Edinburgh), have been discontinued and since 1972 the new series of symposia have been published by Elsevier/Excerpta Medica/North-Holland in Amsterdam and New York

ciba foundation symposia (new series)

published in 1973 by

elsevier
excerpta medica
north-holland

P.O. Box 211, Amsterdam,
The Netherlands

9: Protein Turnover
327 pages US $ 15.95 / Dfl. 41.00

10: Intrauterine Infection
227 pages US $ 10.95 / Dfl. 28.50

11: Hard Tissue Growth, Repair and Remineralization
465 pages US $ 22.50 / Dfl. 58.00

12: Atherogenesis: Initiating Factors
296 pages US $ 14.25 / Dfl. 37.00

13: Haemopoietic Stem Cells
355 pages US $ 16.95 / Dfl. 44.00

14: Locomotion of Tissue Cells
388 pages US $ 18.95 / Dfl. 49.00

15: Corneal Graft Failure
371 pages US $ 17.95 / Dfl. 46.50

16: Medical Care of Prisoners and Detainees
246 pages US $ 11.75 / Dfl. 30.50

17: Law and Ethics of A.I.D. and Embryo Transfer
117 pages US $ 5.95 / Dfl. 15.00

18: Immunopotentiation
365 pages US $ 18.25 / Dfl. 47.50

19: The Human Lens - in Relation to Cataract
336 pages US $ 16.75 / Dfl. 43.50

21: Medical Research Systems in Europe
343 pages US $ 16.50 / Dfl. 43.00

In the USA and Canada these volumes are available from:
Elsevier / North-Holland Inc.
52 Vanderbilt Avenue, New York, N.Y. 10017

ciba foundation symposia (new series)

published in 1972 by

elsevier
excerpta medica
north-holland

P.O. Box 211, Amsterdam,
The Netherlands

1: Civilization and Science: in Conflict or Collaboration? (Paperback)
238 pages US $ 6.50 / Dfl. 17.50

2: Carbon-Fluorine Compounds: Chemistry, Biochemistry and Biological Activities
425 pages US $ 19.95 / Dfl. 52.00

3: Lipids, Malnutrition and the Developing Brain
337 pages US $ 15.50 / Dfl. 40.00
(Microfilm edition only)

4: Peptide Transport in Bacteria and Mammalian Gut
168 pages US $ 7.75 / Dfl. 20.00

5: Ontogeny of Acquired Immunity
292 pages US $ 13.50 / Dfl. 35.00

6: Pathogenic Mycoplasmas
414 pages US $ 19.95 / Dfl. 52.00

7: Polymerization in Biological Systems
324 pages US $ 16.50 / Dfl. 42.50

8: Physiology, Emotion and Psychosomatic Illness
429 pages US $ 20.50 / Dfl. 53.00

Earlier volumes not listed here were published by Churchill and are available from Longmans at the addresses given on the order form.

In the USA and Canada these volumes are available from:
Elsevier / North-Holland Inc.
52 Vanderbilt Avenue, New York, N.Y. 10017

The publisher would be pleased to keep you informed about forthcoming publications in your field. Should you wish to receive an interest profile card, please tick the appropriate box below.

ORDER FORM

Send to your bookseller or

Elsevier · Excerpta Medica · North-Holland

P.O. Box 211, Amsterdam, The Netherlands

For customers in the USA and Canada:
Elsevier/North-Holland Inc.
52 Vanderbilt Avenue, New York, N.Y. 10017

Ciba Foundation Symposia (new series)

Please send me the volumes indicated below:

☐ 1	☐ 10	☐ 19	☐ 28	☐ 37	☐ 46
☐ 2	☐ 11	☐ 20	☐ 29	☐ 38	☐ 47
☐ 3	☐ 12	☐ 21	☐ 30	☐ 39	☐ 48
☐ 4	☐ 13	☐ 22	☐ 31	☐ 40	☐ 49
☐ 5	☐ 14	☐ 23	☐ 32	☐ 41	☐ 50
☐ 6	☐ 15	☐ 24	☐ 33	☐ 42	☐ 51
☐ 7	☐ 16	☐ 25	☐ 34	☐ 43	☐ 52
☐ 8	☐ 17	☐ 26	☐ 35	☐ 44	☐ 53
☐ 9	☐ 18	☐ 27	☐ 36 Hardback	☐ 45 Hardback	☐ 54
			☐ 36 Paperback	☐ 45 Paperback	

☐ The Ciba Foundation: An Analytic History 1949-1974

☐ Writing Scientific Papers in English

Name: ______________________________

Address: ______________________________

____

____

Orders from individuals must be accompanied by a remittance, following which books will be supplied postfree.

I enclose	my personal cheque	bank draft	UNESCO coupons

☐ please send me your interest profile card

Date: ____________________ Signature:

Volumes not listed above may be ordered from:
Longman Group Ltd., Trade Dept., Pinnacles, Harlow, Essex, CM 19 5AA, UK or Longman Inc., 19 W. 44th St., New York, N.Y. 10036, USA.

The Dutch guilder price is definitive. US $ prices are subject to exchange rate fluctuations.

whereas the final step will require a reciprocal reduction by NADH to restore the hydroxyl function.

A summary of many of these reactions is attempted in Fig. 1, which indicates that the nucleotide sugar activation and interconversion reactions are common to many glycoconjugate biosynthesis systems.

The components that create uniqueness in this process are the glycosyl transferases. These enzymes add sugar residues one at a time, each with astonishingly accurate perception of the precursor presented to it. In this way a stepwise elaboration of the glycosyl residues results and it is a frequent finding that the enzymes associated with the synthesis of a certain structure are found in quasi enzyme-complexes.

Elegant work by Roden and co-workers (Schwartz & Roden 1974) gives an attractive example of this aspect of the work. The neutral sugar-attachment region in proteoglycans involves the transfer of a xylose residue to particular serine hydroxyl groups. By preparing the protein core acceptor and immobilizing the acceptor on a column, the initiating xylosyl transferase could be purified from cartilage extracts by affinity chromatography. This transferase is easily solubilized and is found in the high speed supernatant of homogenized cartilage tissue. Down this column containing the bound xylosyl transferase, the solubilized membrane fraction (in detergent and high salt) may be passed. It is then found that the second transferase—the galactosyl transferase—is bound. Since this latter enzyme does not bind to the protein core, it must be concluded that it associates with the xylosyl transferase.

Further significant features which emerge from our studies are that almost all the glycosyl transferases appear to be specifically associated with membrane material when subcellular studies are undertaken, and that they require metal ions, chiefly Mn^{2+}, for full expression of activity in all cases except the sialyltransferase (CMP-*N*-acetylneuraminate-galactosyl-glycoprotein sialyltransferase, EC 2.4.99.1).

The foregoing events might suggest then that the nascent protein core, moving by some agency through the membraneous vaults of the cisternae, encounters a packet of glycosyl transferases which process specific residues on the protein in such a way that the finally 'packaged' or vesiculated product ready for export has a full complement of sugar architecture on it. It may be possible to specify other attributes of the system. Control of the glycosylation can be achieved by a repetition of the principles enunciated above: metabolite or precursor supply and membrane movement (controlling the flux of biosynthetic product). Control may also be effected by modulating the activity of the first enzyme in the pathway—the initial glycosyl transferase—and one may speculate that this may be done in a number of subtle ways, such as

TABLE 2: Some glycosyltransferases involved in *O*-glycosidically linked glycoconjugates

Tissue	*Glycoconjugate*	*Transferase*	*Acceptor*
Cartilage	(D) (C) (B) (A) (disacch)$_n$-βGlcUA(1 → 3)βGal(1 →)βGal(1 → 4)βXylose-Ser	(A) Xylosyl (B) Galactosyl (C) Galactosyl (D) Glucuronyl	Smith degraded protein core Product of A Product of B Product of C
Submaxillary gland	(B) (C) (A) αGalNAc(1 → 3)βGal(1 → 3)βGalNAc – Ser(Thr) (D) ↑ 2 (E) ↑ 6 1 2 αFuc αNGlgNeu	(A) *N*-acetylgalactosaminyl (B) *N*-acetylgalactosaminyl (C) Galactosyl (D) Fucosyl (E) Sialyl	Various protein core acceptors and enzyme-treated mucins
Stomach and other organs	βGal(1 → 3)βGalNAc. . . (A) ↑ 2 ↑ 6 1 1 αFuc βGlcNAc ↑ 4 1 βGal (A) ↑ 2 1 αFuc	(A) Fucosyl (*H* gene)	βGal(1 → 4)Glc GDP fucose βGal(1 → 3)GlcNAc βGal(1 → 4)GlcNAc etc.
	βGal(→ 3)βGlcNAc . . . (A) ↑ 2 ↑ 4 (B) 1 1 αFuc αFuc	(B) Fucosyl (*Le* gene)	de- 'B'- ed substrate GDP fucose
	βGal(1 → 4)βGlcNAc . . . ↑ 3 (C) 1 αFuc	(C) Fucosyl	GDP fucose?
		(D) Presumtive α (1 → 6) fucosyl transferase to βGal	
	(E) or { αGalNAc(1 → 3) – Gal . . . { αGal (1 → 3) ↑ 2 (F) 1	(E) *N*-acetylgalactosaminyl *A* gene	UDP GalNAc
		(F) Galactosyl *B* gene	UDP Gal

altering the activity of the glycosyl transferase between membrane-bound and soluble phases so that activity requires concomitant membrane attachment *and* protein core arrival. Other possibilities include kinetically determined protein folding where glycosyl transferases would be competing against time, for a transition state in the protein which presented the recognition sequences to the glycosyl transferases for glycosylation, and there are clearly many more possibilities.

Table 2 summarizes a few characteristics of some glycosyl transferases involved in *O*-glycosidically-linked saccharide sequences. The experimental enquiry into these systems has been exceedingly difficult and very few fully authenticated enzyme reports exist. One major problem in the past has been the intelligent choice of acceptor molecule. Ideally this should be the authentic glycoconjugate itself which has been pared down by specific glycosidase action to the required extent. This ideal situation has been achieved in only a very few cases. The use of non-cognate substrates, of course, allows measurements of specificity to be made which are not possible with endogenous substrates.

What then? It might appear that the synthetic process is complete and all that remains is the encapsulation within a membrane and the wait for the signal for export. However there are many modifications which can be made to the apparently finished glycoconjugate. These include changes in the number and type of terminal sugars. Examples range from the inclusion of sulphate groups in hexosamine sugar moieties to the modifications of sialate molecules in finished polymers. Fig. 2 shows some of the versatility in the disposition of substituent groups within a single terminal sugar such as sialate. Work by Watkins and associates (see Watkins 1974) summarizes some of the problems of looking at even one apparent enzyme—fucosyl transferase. It is not known how many of these changes are 'deliberate' requirements of the finishing process and how much they reflect carryover of membrane-bound enzyme activity into the secretory vacuole. As will be discussed later, there is the further possibility that the nature of the terminating sugars may alter depending on the physiological stimulus applied to the secreting cell.

All in all a difficult birth for any glycoprotein. But the moment when its development is complete is difficult for outsiders to determine. Operationally we must accept the definition of the molecule as that which emerges from its secretory process. We have a few things to say about that in what follows.

THE PRACTICAL FINDINGS

In our studies we have used the cat submandibular gland *in vivo*. Schematic details of the physiological system are shown in Fig. 3. In the anaesthetized

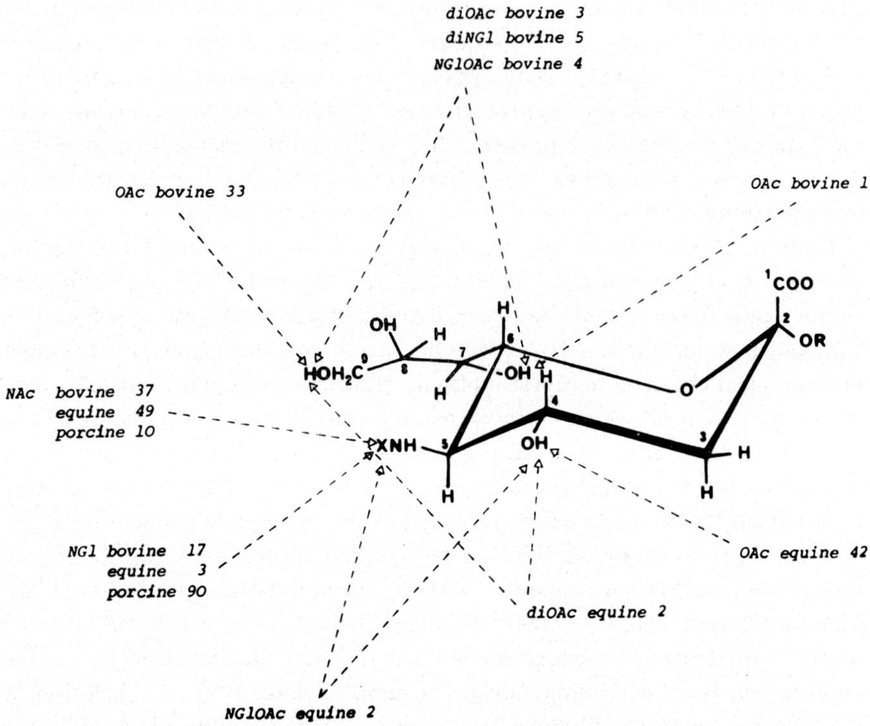

FIG. 2. The variety of positional substituents on terminal sialate molecules. Figures refer to the percentage of each component found in bovine, equine and porcine submandibular mucin. OAc, NAc refer to acetyl substituents, NGl to *N*-glycolyl.

cat, which does not secrete any submandibular mucin, the two submandibular glands are exposed surgically. One gland is cannulated so that the elicited mucin may be collected in sterile cooled tubes containing *p*-phenyl methyl sulphonyl fluoride, to inhibit any expected proteolytic attack. The sympathetic and parasympathetic nerve supplies are exposed and bipolar electrodes are placed on them. Further, the blood supply to the gland can be isolated and thus the preparation is sequestered from outside humoral influence.

This preparation possesses some experimental advantages which may be summarized as follows. *(a)* It is physiological and allows the rate and concentration of mucin to be monitored continuously; *(b)* the glands synthesize only a few proteins, amongst which mucin is the predominant glycoprotein and is produced in a homogeneous aqueous phase; *(c)* the gland is not notably affected by extrinsic factors such as hormonal stress of external

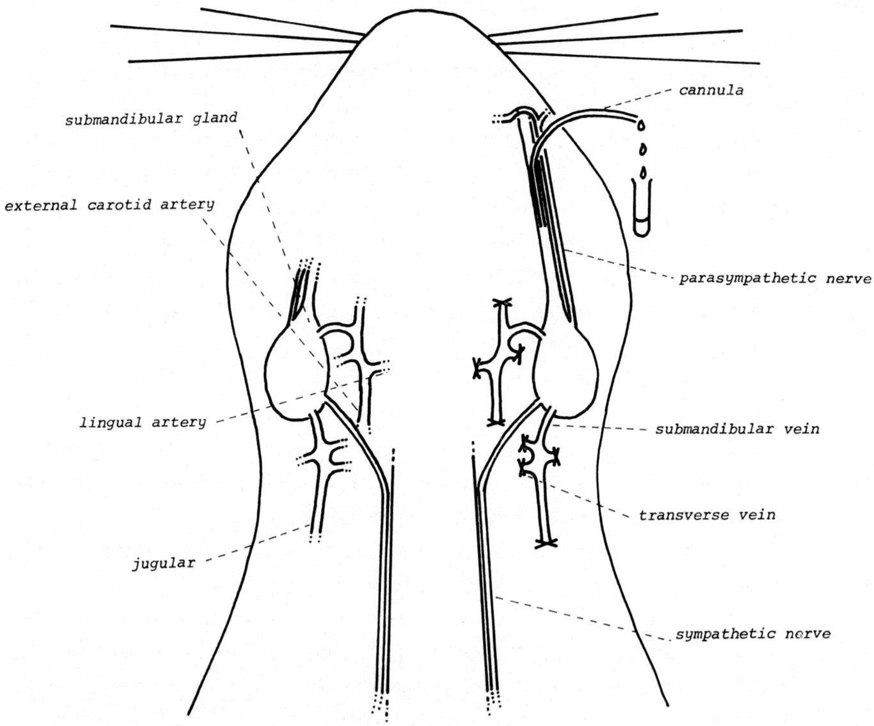

FIG. 3. Schematic diagram of cat submandibular gland preparation.

metabolic changes; *(d)* as it has both sympathetic and parasympathetic innervation, all states of activity from quiescent to maximally stimulated can be sampled; *(e)* in all experiments the contralateral gland is used as a control, so that tissue sampling, measurement of metabolite levels and electron microscopy may be done in a difference mode in the resting and in the exercised gland, thus obviating some of the problems of biological variation between animals.

We have specifically addressed ourselves to a small number of questions: *(i)* Between rest and maximal activity, what happens to the energy economy of the secretory cell? Can it cope? Does it borrow from some 'international fund' of energy? To this end we have embarked on a detailed analysis of the nucleotide potential (Atkinson 1968) of the cell in the maximally exercised and resting states.

(ii) Are there any conditions under which the gland synthesizes an incomplete

glycoconjugate—for instance at the highest rates of synthesis? With parasympathetic stimulation it is possible to obtain from the gland (wet weight 1 g) over 500 μl of fluid per minute, which illustrates the extreme activity of which this tissue is capable.

(iii) What cells do what job? Dische *et al.* (1962) first showed that the sugar composition of the exported mucin in dog submandibular glands varies with the physiological stimulus. Winzler (1973) confirmed these findings and indicated that material produced by parasympathetic and by chemical means (sympathomimetically) differed substantively only in sugar composition. Either different cells do different tasks or there is some kind of electrical witchcraft afoot within a single cell type.

(iv) What is the extent of post-synthetic modifications? This may seem a tautological conundrum—after all what is a modification and what is *in esse?* In this particular question we have attempted to compare what is passively stored in the secretory cell with what is actively secreted both with respect to physical parameters and to chemical composition.

(v) What is the time required for export in the maximally stimulated cell? Here we have looked at the problem of speed of transport of mucin.

Synthesis of a mucin molecule makes heavy demands on nucleotide material, capturing much nucleotide triphosphate potential—examples include amino acid and sugar activation as well as bond synthesis in messenger RNA, protein and carbohydrate. We have attempted to compare the 'balance of payments' in submandibular glands under heavy exercise and at rest. To do this we evolved a separatory technique capable of resolving each and every nucleotide species (A. Stevens, R. Stevens & C. Phelps, unpublished observations). Table 3 shows the differences between two sets of glands where the parasympathetic nerve supply was stimulated. The exercised and the control glands were freeze-clamped immediately after final stimulation and extracted in trichloroacetic acid. The nucleotides were separated on Dowex-1 (HCO_3 form) columns.

An attractive way of documenting the credit-worthiness of a cellular economy has been defined by Atkinson (1968) as

$$0.5\,\frac{\{\mathrm{XDP}\} + \{\mathrm{XTP}\}}{\{\mathrm{XMP}\} + \{\mathrm{XDP}\} + \{\mathrm{XTP}\}}$$

This term varies between zero when all nucleotide is present as monophosphate, and unity when all is present as triphosphate. In addition to this aspect of the work, it will be remembered that many of the key enzymes in nucleotide sugar metabolism are regulated by the XMP/XTP ratio.

It is surprising to observe, from Table 3, that the values for the energy

TABLE 3

Nucleotide concentrations in unstimulated (control) and stimulated cat submaxillary glands

Nucleotide	Condition A				Condition B			
	µmol/g wet wt.		Energy charge		µmol/g wet wt.		Energy charge	
	Control	*Stimulated*	*Control*	*Stimulated*	*Control*	*Stimulated*	*Control*	*Stimulated*
AMP	0.025	0.007			0.038	0.073		
ADP	0.028	0.412	0.91	0.87	0.460	0.780	0.86	0.84
ATP	1.7	1.2			2.200	2.100		
CMP	0.015	0.029			0.027	0.052		
CDP	0.012	0.012	0.63	0.56	0.064	0.034	0.61	0.59
CTP	0.030	0.038			0.060	0.082		
GMP	0.01	0.0121			0.036	0.038		
GDP	<0.01	0.057	0.71	0.52	0.046	0.025	0.64	0.69
GTP	0.049	0.016			0.039	0.101		
UMP	0.064	0.043			0.042	0.107		
UDP	0.021	0.039	0.74	0.77	0.040	0.083	0.85	0.71
UTP	0.2	0.190			0.323	0.325		
Uridine diphosphate sugars	0.296	0.3			0.547	0.6		

Condition A: 60 s stimulation, 20 s rest for 1.5 h duration.
Condition B: 80 s stimulation, 20 s rest for 2 h duration
Energy charge is calculated from the Atkinson equation: see text.

potential are high and unchanged when the exercised and control glands are compared. It appears that whatever duress the cell machinery is subjected to, the energy-conserving machinery is well able to cope.

Question *(ii)* can also receive an optimistic affirmative. It seems, from a detailed analysis of the methanolysed, re-*N*-acetylated and trimethylsilyl derivatized glycoconjugate portion of the mucin after separation by gas-liquid chromatography, that even maximal rates of stimulation (and therefore synthesis) do not perturb the stoichiometry of sugar residues found within the glycoconjugate. This is shown in Fig. 4, which compares the stoichiometry of sugar residues found on the exported mucin (compared to galactose as 6 mol) when the frequency of stimulation is varied from 2 to 20 Hz. It is

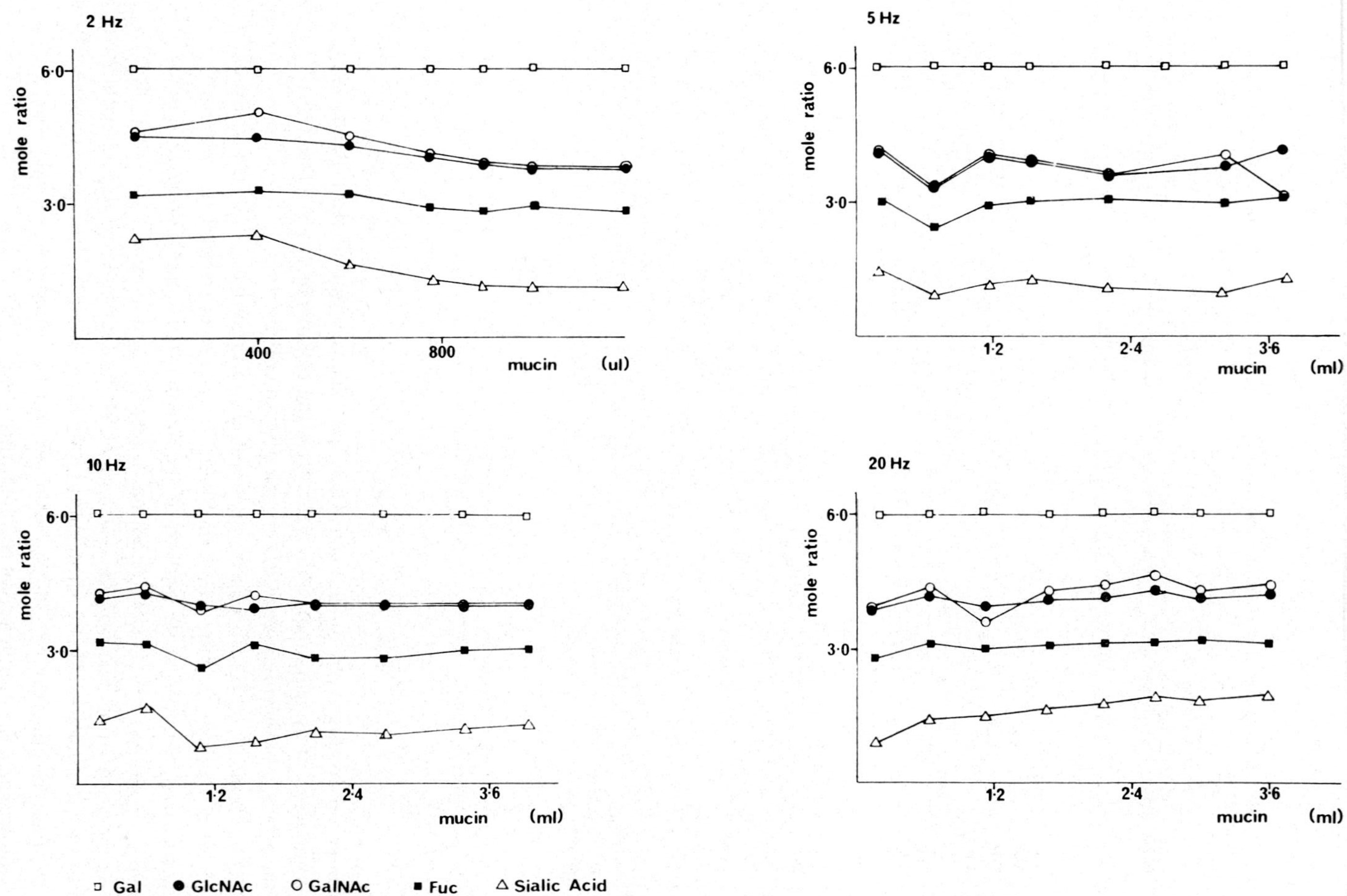

FIG. 4. Mole sugar ratio from hydrolysates of mucin secreted at various frequencies of stimulation (parasympathetic). The ratios are normalized to six residues of galactose.

clear that apart from some minor variation in sialate, the exported molecule always has the correct complement of sugars attached.

This point needs amplification. Whereas our experiments have stressed the homeostasis which results from varying the intensity of stimulus, the effect of varying the type of stimulus can lead to other conclusions. Thus Dische *et al.* (1962) first observed that when the mucin obtained by parasympathetic stimulus was compared with that produced after pilocarpine administration, a reciprocal relationship existed between sialate and fucose, varying over an order of magnitude, whereas the sum of the two remained constant. Dische argued that as both sugars are terminal non-reducing components of glycoconjugates they might compete to terminate a growing oligosaccharide chain and that this competition might be under physiological control.

Winzler and co-workers (Lombart & Winzler 1974) extended this argument with some provocative experimental work in the same system as Dische had used. They showed that pilocarpine and electrical stimulation both produced a mucin whose protein portion as judged by amino acid analysis seemed invariant, but whose sugar complement varied with the type of stimulus. Interestingly, they discovered charge compensation in the glycoconjugate in the form of sulphate ester, so that the oligosaccharides fell into two categories —those with sialic acid but no sulphate and those that had a reciprocal relation.

We have suggested that this could have many bizarre explanations, but a simple one which requires testing is whether different cell types are being differentially stimulated. We have no certain answer to this question (question *iii*) yet, though comparison of the micrographs shown in Fig. 5 suggests that parasympathetic stimulation is specifically depleting only one cell type. We hope to extend this work to document the microscopic appearance of the tissue under a variety of stimuli.

This leaves two of the tabled questions without comment. There is a considerable amount of unsubstantiated opinion which questions whether the material found packaged inside a cell need necessarily be identical in all chemical and physical respects to that found extracellularly after secretion. Most studies on submandibular mucin have been performed on material prepared from frozen glands (Tettamanti & Pigman 1968; Katzman & Eylar 1966). There is little molecular characterization of feline mucin, but work on porcine material, which has a similar chemical composition, suggested a molecular weight for the major component of only 1×10^6 (Katzman & Eylar 1966). Recent evidence favours the existence of still smaller protomers in ovine submandibular mucin, and work by Hill (Hill *et al.* 1977) supports a small apomucin of protein molecular weight 58 000. Addition of sugars would be expected to raise this value to 154 000. In fact the experimentally

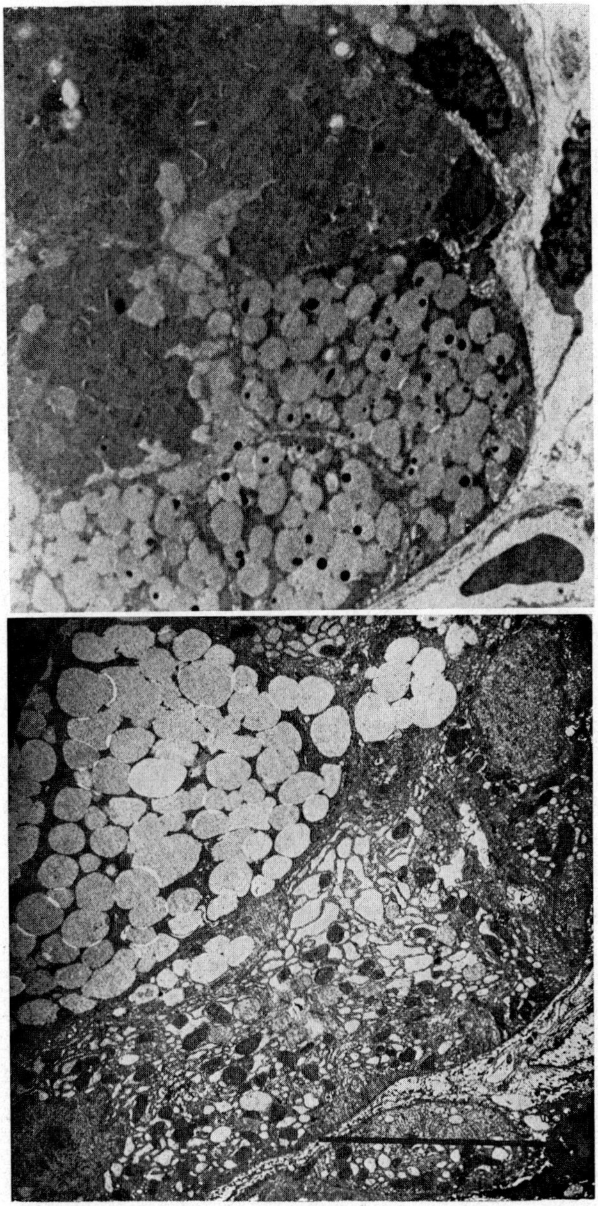

FIG. 5. Electron micrographic comparison of cat submandibular gland before (top) and after (bottom) extensive stimulation via parasympathetic innervation. There is considerable depletion of packaged material in the demilune cells. × 3000.

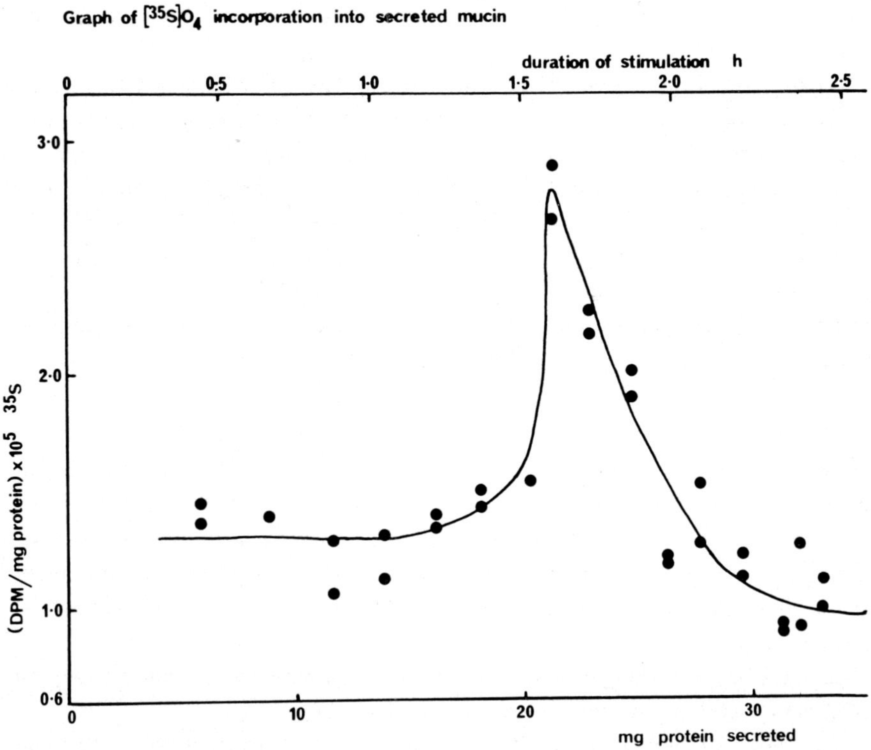

FIG. 6. The time course of appearance of ^{35}S label in parasympathetically elicited mucin after a single pulse of [^{35}S]sulphate.

recorded minimum molecular weight for the mucin is 560 000. The conclusion suggested is the attractive one that the primary gene product is a 'normally'-sized protein which on glycosylation aggregates up to large weights.

It is not unreasonable, however, to imagine that the stored material and the exported material are different. From considerations of minimizing volume and solvation effects inside the cell, it seems that the liberated material has exactly contrary requirements—that of occupying large domains of aqueous solution. We have been surprised, in our own attempts to characterize the submandibular saliva mucin by light scattering, to find that the material is in excess of 40×10^6 when measured in 100 mM-NaCl, 50 mM-sodium phosphate buffer at pH 7.0. It is notoriously true that the apparent molecular weights of mucins are susceptible to a large variety of environmental and experimental effects (ionic strength, concentration, etc.), and we do no more here than draw attention to a likelihood.

Finally, the time taken to export a mucin has been investigated by two methods. In the first, the gland with isolated blood supply is pulsed with radioactive sulphate or fucose and the mucin is collected after stimulation of the gland. A typical profile is shown in Fig. 6, where the time course of export is in the time scale of an hour. Using autoradiography it is possible to show, however, that the isotope moves into the Golgi zone of the synthesizing cell within a very few minutes, and we must conclude that the long delay in appearance of the isotope is caused at the stage of movement of packaged material from the smooth membrane complex to the cell periphery.

CONCLUSION

The distinctive component that endows mucus with its characteristic physical properties is glycoprotein. We know extraordinarily little of the functions of such glycoconjugates. In an attempt to understand more we have devised an experimental system *in vivo* which is under fairly stringent operator control. It has enabled us to stress the role that the biosynthesizing cell plays, which is one of great complexity. Many factors are considered: the timetable of events, the programming of sequences of operations, the geographical dispersion of these processes and the 'financing' of the synthesis.

We have searched for generalizations of behaviour or taxonomy in this field and we may be excused for having felt a little daunted by the 'viscosity of the environment'. There are clear signs of methodological improvements in the separation and chemical characterization of mucus and this presages the advent of a biochemical classification, and with it the prospect of visualizing the steric display of these molecules. Experimental approaches are not lacking either, as this meeting indicates. We believe that the future augurs well for intelligent research into the molecular characteristics of mucin production.

ACKNOWLEDGEMENT

This work was generously supported by the Cystic Fibrosis Research Trust.

References

ATKINSON, D. E. (1968) The energy charge of the adenylate pool as a regulatory parameter. Interaction with feedback modifiers. *Biochemistry 7*, 4030–4034

DISCHE, Z., PALLAVICINI, C., KAVASAKI, H., SMIRNOW, N., CIZEK, L. & CHIEN, S. (1962) Influence of the nature of the secretory stimulus on the composition of the carbohydrate moiety of glycoproteins of the submaxillary saliva. *Arch. Biochem. Biophys. 97*, 459–469

HEMMING, F. W. (1974) Lipids in glycan biosynthesis, in *Biochemistry of Lipids* (Goodwin, T. W., ed.) (*M.T.P. Int. Rev. Sci. Biochem. Ser. One vol. 4)*, pp. 39–98, Butterworth, London

HILL, H. D., REYNOLDS, J. A. & HILL, R. L. (1977) Purification, composition, molecular weight and subunit structure of ovine submaxillary mucin. *J. Biol. Chem. 252*, 3791–3798

KATZMAN, R. L. & EYLAR, E. H. (1966) Physical and chemical studies on glycoproteins. I. Isolation and characterization of glycoproteins from porcine submaxillary gland. *Arch. Biochem. Biophys. 117*, 623–637

LOMBART, C. G. & WINZLER, R. J. (1974) Isolation and characterisation of oligosaccharides from canine submaxillary mucin. *Eur. J. Biochem. 49*, 77–86

SCHWARTZ, N. B. & RODEN, L. (1974) Biosynthesis of chondroitin sulphate. Purification of UDP-D-xylose: core protein β-D-xylosyltransferase by affinity chromatography. *Carbohydr. Res. 37*, 167–180

TETTAMANTI, G. & PIGMAN, W. (1968) Purification and characterisation of bovine and ovine submaxillary mucin. *Arch. Biochem. Biophys. 124*, 41–50

WATKINS, W. M. (1974) Genetic regulation of the structure of blood group specific glycoproteins. *Biochem. Soc. Symp. 40*, 125–146

WINTERBURN, P. J. & PHELPS, C. F. (1972) The significance of glycosylated proteins. *Nature (Lond.) 236*, 147–151

WINTERBURN, P. J. & PHELPS, C. F. (1973) The influence of substrates and modifiers on L-glutamine D-fructose 6-phosphate aminotransferase, in *Enzymes of Glutamine Metabolism* (Prusiner, S. & Stadtman, E. R., eds.), pp. 343–363, Academic Press, New York

WINZLER, R. J. (1973) A model for control of oligosaccharide structure in membrane glycoproteins, in *Membrane Mediated Information* (Kent, P. W., ed.), vol. 1, pp. 3–19, Medical and Technical Publishing, Lancaster

Discussion

Nadel: Increasing frequency of stimulation has two effects: one is the volume obtained (maximum at about 10 Hz); the other is the decreasing concentration of mucins with increased frequency. Why did you choose that particular voltage, Professor Phelps?

Phelps: We asked the physiologists about the voltage we used and I believe it was the correct one. What we did get was enormous dynamics in the amount of mucin produced, but not in mole stoichiometry of sugars added. Very little comes out at 2 Hz and quite a lot comes out at 10 Hz.

We took the dribble that came out of the cannula—the alcohol precipitate—and subjected it to methanolysis, re-*N*-acetylation, and trimethylsialyl derivatization by gas-liquid chromatography. The results are expressed as mole proportions; I have assumed that there are 6 mol galactose present, and worked out the mole ratios of the *N*-acetylglucosamine, galactosamine, fucose and sialate components to the six galactose residues.

Guz: So it is a difference in the proportion of different chemicals coming out.

Allison: The chemistry doesn't change but the quantities do, which is reasonable.

Reid: Does anyone know anything about the amount of enzyme in cells under these different conditions? For example in the hypertrophied gland in the human and in certain animal species, studies have suggested that there is a higher concentration, a higher activity of enzymes. If one went on stimulating these glands in this way, would the weight of enzyme increase?

Phelps: In most of our experiments, we consider two hours as a very long time. Also, the animal is losing so much water through its dribbling that we have to give it a saline or dextran transfusion to counteract dehydration. So we tend to say that, after two hours, the animal has done quite enough work through its gland. To answer your question one would have to go on for many more hours.

Cumming: As secretion continues without there being any further addition of galactose isn't it becoming more dilute?

Phelps: Yes. One has to pause because it seems that water transport is a main determinant. There is a cycle of stimulation and then rests.

Douglas: What picture do you see with adrenergic stimulation?

Phelps: We have only documented experiments using parasympathetic stimulation because it works well. With sympathetic stimulation massive vasoconstriction takes place which has the outward consequence of producing just one single gob of saliva in what looks like very concentrated form. It is quite difficult to get anything out thereafter. One can override this by using α-blockers, for example, but we haven't done that yet.

Douglas: I asked because it is the sympathetic which normally produces the sticky mucinous spit and one can certainly get rid of the constrictive effects with an α-blocking agent.

Phelps: Would you then be totally happy that you had created a biochemically non-interventional system and that the agents that you were using were directed purely towards overcoming vasoconstriction and not having any secondary effect on the cell mass?

Douglas: No, but I think I should worry about that afterwards.

Nadel: Or you could use a low level of cholinergic stimulation. I would agree with you because the evidence in the salivary gland and other glands and now in this gland is that parasympathetic stimulation primarily secretes water, so it is not surprising that the ratio of sugars doesn't change and the secretion becomes more diluted. However, adrenergic stimulation might selectively increase the secretion of one type of sugar.

Phelps: I am sure you all know Winzler's (1973) experiments, derived from Dische's experiment (Dische *et al.* 1962). In the dog, if parasympathetic electrically produced mucin is compared with that produced by chemical agents such as pilocarpine, the total amounts of capping sugars (fucose and sialic acid) remain constant but the ratio of each to each goes through a complete reversal from fucose to sialate ratios of 0.2 to 2.0. Dische found that there were reciprocal relations between the fucose and the sialate. Winzler demonstrated that Dische's essential findings were right but there was a charge compensation in the mucin low in sialate. The sulphur mucin that we are talking about possesses a charge as a sulphate ester on position 4 of the galactose moiety, which is why Winzler was not able to separate the mucin components electrophoretically. We tried pilocarpine, 5 μg/ml, and the nose and gut and everything went into total dissolution. Something curious happens early in the pilocarpine experiments because the system soon relaxes back to what one sees after electrical stimulation. I don't know what it is but it must be happening on a fast time-scale.

Douglas: How much of the spit is composed of the mucinous material and how much of kallikreins and other substances? If there is a mixture are you implying that it is all coming out of the one cell?

Phelps: This is the whole question—how much mucin is there? There is 60% sugar, 40% protein, and there is up to about 200–400 μg protein/ml in a sample stimulated at 5–10 Hz.

Douglas: But is mucin the principal component?

Phelps: Presumably there will be growth factor there in minute amounts, but probably 97% or 98% of what is coming out is water, although there are these macromolecular components.

Douglas: But if I were attempting to measure the principal macromolecule this gland is secreting, what should I choose?

Phelps: The glycoprotein, the glycoconjugate, without a doubt—by an order and a half of magnitude.

Reid: You were claiming that with your stimulation you emptied only the demilunes and not the mucous cells. Is the dog submaxillary gland like the cat's in this respect? Did Winzler report any difference in cell types that could account for this?

Jeffery: Garrett & Parsons (1976) found very marked species differences when they compared the salivary glands of the rabbit with those in the cat. They haven't looked at the dog.

Allison: Suppose, for example, that you have a high sialate, low sulphate-containing material in glands and low sialate, high sulphate conjugates in the demilunes, surely there might be selective discharge. This could be sorted out morphologically.

Reid: You want both together, don't you?

Allison: Alternatively you could have a difference in the amount of sialic acid or sulphate transferred onto the macromolecules but that is more complex and less likely to be right, because of the short time involved.

Nadel: What are the resting levels of secretion?

Phelps: There are no resting levels. The anaesthetized cat does not secrete at all; it only starts dribbling after stimulation but I don't know about the dog.

R. Jones: Most of the unstimulated mucous cells in the submaxillary salivary gland of the dog contain sialylated glycoprotein but a fair proportion also contains sulphate. Some have sialylated glycoproteins only and some have sialylated combined with sulphated glycoprotein.

Allison: Is there any difference in different areas of the gland?

R. Jones: I don't know.

Phelps: You say that there are sialomucin-containing cells and cells with sialosulphate mucin. Do you see any that are purely sulphate?

R. Jones: Not in the mucous cells.

Reid: Are there mucous and serous cells in the submaxillary?

R. Jones: Yes, both cell types are present. But we have not looked in any detail at the glycoproteins of the serous cells.

Phelps: Have you looked at the cat?

R. Jones: No. But from our studies we know that in the serous cells of the dog gland at least sialomucin is present.

Allison: It would be interesting to look at these glands after, say, pilocarpine stimulation to see whether there are any differential effects.

Nadel: There could be differences between a cholinergic agonist (e.g. pilocarpine) given via the bloodstream and electrical stimulation of the vagus nerves. For example, receptors may be more accessible to nerves or to the blood vessels.

References

DISCHE, Z., PALLAVICINI, C., KAVASAKI, H., SMIRNOW, N., CIZEK, L. & CHIEN, S. (1962) Influence of the nature of the secretory stimulus on the composition of the carbohydrate moiety of glycoproteins of the submaxillary saliva. *Arch. Biochem. Biophys. 97*, 459–469

GARRETT, J. R. & PARSONS, P. A. (1976) Movement of horseradish peroxidase in rabbit submandibular glands after ductal injection. *Histochem. J. 8*, 177–189

WINZLER, R. J. (1973) A model for control of oligosaccharide structure in membrane glycoproteins, in *Membrane Mediated Information* (Kent, P. W., ed.), vol. 1, pp. 3–19, Medical and Technical Publishing, Lancaster

The roles of mediators, irritants and allergens in causing mucin secretion from the trachea

P. S. RICHARDSON, R. J. PHIPPS, K. BALFRE and R. L. HALL

Department of Physiology, St George's Hospital Medical School, London

Abstract Two species, the cat and the goose, have been investigated to determine whether a variety of pharmacological mediators, irritants and allergens change the rate at which mucins (mucus glycoproteins) are secreted into the trachea. Mucins were labelled by the administration of radioactive precursors which the mucous cells took up and incorporated into glycoproteins. These were periodically washed out of a segment of trachea with physiological saline solution. Changes in the amount of mucin secreted were estimated from measurements of the amount of bound radioactivity in tracheal washings.

Histamine increased mucin secretion but the effects were stronger and more consistent in the goose than in the cat. A variety of prostaglandins increased the secretion in both species. 5-Hydroxytryptamine failed to stimulate mucin output in the cat. Ammonia and cigarette smoke both increased mucin secretion in the cat and preliminary results suggest that this was by a combination of local and reflex mechanisms.

O-Chlorobenzilidine malononitrile increased secretion from the goose trachea entirely by a local mechanism. Preliminary experiments in which sensitized cats were challenged by various routes have given equivocal results on whether anaphylaxis increases airway mucin secretion. It is concluded that irritants cause mucin secretion both by reflexes and local mechanisms. The mechanisms for the latter may well include release of pharmacological mediators.

The work described here was done to answer three questions: do pharmacological mediators cause mucin secretion from the respiratory tract; do common irritants increase mucin secretion and if so what is the mechanism; and, can allergens increase mucin output into the airway?

Irritants and allergens can precipitate asthma in susceptible people and it is known that, at least in some asthma attacks, secretion of excessive mucus blocks airways which are already narrowed by smooth muscle contraction. Mediators such as histamine, 5-hydroxytryptamine, slow-reacting substance A (SRS-A) and prostaglandins are suspected of causing, either directly or via reflexes, the smooth muscle contraction of asthma. Can they also clog the airways with mucus?

We have done these experiments in two species, the cat and the goose. Cats have a well-developed mucus-secreting apparatus in their trachea. It is anatomically similar to that in humans, with mucus coming from epithelial goblet cells and also from acinar glands which lie in the submucosa. The goose was used because it has a long trachea which secretes copious mucus when stimulated. Unlike the cat it has mucus-secreting cells only in the epithelium and no submucosal glands; thus it provides an opportunity to study mucus secretion from epithelial goblet cells alone.

Much is already known about the control of mucin secretion in these two species. In the goose there is a parasympathetic innervation of the mucous cells from the descending oesophageal nerves, derived from cranial nerves IX and X. Stimulation of these nerves augments mucin production and atropine blocks most, but not all, of this effect. A significant proportion of the effect seems to be mediated by some transmitter other than acetylcholine. Stimulation of segmental nerves, which innervate the trachea in birds and might be expected to carry sympathetic nerve fibres, and administration of sympathomimetic drugs had no effect on mucin secretion so we think that the secretion is independent of that division of the nervous system (Phipps *et al.* 1977).

In the cat, parasympathetic nerve stimulation and parasympathomimetic drugs excite mucin secretion—effects which atropine blocks. Sympathetic nerves and sympathomimetic drugs also cause mucin secretion and this appears to be mediated through β-receptors (Gallagher *et al.* 1975).

METHODS

We have developed a method of collecting mucins (mucus glycoproteins) which have been secreted into the trachea of anaesthetized animals. Three cannulae are inserted into the trachea of an anaesthetized cat or goose; the most caudal of them points down towards the lungs and the animal breathes through this, while the more cranial two enclose a segment of trachea with its nerves and blood supply intact. This segment is then filled with a physiological saline solution (Ringer–bicarbonate) and any mucins secreted can be washed out periodically. Because of the difficulty in measuring, by chemical methods, the very small concentrations of mucins which appear in the tracheal washings, we have labelled them with radioactive precursors which are taken up by the mucous cells, incorporated into mucins and then secreted. Measurements of the protein-bound radioactivity in successive samples reflect changes in mucin output. [^{35}S]Sodium-sulphate (given either intravenously or into the segment) and [^{3}H]glucose (given into the segment) are the precursors which we have used in most experiments, but others, such as [^{3}H]fucose, [^{3}H]glucosamine and [^{3}H]mannosamine, have also been tested. In geese the precursors were taken up mainly by the epithelial mucus-secreting cells. Autoradiographs of sections through tracheas of cats showed that the mucous and serous acini of the submucosal gland always took up the precursors but few of the surface epithelial goblet cells became labelled. There were differences, however, between the patterns of uptake of different precursors: the luminal edge of the ciliated cells—probably the microvillus border—became heavily labelled with [^{3}H]glucose, much less so with [^{35}S]sulphate, and did not take up [^{3}H]fucose. A mucosubstance at the luminal edge of ciliated cells in human and dog trachea has been described elsewhere (Spicer *et al.* 1971).

In most of the experiments described here two radioactive precursors were given, usually [^{3}H]glucose and [^{35}S]sulphate. Stimuli which increased ^{3}H output but had little effect on the ^{35}S were thought to be acting mainly on release of glycoproteins from the luminal edge while those that altered ^{35}S more than ^{3}H output had their main effect on secretion from the submucosal glands. Because the goblet cells of the cat took up little of the radioactivity we have less information about the control of goblet cell secretion in that species.

One of the drawbacks of measuring the output of bound radioactivity is that it only gives results in terms of a percentage change in output rather than in absolute terms. Recently we have developed a method of measuring the quantity of mucins in tracheal washings (after a method by Whiteman 1973). This involves precipitating the glycoproteins in each sample with Alcian blue, a dye which binds to the acidic groups of the glycoprotein molecules and renders them insoluble. After the precipitate has been centrifuged and washed, it can be re-dissolved in Manoxol 1B (sodium dibutyl sulphosuccinate) and the amount of precipitated dye, which is proportional to the mass of glycoprotein, can be estimated colorimetrically. A preliminary experiment (see Fig. 1) suggests that, at least when the stimuli given affect mainly the gland secretion, the output of mucins correlates well with the ^{35}S label and more poorly with the [^{3}H]glucose.

RESULTS

Effects of mediators

Histamine. Histamine acid phosphate was given in two ways; by aerosol into the lungs (to cats) and as a solution directly into the tracheal segments (to cats and geese). It was given as an aerosol into the lungs of nine cats

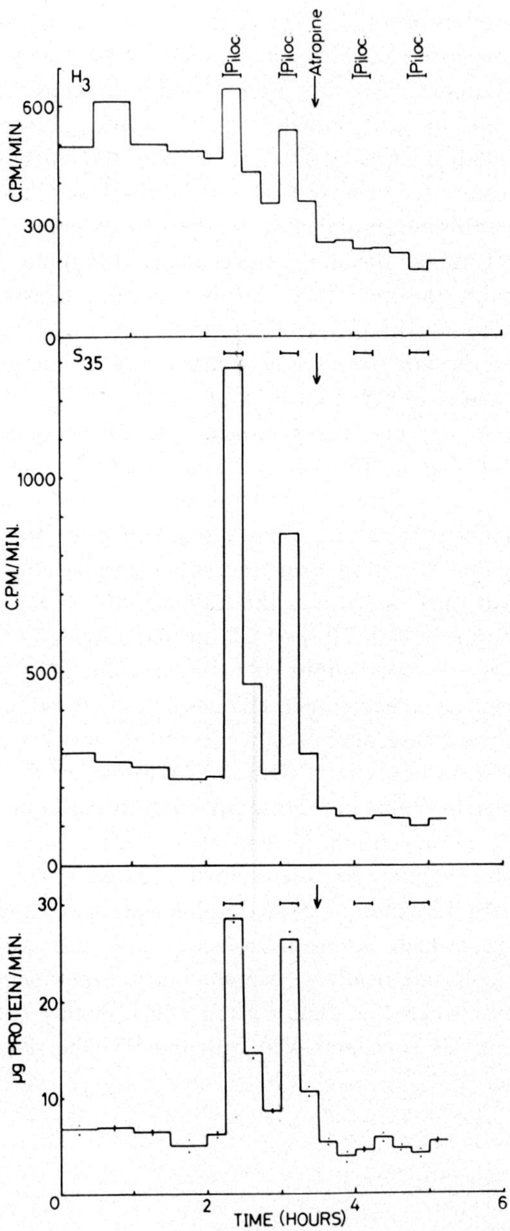

FIG. 1. Histogram showing the output of ^{3}H-labelled glycoprotein (top panel), ^{35}S-labelled glycoprotein (middle) and total glycoprotein (in μg/min., bottom panel) from the trachea of a cat, as determined by the Alcian blue method.

and always caused rapid shallow breathing, presumably by excitement of irritant receptors (Mills *et al.* 1969). However it failed to change mucin secretion from the tracheal segment (mean change $\pm$ S.E. $= 2 \pm 12\%$, $n = 9$, ^{35}S label).

When histamine was given as a solution (10 μg/ml) into the tracheal segment of cats, ^{35}S-labelled mucin secretion increased by a mean of $+ 101 \pm 46.3\%$ (11 trials). The effects were very variable and ranged from a decrease of 24% in secretion to an increase of 418%. In two animals we gave a range of concentrations from 1 μg/ml to 30 μg/ml, but the effects did not increase with dosage as we had expected. The lower doses (1 and 3 μg/ml) had negligible effects, and the dose of 10 μg/ml had a larger effect than that of the 30 μg/ml given afterwards. It may be that histamine can only give one 'all-or-nothing' stimulation of mucins (Fig. 2).

In five cats histamine was given into the trachea to which both [^{3}H]glucose and [^{35}S]sulphate had been administered as precursors. With one exception, the effects on the ^{35}S-labelled mucins were proportionately greater than those on the ^3H-labelled mucins. We interpret this as meaning that histamine releases mucins mainly from the mucous glands rather than the luminal border of the epithelial cells. The results do not indicate whether the epithelial goblet cells discharged their contents; histological studies are planned which should answer this question.

How does histamine act? Our results indicate that it is not by a reflex involving the central nervous system (CNS), because the aerosol given into the lower trachea and lungs failed to cause secretion from the segment. It could be by a local reflex (and one experiment we have done, in which histamine had no effect when given into the tracheal segment of a cat treated with propranolol and atropine, goes a little way to support this idea). It might be by a direct action on the mucus-secreting cells. Another possible action we have considered is that histamine caused contraction of tracheal smooth muscle (either myoepithelial cells in the submucosal glands [Meyrick & Reid 1970], or the smooth muscle of the tracheal wall) and so squeezed extra mucus from the acinar ducts. While we cannot exclude this possibility altogether we think it unlikely on three grounds: (*i*) If it had occurred there would have been a corresponding depression of mucin secretion when histamine was removed, the smooth muscle should have relaxed and the acinar ducts should have regained their capacity: this was not seen. (*ii*) Though it was not measured directly, we should have expected histamine aerosol, given into the lungs, to cause a reflex constriction of the tracheal segment which might have squeezed the glands. As histamine aerosol failed to increase mucus output into the trachea we doubt whether smooth muscle contraction squeezes mucus from

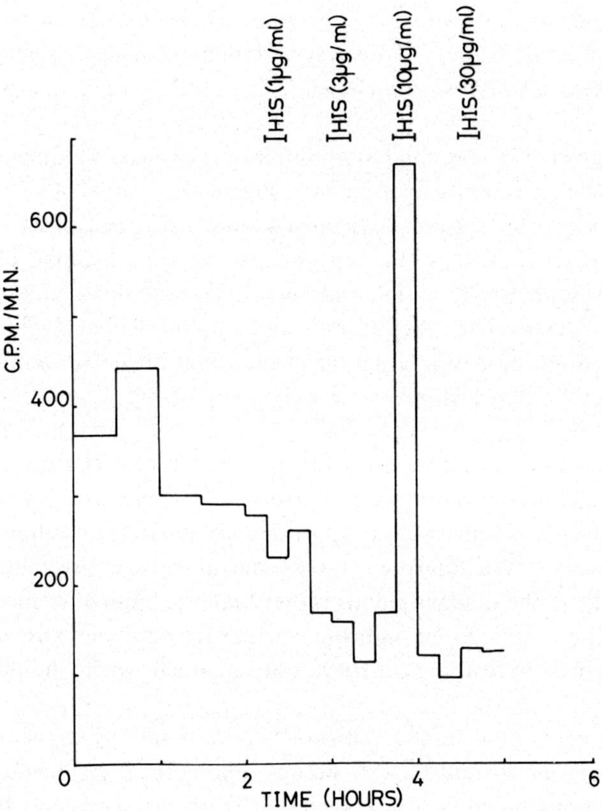

FIG. 2. Histogram showing the output from a cat's trachea of ^{35}S-labelled mucin against time. Of the four doses of histamine given, only one (10 μg/ml) increased secretion significantly.

glands. (*iii*) Histamine had a strong effect on mucus secretion from the goose trachea which contains little smooth muscle (P. K. Jeffery, personal communication).

We were rather surprised that histamine had any effect in these experiments. Other workers who have given it to mammalian airway tissue (Sturgess & Reid 1972; Chakrin *et al.* 1973) have reported negative results only.

Histamine given into the tracheal segment of the goose caused no change in the pattern of breathing but consistently and strongly excited mucin output. Doses ranging from 0.1–10 μg/ml all increased mucin output (mean for ^{35}S-labelled mucin, $\Delta = +185 \pm 75\%$, $n = 6$; for ^{3}H-labelled mucin, $\Delta =$

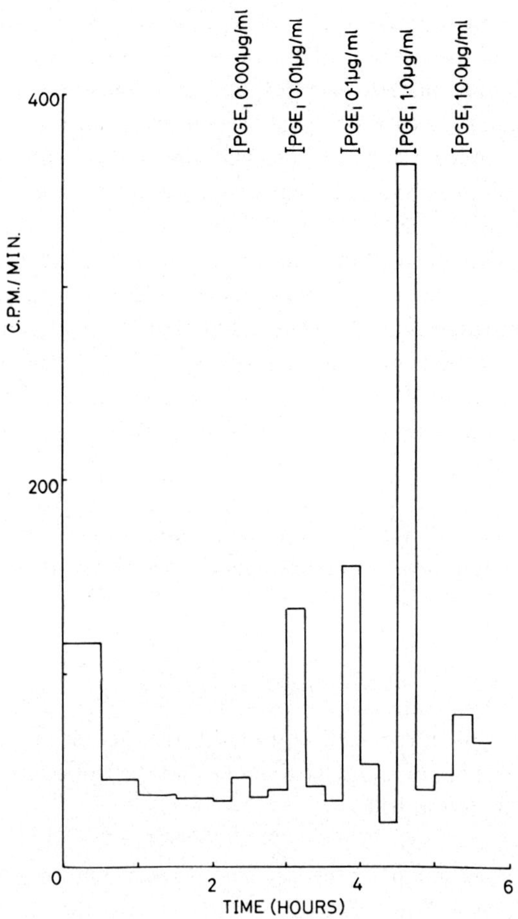

FIG. 3. Histogram showing the effects of five doses of prostaglandin E_1 on ^{35}S-labelled mucin output of a cat's trachea.

$118 \pm 41\%$, $n = 7$). Where different doses were given to the same animal the higher doses in general had the greater effects.

Prostaglandins. A variety of prostaglandin solutions were given into the tracheal segment of the cat. Prostaglandins A_2, E_1, E_2, $F_{1\alpha}$ and $F_{2\alpha}$ all increased mucin output. Those with the strongest effects were $F_{2\alpha}$ and E_1. In general, prostaglandins had stronger and more consistent effects on mucin output than did histamine. When these were given in ascending doses E_1 had an effect at 1 ng/ml while the threshold dose for $F_{2\alpha}$ was between 10 and 100 ng/ml.

Fig. 3 shows the effect of increasing doses of PGE_1. The largest doses of such a series often had smaller effects than intermediate ones, probably because, by the time they were given, the mucous cells were exhausted.

When prostaglandins were given to cats which had been given both [^{3}H]-glucose and [^{35}S]sulphate mucin precursors, the prostaglandins had a stronger effect on the [^{35}S]mucins. We think that this is evidence that the prostaglandins were causing release of glycoproteins mainly from the mucous glands rather than from the luminal border. Our experiments on the mechanism of effects have not yet progressed very far but in one experiment $PGF_{2\alpha}$ increased mucin output from an animal treated with atropine. Although it is possible that prostaglandins were working through reflex pathways to release mucus we think that a direct effect is more likely.

One experiment with prostaglandins E_1 and $F_{2\alpha}$ in the goose trachea suggests that they have a similar effect.

5-Hydroxytryptamine. 5HT was given into the tracheal segments of two cats in doses from 0.1–100 μg/ml but failed to increase mucin secretion at any concentration.

Irritant agents

We have investigated the effects of three respiratory tract irritants on mucin output from the trachea; ammonia vapour, cigarette smoke and the riot control agent CS (*O*-chlorobenzilidine malononitrile).

Ammonia vapour. Ammonia was given to the cat as a vapour (molecular concentration of ammonia between 1 in 300 and 1 in 1000) into the lungs (i.e. it did not pass through the tracheal segment from which we collected mucins). When given in this way it caused coughing and rapid breathing which was either deeper or shallower than in the control period. At the same time ^{35}S-labelled mucin output from the tracheal segment increased ($\Delta = +74 \pm 21.2\%$, $n = 13$). Both the effects on breathing and those on mucin output depended on the integrity of the vagus nerves. Once those in the neck had been cut no changes in mucin secretion were seen ($\Delta = -5 \pm 12.0\%$, $n = 6$), so the reaction to ammonia seems to have been by way of reflexes.

As vagal section would interrupt both the afferent and efferent pathways of the reflex we tested the effects on the reflex of the muscarinic blocking agent atropine (1 mg/kg i.v.) and the β-adrenergic blocker propranolol (10 μg/ml into the tracheal segment). On the three occasions it was tried, atropine almost abolished the reflex, while on the two occasions propranolol was given it made little difference to the strength of the reflex. It seems, therefore, that the efferent part of the reflex depends mainly on the parasympathetic nervous system.

In another series of experiments ammonia vapour was given directly into the tracheal segment. For these and other experiments in which vapours were given directly into the segment from which mucins were being gathered, we drained all the Krebs–Henseleit solution from the trachea in between washes and so were able to puff the irritant gases through an air-filled trachea. The segment was similarly drained in the control periods between gas administrations. When air was passed through the trachea in the same way it did not stimulate mucin secretion. Dilute ammonia vapour caused a considerable increase in the mucin output ($\Delta = +110 \pm 17\%$, $n = 26$ for ^{35}S-labelled mucins; $\Delta = +84 \pm 10\%$, $n = 22$ for ^{3}H-labelled mucins). When repeated doses of the irritant were given, in nine experiments the responses to the first three or four doses were similar in size, but subsequent administrations caused less effect.

It seemed likely from the experiments described above, in which ammonia had been given into the lungs, that all or part of the response was nervously mediated. This was confirmed by four experiments in which ammonia was given into the tracheal segment before and after administration of atropine and propranolol (Fig. 4). In these the effects were larger before the blockers had been given; $\Delta = +83 \pm 13\%$, $n = 4$ before, compared with $\Delta = 39 \pm 25\%$, $n = 4$ after autonomic nerve blockade. All had ^{35}S-labelled secretions.

In another experiment (done for a different purpose) two tracheal segments were prepared in the neck and ammonia vapour was given to one of them. This caused an increase in mucin output from the ammonia-treated segment and a smaller increase from the other segment which had had no contact with the vapour (Fig. 5).

These results suggest, then, that part of the response is nervously mediated but that another part, perhaps half, depends on some local excitation.

Florey *et al.* (1932) found that ammonia solution increased the volume of mucus secreted into the cat trachea and that at least part of the response remained after they had treated the cat with atropine. They too concluded that there was a local mechanism which controlled mucus output.

We are interested in what this local mechanism might be. Possibly ammonia, a soluble gas which gives a strongly alkaline solution, can stimulate mucin release by a direct action on the secretory cells. Another possibility is that it causes local release of some mediator which in turn causes mucus secretion. Preliminary results, from experiments in which a prostaglandin synthesis inhibitor—indomethacin, 2 mg/kg—was given (Vane 1971), suggest that there

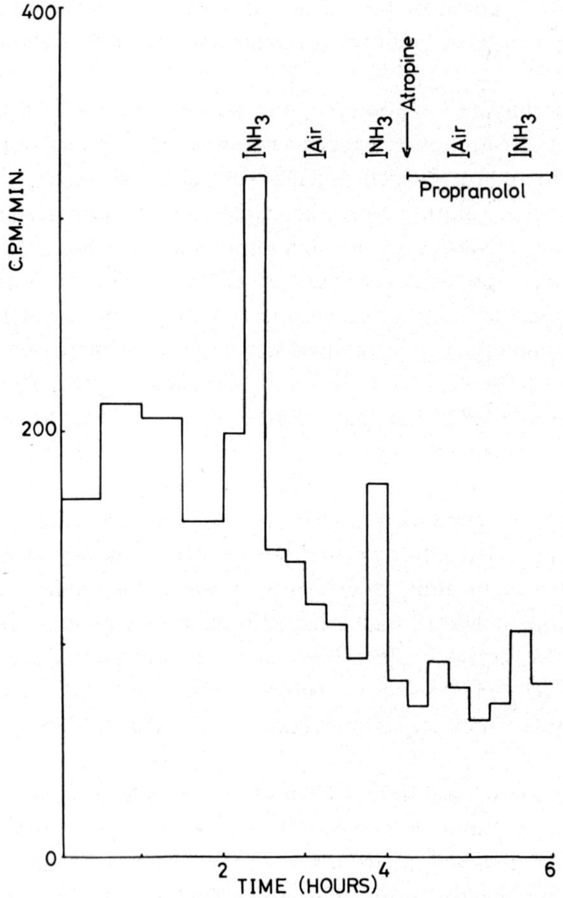

FIG. 4. The effect of 100 ml of 1 in 500 (2000 parts/10^6) ammonia insufflated through the trachea on three occasions. On the first two occasions this increased ^{35}S-labelled mucin output by 86% and 94% respectively and on the third, after atropine and propranolol had been given, the effect was + 38%. Control insufflations of air failed to stimulate secretion.

may be some weakening of the response to ammonia after administration of the drug. The initial responses to ammonia were $+ 100 \pm 38\%$ ($n = 6$) for the ^{35}S-labelled mucins and $+ 93 \pm 19\%$ ($n = 6$) for the [^{3}H]glucose-labelled mucins, while after indomethacin the responses were $+ 75 \pm 23\%$ ($n = 6$) for the ^{35}S and $+ 51 \pm 13\%$ ($n = 6$) for the ^{3}H. Prostaglandins may therefore act as intermediaries between the irritant and the secretion.

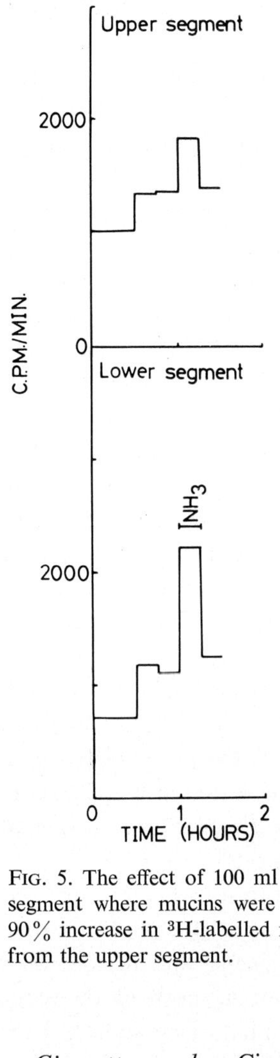

FIG. 5. The effect of 100 ml of 2000 parts/10^6 ammonia vapour given through the lower segment where mucins were being collected from two tracheal segments. This caused a 90% increase in ^{3}H-labelled mucin secretion from the lower segment and a 24% increase from the upper segment.

Cigarette smoke. Cigarette smoke was given into the drained tracheal segment in various concentrations. In the first experiments, undiluted smoke from a cigarette was drawn through the segment by a pump at 1 litre/min. This increased ^{35}S-labelled mucin output ($\Delta = 186 \pm 39\%$, $n = 9$) but when the stimulus was repeated the changes tended to fall off.

In later experiments 300 ml diluted cigarette smoke (1 part of smoke with 9 volumes of air) was given. Smoke given in this way still stimulated mucin secretion ($\Delta = +61 \pm 9\%$, $n = 10$ for ^{35}S-labelled mucins; $\Delta = +35 \pm 6\%$, $n = 16$ for ^{3}H-labelled secretions). Where both [^{3}H]glucose and [^{35}S]sulphate were given as precursors smoke had a greater effect on the ^{35}S-labelled mucins and the difference was highly significant. We suggest, therefore, that the dilute cigarette smoke excites secretion mainly from the mucous glands, and rather less from the highly glycosylated luminal edge.

At the same dilution successive doses of smoke caused increases in mucin output which were, in general, repeatable over three successive stimulations, so we did a few experiments in which we gave diluted cigarette smoke both before and after the blocking agents were given.

The effects of atropine and propranolol on changes in mucin output induced by cigarette smoke have been investigated in three experiments, one with [^{35}S]sulphate and two with [^{3}H]glucose as the precursor. The changes in the ^{35}S-labelled mucins were —17% and + 3% after the nerve blockers compared with + 99% and + 61% before. With [^{3}H]glucose as the precursor, cigarette smoke increased ^{3}H-labelled mucin secretion by 13% and 10% after propranolol and atropine respectively, compared with 34% and 53% before these substances were given in one experiment and by 29% and 11% compared with 42% and 10% in the other. These preliminary experiments do not prove that nerves caused the responses but suggest that they might have done.

In another experiment indomethacin appeared to have no effect on secretion.

The effects of CS. CS solution, given directly into the trachea of cats at a concentration of 0.2 mM, had little effect on mucin output. However when it was given in the same way to geese it increased the output of mucin by a mean of $356 \pm 49.5\%$ ($n = 23$), and at the same time it caused hypertension, tachycardia and rapid irregular breathing. Neither atropine nor cutting of the oesophageal nerves appeared to diminish these effects.

Two types of experiments were done in an attempt to see whether there was a reflex component. In one experiment local anaesthetic (0.25% lignocaine) was given along with the CS solution into the segment, and in the other experiment two tracheal segments were prepared in the neck of the same goose and the irritant was given into one segment. Lignocaine abolished the effects of CS on circulation and breathing and also on the mucin output. These responses could be restored by repeating the stimulus after lignocaine had been washed out of the trachea. However, it turned out that the local anaesthetic was not acting solely by blocking conduction in nerves; it caused an appreciable excitement of mucin output and also abolished increases in mucin secretion normally seen in response to acetylcholine (Phipps *et al.* 1977). We think that lignocaine has a direct action on the mucous cells but that these results do not in themselves indicate a reflex basis for the action of CS.

When CS was given to one of a pair of tracheal segments it increased the mucin secretion from that one ($\Delta = + 358 \pm 48.17\%$, $n = 8$) but not from the innervated control segment ($\Delta = -8 \pm 3.5\%$, $n = 8$).

The integrity of the innervations of the two segments was checked by stimulating the oesophageal nerves and in each case this increased secretion from both segments.

We conclude, therefore, that CS had a direct effect on mucin secretion from the goose trachea but we have no evidence for any reflex component to the effect. In two experiments we tested whether the prostaglandin-synthesis blocker indomethacin would quench the effect, but it did not. (Changes were + 148% and + 240% before indomethacin and + 195% and + 167% afterwards.)

THE EFFECTS OF ANTIGEN CHALLENGE IN SENSITIZED CATS

Three cats had been sensitized to the protein horseradish peroxidase (HRP) (method of L. A. Engel and J. Colebatch, personal communication), and then the effect of a challenge was investigated. Three routes of challenge were used: HRP solution was first given into the lungs as an aerosol (0.1–0.2% solution from a de Villbis generator), then as a solution (0.1–0.2%) into the tracheal segment and finally, in two cats, intravenously.

Administration of the aerosol changed neither breathing pattern nor mucin output. When HRP was given into the tracheal segment mucin output increased but no more than it had when HRP was given in the same concentration into the tracheas of non-sensitized cats.

In two cats, the challenge was also given intravenously, which resulted in anaphylactic reaction (blood pressure dropped sharply, breathing became rapid and shallow with frequent augmented breaths). In one of these there was no appreciable change in secretion of ^{3}H- or ^{35}S-labelled mucins from the tracheal segment but in the other mucin production increased (see Fig. 6).

CONCLUSIONS

Histamine and prostaglandins increase mucin secretion from the trachea in both of the species we have studied. Their role, if any, in causing the plugging of the airways in human asthma remains to be determined, but recent experiments with $PGF_{2\alpha}$ (M. T. Lopez-Vidriero *et al.*, personal communication) show that this mediator, at least, has a similar action in humans.

The experiments we have described show that the respiratory tract irritants, ammonia and cigarette smoke, probably excite secretion from the submucosal

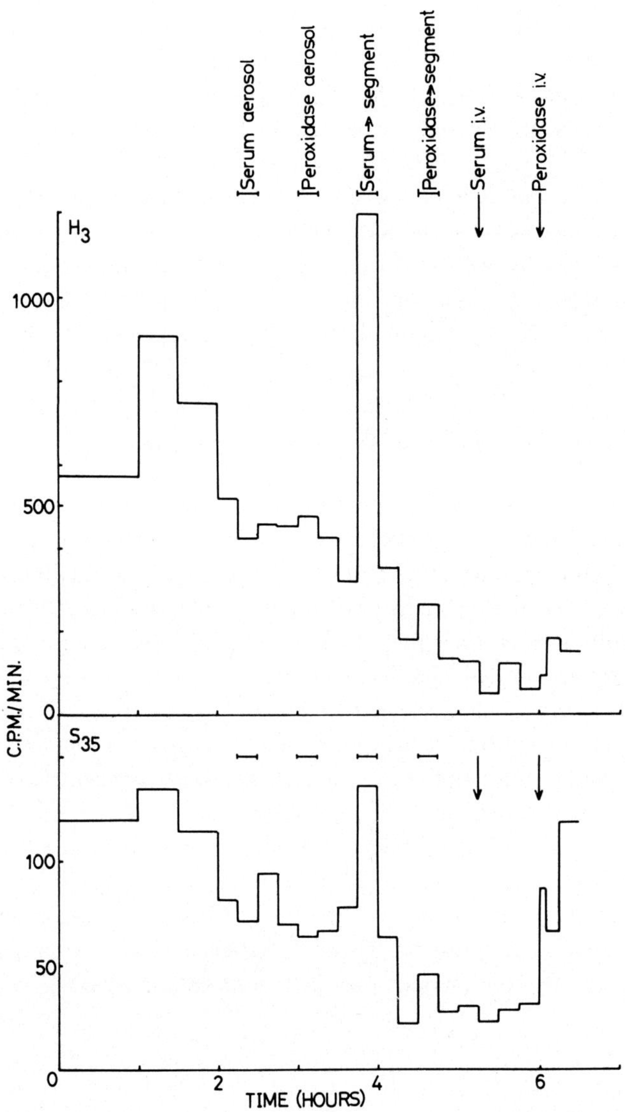

FIG. 6. Histogram showing the effects of antigen challenge by aerosol, administration into the tracheal segment and intravenously to a cat sensitized to horseradish peroxidase (HRP). Upper panel, ^{3}H-labelled mucin output; lower panel, ^{35}S-labelled mucins. Diluted horse serum was used as a control in this experiment. Note that challenge with HRP by aerosol and direct administration to the tracheal segment had trivial effects. The 'control' challenge into the tracheal segment increased secretion greatly. The intravenous challenge with HRP, which caused an anaphylactic reaction, also increased the output of mucins, particularly the ^{35}S-labelled mucins.

glands by way of nerves. It is likely that any stimulus which causes coughing will do this (Phipps & Richardson 1976). Soluble irritants would first be diluted and then expelled by coughing. The thicker the layer of mucus, the more effective a cough would be in shearing the mucus from the airway wall (Clarke 1973).

Although nervous pathways are involved it is likely that irritants cause part of their effect by some more direct mechanism. CS, in the goose, acts entirely in such a way, but ammonia and cigarette smoke also seem to excite secretion by a mechanism not involving nerves. Our experiments have so far not established whether this is by way of mediators or by some direct effect of the irritant.

Mucus consists of a mixture of components: water, salts and glycoproteins. There is evidence that the glycoproteins themselves are heterogeneous; of the secretory cells in airways some will stain one way, some another (Spicer *et al.* 1971; Lamb & Reid 1969, 1970; Jones & Reid 1973*a*, *b*), and there are differences in the appearance of the secretory granules of different cells which can be seen under the electron microscope (Phipps *et al.* 1977; Meyrick & Reid 1970). It is arguable whether the luminal edge glycoprotein whose output was stimulated by ammonia is a real secretion; it might be a part of the cell which detaches itself when the cell is damaged. We think it more likely that it is a secretion and our evidence for this is as follows: (*a*) even when no irritants are present the luminal edge incorporates radioactive precursors very rapidly. This suggests that it has a high rate of turnover. *(b)* Agents which stimulate gland secretion cause a much larger percentage increase in the ^{35}S output than in the ^{3}H output when both labelled sulphate and glucose are given as precursors (see Fig. 1). This is most easily explained if there is a background output of ^{3}H-labelled material from the luminal edge. Again this argues for a secretion from the luminal edge even in the absence of cell damage. *(c)* Chemical evidence shows that the glycoprotein is relatively homogeneous and that it behaves less like a fragmented cell wall than a secretion.

In future research we intend to investigate whether there are separate controls for the different glycoprotein components of mucus, how the various mucins interact to determine the physical and chemical properties of mucus, and how water and salts are added to the mucus.

ACKNOWLEDGEMENT

We wish to thank Dr I. Lampert, who suggested the Alcian blue method of measuring mucins.

References

CHAKRIN, L. W., BAKER, A. P., CHRISTIAN, P. & WARDELL, J. R. (1973) The effect of cholinergic stimulation on the release of macromolecules by canine trachea *in vitro*. *Am. Rev. Respir. Dis. 108*, 69–76

CLARKE, S. W. (1973) The role of two-phase flow in bronchial clearance. *Bull. Physio-Pathol. Respir. 9*, 359–372

FLOREY, H., CARLETON, H. M. & WELLS, A. Q. (1932) Mucus secretion in the trachea. *Br. J. Exp. Pathol. 13*, 269–284

GALLAGHER, J. T., KENT, P. W., PASSATORE, M., PHIPPS, R. J. & RICHARDSON, P. S. (1975) The composition of tracheal mucus and the nervous control of its secretion in the cat. *Proc. R. Soc. Lond. B Biol. Sci. 192*, 49–76

JONES, R. & REID, L. (1973*a*) The effect of pH on Alcian blue staining of epithelial acid glycoptoteins. I. Sialomucins and sulphomucins (single or in simple combinations). *Histochem. J. 5*, 9–18

JONES, R. & REID, L. (1973*b*) The effect of pH on Alcian blue staining of epithelial acid glycoproteins. II. Human bronchial submucosal gland. *Histochem. J. 5*, 19–27

LAMB, D. & REID, L. (1969) Histochemical types of acidic glycoprotein produced by mucous cells of the tracheobronchial glands in man. *J. Pathol. 98*, 213–229

LAMB, D. & REID, L. (1970) Histochemical and autoradiographic investigation of the serous cells of the human bronchial glands. *J. Pathol. 100*, 127–138

MEYRICK, B. & REID, L. (1970) Ultrastructure of cells in the human bronchial submucosal glands. *J. Anat. 107*, 281–299

MILLS, J. E., SELLICK, H. & WIDDICOMBE, J. G. (1969) Activity of lung irritant receptors in pulmonary microembolism, anaphylaxis and drug-induced bronchoconstrictions. *J. Physiol. (Lond.) 203*, 337–357

PHIPPS, R. J. & RICHARDSON, P. S. (1976) The effects of irritation at various levels of the airway upon tracheal mucus secretion in the cat. *J. Physiol. (Lond.) 261*, 563–581

PHIPPS, R. J., RICHARDSON, P. S., CORFIELD, A., GALLAGHER, J. T., JEFFERY, P. K., KENT, P. W. & PASSATORE, M. (1977) A physiological, biochemical and histological study of goose tracheal mucin and its secretion. *Phil. Trans. R. Soc. Lond. B Biol. Sci. 279*, 513–543

SPICER, S. S., CHAKRIN, L. W., WARDELL, J. R. & KENDRICK, W. (1971) Histochemistry of mucosubstances in the canine and human respiratory tract. *Lab. Invest. 25*, 483–490

STURGESS, J. & REID, L. (1972) An organ culture study of the effect of drugs on the secretory activity of human bronchial submucosal gland. *Clin. Sci. (Oxf.) 43*, 533–543

VANE, J. R. (1971) Inhibition of prostaglandin synthesis as a mechanism of action for aspirin-like drugs. *Nat. New Biol. 231*, 232–235

WHITEMAN, P. (1973) The quantitative determination of glycosaminoglycans in urine with Alcian Blue 8 GX. *Biochem. J. 131*, 351–357

Discussion

Guz: How far can you push this method along classical pharmacological lines? Can one in fact document a log dose-response curve and get the sort of information that pharmacologists are interested in?

Richardson: It is difficult to express results in terms of a log dose-response curve as long as we are restricted to expressing our results in terms of percentage increases in the amount of radioactively labelled mucins coming out. I hope we shall soon be able to express results usefully as a log dose-response curve when we can measure the actual mass of glycoproteins being secreted per minute and analyse each specimen that we collect in those terms. At the moment we cannot.

Widdicombe: You and Dr Jeffery described a distinction between surface secretion and gland secretion and I think you implied that you could study the distinction between the two by comparing tritium and ^{35}S. To what extent have you applied this to your results with these irritants, in particular *O*-chlorobenzilidine malononitrile (CS)? As I understand it, CS is effective in causing intense pain and not killing people since it is so insoluble that it sticks to the surface. That might be an ideal chemical tool for looking at the surface secretion.

Richardson: I am not sure that it would be, because in the cat its effect on mucin output was small; it increased only by a mean of 30%. In the goose it had large effects, but the goose has very little luminal surface glycoprotein that we can label with the precursors that we have tried so far.

Jeffery: The goose airway has a lot of surface mucosubstance but it doesn't seem to label very well with tritiated compounds, particularly the glucose. How did you measure the protein output in these experiments?

Richardson: We used an Alcian blue method. Alcian blue combines with the acid terminals of the glycoprotein molecules so that they form an insoluble complex which can be centrifuged into a pellet. Under the right conditions this will precipitate 97% of the radioactivity. Then the pellet can be resuspended in Manoxol 1B and the amount of glycoprotein present can be estimated colorimetrically. When R. L. Hall (personal communication) tested the method on tracheal glycoproteins at different dilutions he found that it was a quantitative reaction: the amount of dye precipitated was proportional to the quantity of glycoprotein in the solution.

J. G. Jones: Can you tell us something about the appearance time of the isotope? It wasn't clear to me whether the baseline changes in your results reflected the way the isotope was appearing, and I wondered whether we were seeing a mixture of incorporation times or some other reflex effects of the washings on which you superimpose your experiment. Could it be that after introducing a single dose of the isotope, you are exhausting the system if the isotope takes, say, an hour or so to be incorporated and actually appear in the mucus?

Richardson: There were various different patterns of the emergence of the isotope. In experiments where we gave the radioactive isotope intravenously, very little bound radioactive material appeared in the first sample of tracheal washings and there was a gradual increase over the first $1\frac{1}{2}$ or 2 hours after the pulse label. Where we gave the dose of radioactively labelled precursor directly into the tracheal segment, we discarded the first tracheal wash sample which was obviously grossly contaminated with unbound radioactivity. Graphs from those experiments started after the pulse label had been in the trachea for one hour. In the latter experiments the amount of radioactive material secreted per unit time tended to diminish during the experiment. As to whether the actual procedure of the washing had a big effect on the mucin output, Dr Jeffery has looked at that by comparing the appearance of the tracheal segment after the experiment with that of the trachea below the segment, which had not been washed repeatedly. There was little difference in the histological appearance of the two parts of the trachea.

J. G. Jones: Are you exhausting the isotope from the system?

Richardson: Yes; with a pulse label I think it is inevitable that there is less isotope in the system at the end of the experiment than there was at the beginning. So the specific activity of the glycoproteins that are being washed out is less after, say, 6 or 8 h than near the beginning of the experiment.

J. G. Jones: Couldn't you have given a continuous intravenous infusion to maintain a blood level so that you could look at the incorporation and elimination?

Richardson: Yes, but that puts up the expense of the experiment.

Nadel: Can we consider the role of the epithelial damage in some of your experiments? The responsiveness of airway smooth muscle to mediators such as histamine and prostaglandin $F_{2\alpha}$ is increased by damage to the airway epithelium by respiratory virus infection (Empey *et al.* 1976; Laitinen *et al.* 1976) and by inhalation of ozone (Lee *et al.* 1977). This increased responsiveness of the airway smooth muscle is abolished by atropine or by blocking conduction in the cervical vagus nerves, implicating cholinergic vagal pathways in the exaggerated responses. Perhaps damage to the airway epithelium has a similar effect on cholinergically mediated airway secretion. Could changes in the airway epithelium increase the ability of horseradish peroxidase to reach and be bound to antigen?

Richardson: That might be possible. We were surprised that we didn't get an increase in the mucin output when we challenged sensitized cats with horeseradish peroxidase directly into the tracheal segment and I think that may have been because the horseradish peroxidase didn't get in through the tight junctions to the underlying mast cells.

Allison: You imply that you produced immediate hypersensitivity in these cats. Do you know whether IgE was produced, or IgG? The intravenous effects you described sound very much like a serum sickness reaction which is typical of IgG-dependent allergy rather than IgE-mediated immunopathology.

Richardson: I don't know which immunoglobulin was produced.

Reid: In organ cultures of human glands we have looked at precursor uptake, synthesis and discharge from individual cells. We haven't found any stimulatory effect from the sympathetic system. On the other hand we know that giving isoprenaline (isoproterenol) over a matter of days to the living animal will produce an effect, but, in the short term, which we are discussing now, we can show only that the parasympathetic controls the secretion, at least in human material. We get a degree of inhibition but we never abolish secretion altogether. When you look at the sympathetic system, are you in fact looking at what is essentially an effect on the myoepithelial cells?

After giving ourselves prostaglandins we were able to collect sputum after about seven puffs of $PGF_{2\alpha}$. This secretion contains epithelial glycoprotein but very little of the markers of sputum, such as mannose, that are present in small amounts even in sputum from a mucoid bronchitic (Lopez-Vidriero *et al.* 1977). The fact that we can pick up a difference, as it were, in the total bronchial fluid that is produced suggests that prostaglandin may have squeezed from the glands a secretion that was already there—or that it has a different effect. Can you pick up a difference in the nature of the secretion or the timing of the emptying of glands or of cells by the sympathetic as compared with the parasympathetic?

Richardson: We asked Paul Kent and his colleagues, who are analysing the mucins we collect, whether the secretions produced by the sympathomimetic amines are the same as those produced by acetylcholine and vagal stimulation. So far they cannot detect any differences. That doesn't mean that there isn't a difference but these substances are very difficult to deal with biochemically and it is possible that minor differences in the secretions would have been missed. We wondered whether the sympathomimetic amines were causing contraction in the myoepithelial cells and squeezing the mucins out of glands, as you suggest. That is unlikely, though, on two grounds. First, we find that they act through β-adrenoceptors (Gallagher *et al.* 1975) and we would expect these to relax myoepithelial cells, if anything. Secondly, if the gland was being squeezed, it would be unlikely that there could be several squeezes in fairly quick succession; but when we gave three doses of sympathomimetic amines one after another we got three consecutive responses. Similarly one would expect that after the squeeze the myoepithelial cells would relax, the ducts of the acinar glands would regain their capacity, and the secretion would be reduced. When the sympathomimetic amines were given there would be an increased secretion but then one would expect to find a drop below the control rate of secretion as the ducts filled up again. We have looked very carefully through our results and could not find a biphasic response of this sort.

Reid: It could be a species difference of course, but it could even be that you are detecting a pre-gland effect of the sympathetic, although ultimately the pathway is still going to be through the cholinergic system. After all, you are using an intact nervous system whereas ours is tissue and organ culture.

Richardson: What you are suggesting is that sympathetic nerves excite post-ganglionic cholinergic nerves to the mucous glands. However atropine, which blocks the effect of parasympathetic nerve stimulation, does not prevent sympathetic nerves and sympathetic drugs from causing mucin secretion (Gallagher *et al.* 1975).

Nadel: It normally acts the other way round in systems such as the gut, where the sympathetic nervous output modulates the parasympathetic system. Those who have studied it have shown that it is an α-adrenergic effect and is inhibitory to parasympathetic ganglionic transmission.

Richardson: There is, I agree, quite a big gap in our argument in that so far we haven't shown where the sympathetic nerves are going and whether there are sympathetic axons going to the glands we are looking at. We intend to study this.

Guz: Some of the drugs you are using in your histamine experiments are extremely vasoactive. Histamine is bound to be vasodilatory; the venules become permeable to plasma proteins. Can you tell us what the specimen looks like under the light microscope after application of histamine in the concentrations you used? Secondly, is secretion at all dependent, critically or otherwise, on blood flow?

Richardson: I can't satisfy you on either of those questions. We haven't measured blood flow, and we haven't examined the trachea histologically after it had been treated with histamine.

Jeffery: What would the histologists be looking for?

Guz: Some years ago Fishman's group described the effect of putting a histamine aerosol down the airways and the effect on the veins was quite devastating (Pietra *et al.* 1971). There was venodilatation and tremendous oozing and oedema. I have put histamine down a bronchoscope into the airways of man in much smaller concentrations than you used, and the mucosal surface immediately becomes red.

Godfrey: An obvious example in man is hay-fever. A very small dose of pollen in a sensitive subject will produce an immediate redness, oedema and profuse watery discharge.

Richardson: I don't think the radioactively labelled material in tracheal washings was plasma protein because when we put the isotopic labels into the trachea only minute amounts of labelled proteins actually appeared in the bloodstream.

Guz: I was more concerned with the possibility that the vascular actions might explain some of the results with secretions.

Richardson: Your point is a good one. Histamine may have made blood vessels very permeable to water and allowed transudate to flush secretions from the gland ducts into the trachea. That might explain the single response that we found to repeated large doses of histamine.

Jeffery: But in fact that area of the airway is not really very vascular.

References

EMPEY, D. W., LAITINEN, L. A., JACOBS, L., GOLD, W. M. & NADEL, J. A. (1976) Mechanisms of bronchial hyperreactivity in normal subjects after upper respiratory tract infection. *Am. Rev. Respir. Dis. 113*, 131–139

GALLAGHER, J. T., KENT, P. W., PASSATORE, M., PHIPPS, R. J. & RICHARDSON, P. S. (1975) The composition of tracheal mucus and the nervous control of its secretion in the cat. *Proc. R. Soc. Lond. B Biol. Sci. 192*, 49–76

LAITINEN, L. A., ELKIN, R. B., EMPEY, D. W., JACOBS, L., MILLS, J., GOLD, W. M. & NADEL, J. A. (1976) Changes in bronchial reactivity after administration of live attenuated influenza virus. *Am. Rev. Respir. Dis. 113*, 194

LEE, L.-Y., BLEECKER, E. & NADEL, J. A. (1977) Ozone-induced airway hyperirritability in dogs. *Fed. Proc. 36*, 616

LOPEZ-VIDRIERO, M. T., DAS, I., PICOT, R., SMITH, A. P. & REID, L. (1977) Bronchial secreiont from normal airways after inhalation of prostaglandin F2α, acetylcholine, histamine and citric acid. *Thorax*, in press

PIETRA, G. G., SZIDON, J. P., LEVENTHAL, M. M. & FISHMAN, A. P. (1971) Histamine and interstitial pulmonary edema in the dog. *Circ. Res. 29*, 323–337

Regulation of Na^+ and Cl^- transport and mucous gland secretion in airway epithelium

JAY A. NADEL and BRIAN DAVIS

Cardiovascular Research Institute and Departments of Medicine and Physiology, University of California, San Francisco

Abstract Ussing's short-circuit technique was applied to canine airway epithelium *in vitro* and a net flux of Cl^- towards the airway lumen was demonstrated, with a smaller net flux of Na^+ in the opposite direction. Furosemide decreased and acetylcholine, terbutaline, and histamine increased net ion transport towards the airway lumen. Associated changes in water content in the airway lumen could affect mucociliary clearance, and therefore inhibition of ion transport may play a role in disease states.

To study secretions from submucosal glands *in vivo*, two techniques were used to identify the duct openings in the exposed canine tracheal epithelium. (*a*) The exposed mucosal surface was coated with powdered tantalum; accumulated secretions produced elevations under which the duct openings were located. (*b*) A vital dye (0.1% Neutral red) was placed on the exposed mucosal surface; the dye stained the duct openings. With these techniques, the innervation of the submucosal glands and the autonomic regulation of their secretions were studied. Micropuncture techniques were used to sample the secretions from the glands and ducts.

The title of this symposium, 'Respiratory Tract *Mucus*', reflects the major concern of scientists in the field of airway secretions with mucus: its chemistry, its mechanism of secretion, and its physical properties. The mucus is propelled mouthward by cilia and these cilia must move through a *watery* periciliary fluid to contact and propel the surface gel-like mucous blanket. Our premise is that the regulation of the *watery* layer is of utmost importance to the normal mucociliary clearance mechanism and may be linked to active ion transport. We suggest that 'Respiratory Tract *Secretion*' is a more appropriate title for the materials which leave airway epithelial cells and contribute to the surface fluid in the airway lumen.

Since the airways contain many types of cells, we attempted to isolate them in physiological subunits *in vivo* and to study them separately. Thus, we developed methods for identifying mucous gland duct openings *in vivo* and we used micropuncture techniques to sample gland secretions.

ACTIVE ION TRANSPORT

Cilia move through a layer of thin 'periciliary' fluid to propel secreted mucus up the airways and thus clear the airways of inhaled insoluble particles. Water may facilitate coupling between the superficial layer of mucus and the cilia by forming a layer beneath the mucus (Lucas & Douglas 1938). Our hypothesis is that abnormal mucociliary clearance in diseases such as status asthmaticus and cystic fibrosis may be due to a loss of normal water flow into the airways (Nadel & Davis 1977). Since water flow is linked to active ion transport in other epithelia, we set out to determine whether active ion transport exists in airway epithelium. We applied Ussing's short-circuit technique to canine airway epithelium *in vitro* (Olver *et al.* 1975). We anaesthetized dogs, excised the trachea, dissected off the muscle layer from the posterior membranous portion of the trachea and mounted the remaining epithelium between the two halves of an Ussing chamber. We measured electrical potential difference and short-circuit current via two electrical circuits connected to the chamber via agar bridges. We used radioisotopes (^{22}Na, ^{24}Na, ^{36}Cl) to measure unidirectional ion fluxes. We found a stable electrical potential difference (30.7 ± 2.7 mV) with the lumen negative to submucosa and a short-circuit current of 108 ± 8 $\mu A/cm^2$. Analysis of unidirectional ion fluxes showed that the short-circuit current is largely due to a net Cl^- flux towards the lumen (2.7 ± 0.6 μequiv. cm^{-2} h^{-1}), while the remaining short-circuit current is accounted for by a net Na^+ flux in the opposite direction (0.8 ± 0.2 μequiv. cm^{-2} h^{-1}). There was no significant difference between the short-circuit current and the sum of the net Na^+ and net Cl^- fluxes so there can be no other major electrogenic system for ion transport.

Thus the tracheal epithelium pumps Cl^- toward the lumen and this may provide the means for secreting the fluid that lies beneath the 'mucous blanket'. Because furosemide inhibits Cl^- transport in the thick ascending limb of the nephron, we studied the effect of this drug on the airway epithelium (Davis *et al.* 1977). Adding furosemide (10^{-4}M) to the luminal side of the chamber produced no significant changes, but adding the drug to the submucosal side resulted in a decrease in short-circuit current from 68 ± 9 $\mu A/cm^2$ to 36 ± 6 $\mu A/cm^2$ ($P < 0.0001$; $n = 12$) and a decrease in net Cl^- transport towards the lumen from 1.84 ± 0.55 μequiv. cm^{-2} h^{-1} to 0.81 ± 0.26 μequiv. cm^{-2} h^{-1} ($P < 0.03$; $n = 6$). This evidence suggests that the Cl^- pump is located on the submucosal surface of the cells. More recently Jonathan

Widdicombe has provided the following experimental model (based on studies utilizing ouabain, Na^+-free and K^+-free media) which links Cl^- transport to active Na^+ transport: Na^+ is driven across the submucosal membrane by a Na^+ pump and creates a transmembrane Na^+ gradient. This allows Cl^- to enter the cells from the submucosa together with Na^+ on a neutral carrier molecule. The Na^+ that enters the cells is carried back out of the cells by the Na^+ pumps on the submucosal cell membrane. Cl^- passes down an electrochemical gradient across the luminal cell membrane. The energy for the net Cl^- movement is thus provided by the transmembrane Na^+ gradient (J. H. Widdicombe, personal communication).

There is evidence that both the parasympathetic and sympathetic nervous systems affect mucociliary transport. Cholinergic agonists have been reported to increase mucous transport (Camner *et al.* 1974) and some workers report that cholinergic antagonists slow mucociliary clearance (Pavia & Thomson 1971; Foster *et al.* 1976). The time course of this slowing is consistent with a change in the watery periciliary layer (Denton *et al.* 1968). Furthermore, in a patient with severe bronchorrhoea (production of watery secretions) a cholinergic antagonist delivered into the airways by aerosol resulted in a marked reduction in the volume of secretions (Wick & Ingram 1976). We postulated that active ion transport might account for the cholinergic secretory effects in airways (Marin *et al.* 1976). Under short-circuit conditions, acetylcholine (5×10^{-5}M) increased the net flux towards the lumen of Cl^- ($n = 7$) from 1.7 ± 0.5 to 3.3 ± 0.5 μequiv. cm^{-2} h^{-1} and of Na^+ from -0.8 ± 0.2 to $+ 0.5 \pm 0.2$ μequiv. cm^{-2} h^{-1}. Under open-circuit conditions, acetylcholine (5×10^{-5}M) increased the unidirectional flux of Cl^- towards the lumen from 4.7 ± 1.3 to 5.9 ± 1.4 μequiv. cm^{-2} h^{-1}, but the other measured fluxes did not change significantly. All of these responses were prevented by atropine sulphate (10^{-8}M). From these studies we conclude that the cholinergic system has potent effects on ion transport and may mediate water secretion.

Adrenergic agonists are also reported to increase mucociliary clearance (Kordik *et al.* 1952; Laurenzi *et al.* 1968). We found that a β_2-adrenergic agonist (terbutaline; 10^{-5}M) on the submucosal side increased short-circuit current from 62 ± 6 μA/cm^2 to 90 ± 7 μA/cm^2 ($n = 12$). In each of seven studies, terbutaline (10^{-5}M) increased the unidirectional Cl^- flux towards the lumen from 4.44 ± 1.00 to 5.74 ± 1.02 μequiv. cm^{-2} h^{-1} but did not affect the unidirectional fluxes of Cl^- towards the submucosa or either unidirectional flux of Na^+. Propranolol (10^{-5}M) prevented the changes in short-circuit current and in Cl^- flux, indicating that the effect was due to β-adrenergic receptor stimulation (Davis *et al.* 1975). These findings have been recently confirmed (Al-Bazzaz *et al.* 1977). Thus, the effect of β-adrenergic agonists on mucociliary transport could be secondary to their stimulating effects on Cl^- transport with subsequent increased formation of periciliary fluid. Perhaps the increased transport rates observed with adrenergic drugs in patients with chronic obstructive airway disease (Santa Cruz *et al.* 1974) and in patients with cystic fibrosis (Wood *et al.* 1975) is due to the stimulation of water secretion which facilitates movement of the previously trapped gel-like blanket.

Histamine, a mediator of the allergic response of airways, also increased net flux of Cl^- towards the airway lumen from 1.7 ± 0.5 to 2.4 ± 0.6 μequiv. cm^{-2} h^{-1}. The response to histamine was inhibited by diphenhydramine (10^{-6}M), an H_1-receptor antagonist, but not by burimamide (10^{-4}M), an H_2-receptor antagonist (Marin *et al.* 1977).

Our studies indicate that active ion transport exists in the airway epithelium and provides a mechanism for secretion and reabsorption of water. Others have assumed that all airway secretions must be transported mouthward by ciliary action; some investigators have even calculated the total volume of secreted fluid from the amount cleared. However, there is evidence that two layers of secretion exist on the airway luminal surface: a superficial gel which is propelled by the cilia and a watery 'periciliary' layer underneath, through which the cilia move. Movement of this periciliary layer is poorly understood. To a large extent, this could be a standing layer of fluid whose thickness is regulated to provide the most efficient movement of the cilia in relation to the gel-like mucous blanket. We also suggest that abnormal mucociliary clearance in disease (e.g. cystic fibrosis, status asthmaticus, chronic bronchitis) may be due to a loss of normal water flow into the airway lumen because of inadequate Cl^- transport. Furthermore, we suggest that studies of active ion transport may be useful in evaluating new drugs which may act as secretagogues or inhibitors of secretion. Drugs which affect active ion transport may provide a rational treatment for patients with abnormal mucociliary clearance.

Our tracheal preparation has a pseudostratified columnar, ciliated epithelium, submucosal glands and a fibrous tissue layer. Many sites exist where active ion transport may occur. Some species (e.g. goose) lack submucosal glands. It would be of interest to determine whether active ion transport occurs in the airway epithelium of such species, especially as it is likely that the serous component of mucus is derived entirely from the submucosal glands (Rhodin 1966). Of particular interest in relation to ion transport are the microvilli of surface cells which are about 2 μm in length and whose extensive surface area is ideally suited for active transport.

MUCOUS GLAND SECRETION

The airway epithelium is a complex structure containing many cell types (e.g. mucous gland and duct cells, goblet cells, ciliated cells). To understand the functions and regulation of these structures we need to isolate them in biological subunits. This has been done successfully in other organs (e.g. salivary glands, kidneys). Previous studies of mucous secretion involved collection of either sputum or total respiratory tract fluid (Perry & Boyd 1941; Gallagher *et al.* 1975; Adams *et al.* 1976). These collections came from undetermined areas and were collected only after an unknown delay.

To study the contribution of mucous glands and ducts to airway secretions in anaesthetized dogs and cats, we incised the anterior surface of the cervical trachea vertically and pulled the cut edges widely apart. Blood vessels were visible through the transparent epithelial layer, but gland duct openings were not seen. To identify the openings, we coated the tracheal epithelium with

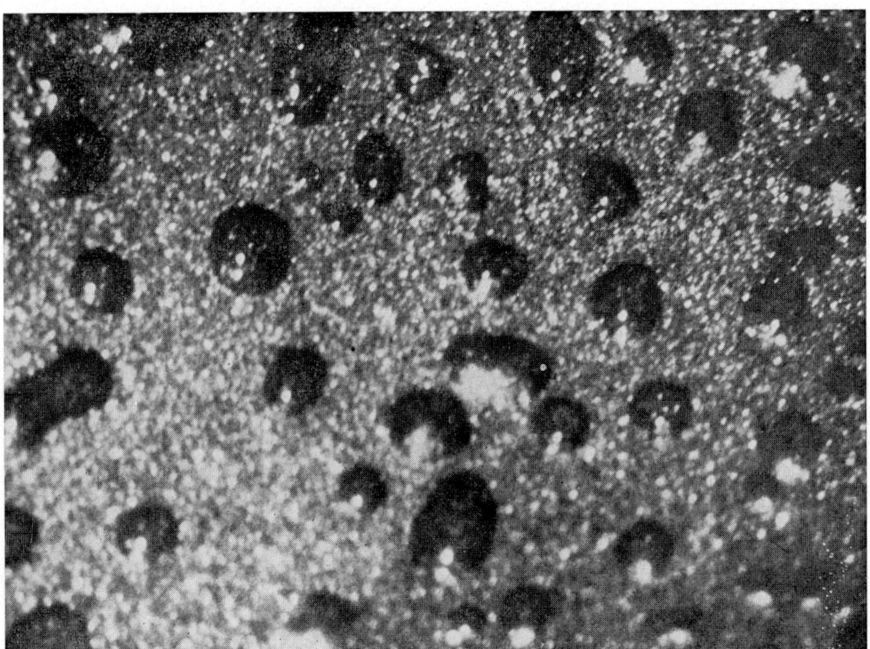

FIG. 1. Photograph obtained through a dissecting microscope of elevations in canine airway epithelium produced by electrical stimulation of the cervical vagus nerves. The airway epithelium was exposed and coated with powdered tantalum. The elevations due to accumulated secretions averaged 0.2 mm in diameter. × 50.

a fine layer of powdered tantalum (Davis *et al.* 1976). Anatomical studies suggest that cholinergic nerves supply the glands (El-Bermani & Grant 1975). We stimulated the peripheral ends of the cut vagus nerves (5–15 V; 10–30 Hz; 3 ms). The particles of tantalum on the surface prevented the dispersion of fluid secreted from the gland duct openings, so small elevations or 'hillocks' appeared in the tantalum layer (Fig. 1). To establish that these hillocks were accumulations of secretions from gland ducts, we fixed the tracheal tissue *in vivo* with Bouin's solution, gently removed the hillocks and examined the underlying areas through a dissecting microscope. Beneath each removed hillock, we found duct openings (Fig. 2), but we found none in other locations. Serial sections obtained from a punch biopsy of one of the fixed hillocks showed typical gland duct epithelium lining a conducting tube from the airway surface to the mucous gland cells. Scanning electron micrographs of duct openings made on the opposite side of the trachea showed that the

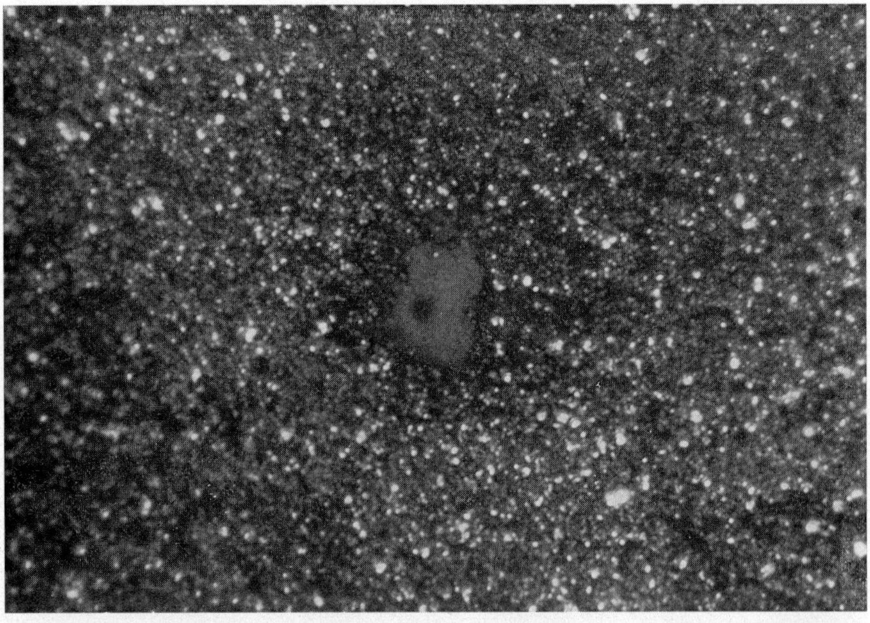

FIG. 2. Photograph of gland duct opening in canine tracheal epithelium. The airway epithelium was exposed and coated with powdered tantalum, the vagus nerves were stimulated to produce elevations (seen in Fig. 1), the trachea was fixed *in vivo*, and one of the elevations was removed with a fine cotton swab. Photograph shows gland duct opening (black circular area, approximately 30 μm in diameter) in the area of epithelium exposed by removal of the elevation. The remainder of the epithelium is coated with powdered tantalum.

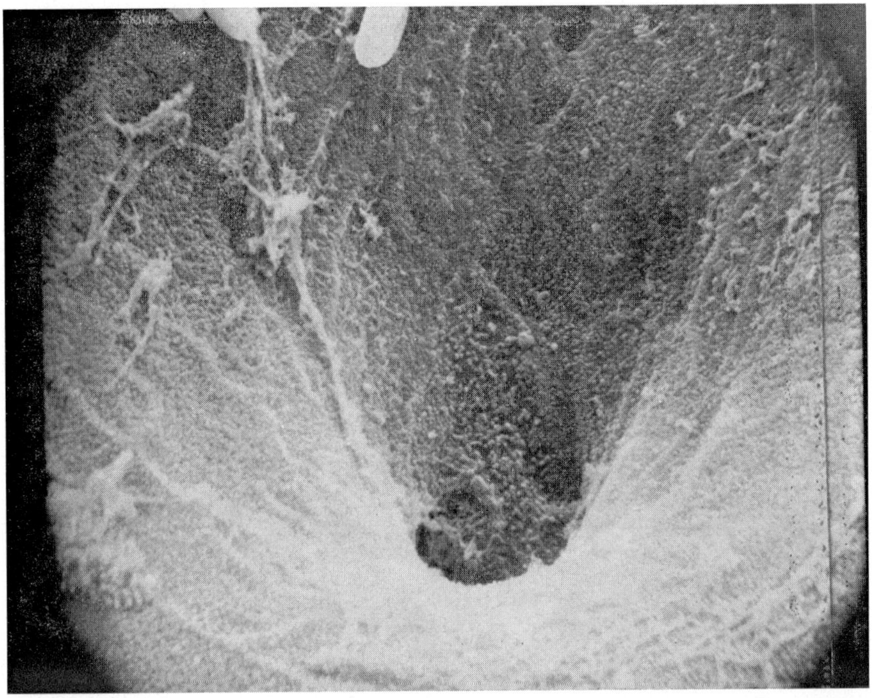

FIG. 3. Scanning electron micrograph of duct opening, showing a border of airway lining cells continuous with cells of the funnel-shaped opening of gland duct. A few red blood cells are seen at the top of the photograph, and secretions can be seen emanating from the gland duct opening (on the left). × 7000.

airway lining epithelium was intact and continuous with the gland duct epithelium (Fig. 3).

Using this technique, we showed that the efferent cholinergic nerve supply to the glands was via the homolateral vagus nerve: the superior laryngeal nerve innervated the glands in the upper trachea and the recurrent laryngeal nerve supplied the glands in the lower trachea. These responses were prevented by atropine sulphate (0.2–0.5 mg/kg, i.v.) (Davis *et al.* 1976). Patients with asthma and some patients with chronic bronchitis have hypertrophy of mucous glands (and airway smooth muscle). Chronic activation of cholinergic reflexes, e.g. by damage to the airway epithelium (Empey *et al.* 1976), could chronically overstimulate both the glands and smooth muscle and cause them to hypertrophy (Nadel 1977). Chronic administration of sulphur dioxide and cigarette smoke in animals results in hypertrophy of the mucous glands (Lamb & Reid 1968; Mawdesley-Thomas *et al.* 1971). These agents also activate vagal reflexes by stimulating rapidly adapting vagal nerve endings (Nadel 1977). Perhaps this reflex pathway is responsible for the glandular hypertrophy that occurs in the airways with chronic inhalation of these irritants.

Tantalum may interfere with the collection of the fluid from the submucosal glands so we looked for a vital dye to outline the gland duct openings. We found that a 0.1% solution of Neutral red placed on the luminal surface of the exposed trachea stained gland ducts and gland duct openings and thus allowed us to sample fluid directly from individual gland duct openings (Nadel 1977). We have not determined the exact sites of staining, but it has been shown that Neutral red granules in pancreatic cells were in lysosomes (reviewed in Allison & Young 1969). Neutral red also stains the submucosal gland cells and this should assist in identifying and removing the glands for later study of isolated cell function and for cell culture.

ACKNOWLEDGEMENTS

These studies were supported in part by a grant from the U.S. Public Health Service: Program Project HL-06285 and by a National Cystic Fibrosis Fellowship (B. Davis). The studies on ion transport were performed with M. G. Marin, R. E. Olver, J. H. Widdicombe, and I. Bruderman; on mucous gland secretion with M. G. Marin, I. Ueki, and P. Graf; and on staining airway glands with I. Ueki.

References

ADAMS, G. K., AHARONSON, E. F., REASOR, M. J. & PROCTOR, D. F. (1976) Collection of normal canine tracheobronchial secretions. *J. Appl. Physiol. 40*, 247–249

AL-BAZZAZ, F. J., KHAN, A. & CHENG, E. (1977) Stimulation of chloride secretion across canine tracheal epithelia by theophylline and epinephrine. *Clin. Res. 25*, 414A

ALLISON, A. C. & YOUNG, M. R. (1969) Vital staining and fluorescence microscopy of lysosomes, in *Lysosomes in Biology and Pathology* (Dingle, J. T. & Fell, H. B., eds.), pp. 600–628, North-Holland, Amsterdam

CAMNER, P., STRANDBERG, K. & PHILIPSON, K. (1974) Increased mucociliary transport by cholinergic stimulation. *Arch. Environ. Health 29*, 220–224

DAVIS, B., MARIN, M. G. & NADEL, J. A. (1975) β-Adrenergic receptor in canine tracheal epithelium. *Am. Rev. Respir. Dis. 111*, 947

DAVIS, B., MARIN, M., FISCHER, S., GRAF, P., WIDDICOMBE, J. & NADEL, J. A. (1976) New method for study of canine mucus gland secretion *in vivo*: cholinergic regulation. *Am. Rev. Respir. Dis. 113*, 257

DAVIS, B., MARIN, M. G., UEKI, I. & NADEL, J. A. (1977) Effect of furosemide on chloride ion transport and electrical properties of canine tracheal epithelium. *Clin. Res. 25*, 132A

DENTON, R., FORSMAN, W., HWANG, S. H., LITT, M. & MILLER, C. E. (1968) Viscoelasticity of mucus. Its role in ciliary transport of pulmonary secretions. *Am. Rev. Respir. Dis. 98*, 380–391

EL-BERMANI, A.-W. & GRANT, M. (1975) Acetylcholinesterase-positive nerves of the rhesus monkey bronchial tree. *Thorax 30*, 162–170

EMPEY, D. W., LAITINEN, L. A., JACOBS, L., GOLD, W. M. & NADEL, J. A. (1976) Mechanisms of bronchial hyperreactivity in normal subjects after upper respiratory tract infection. *Am. Rev. Respir. Dis. 113*, 131–139

FOSTER, W. M., BERGOFSKY, E. H., BOHNING, D. E., LIPPMANN, M. & ALBERT, R. E. (1976) Effect of adrenergic agents and their mode of action on mucociliary clearance in man. *J. Appl. Physiol. 41*, 146–152

GALLAGHER, J. T., KENT, P. W., PASSATORE, M., PHIPPS, R. J. & RICHARDSON, P. S. (1975) The composition of tracheal mucus and the nervous control of its secretion in the cat. *Proc. R. Soc. Lond. B Biol. Sci. 192*, 49–76

KORDIK, P., BULBRING, E. & BURN, J. H. (1952) Ciliary movement and acetylcholine. *Br. J. Pharmacol. 7*, 67–79

LAMB, D. & REID, L. (1968) Mitotic rates, goblet cell increase and histochemical changes in mucus in rat bronchial epithelium during exposure to sulfur dioxide. *J. Pathol. Bacteriol. 96*, 97–111

LAURENZI, G. A., YIN, S. & GUARNERI, J. J. (1968) Adverse effect of oxygen on tracheal mucus flow. *N. Engl. J. Med. 279*, 333–339

LUCAS, A. M. & DOUGLAS, L. C. (1938) Principles underlying ciliary activity in the respiratory tract. II. A comparison of nasal clearance in man, monkey and other mammals. *Arch. Otolaryngol. 20*, 518–541

MARIN, M. G., DAVIS, B. & NADEL, J. A. (1976) Effect of acetylcholine on Cl^- and Na^+ fluxes across dog tracheal epithelium *in vitro*. *Am. J. Physiol. 231*, 1546–1549

MARIN, M. G., DAVIS, B. & NADEL, J. A. (1977) Effect of histamine on electrical and ion transport properties of tracheal epithelium. *J. Appl. Physiol. 42*, 735–738

MAWDESLEY-THOMAS, L. E., HEALEY, P. & BARRY, D. H. (1971) Experimental bronchitis in animals due to sulphur dioxide and cigarette smoke. An automated quantitative study, in *Inhaled Particles III* (Walton, W. H., ed.) *(Proc. Int. Symp. Br. Occup. Hyg. Soc.)*, pp. 509–525, Unwin, London

NADEL, J. A. (1977) Autonomic control of airway smooth muscle and airway secretions. *Am. Rev. Respir. Dis. 115(6) (suppl.)*, 117–126

NADEL, J. A. & DAVIS, B. (1977) Autonomic regulation of mucous secretion and ion transport in airways, in *Asthma: Physiology, Immunopharmacology and Treatment* (Lichenstein, L. M. & Austen, K. F., eds.), pp. 197–210, Academic Press, New York

OLVER, R. E., DAVIS, B., MARIN, M. G. & NADEL, J. A. (1975) Active transport of Na^+ and Cl^- across the canine tracheal epithelium *in vitro*. *Am. Rev. Respir. Dis. 112*, 811–815

PAVIA, D. & THOMSON, M. L. (1971) Inhibition of mucociliary clearance from the human lung by hyoscine. *Lancet 1*, 449–450

PERRY, W. F. & BOYD, E. M. (1941) A method for studying expectorant action in animals by direct measurement of the output of respiratory tract fluids. *J. Pharmacol. Exp. Ther. 73*, 65–77

RHODIN, J. A. G. (1966) Ultrastructure and function of the human tracheal mucosa. *Am. Rev. Respir. Dis. 93*, 1–15

SANTA CRUZ, R., LANDA, J. F., HIRSCH, J. & SACKNER, M. A. (1974) Tracheal mucous velocity in normal man and patients with obstructive lung disease; effects of terbutaline. *Am. Rev. Respir. Dis. 109*, 458–463

WICK, M. M. & INGRAM, R. H. (1976) Bronchorrhea responsive to aerosolized atropine. *J. Am. Med. Assoc. 235*, 1356

WOOD, R. E., WANNER, A., HIRSCH, J. & FARRELL, P. M. (1975) Tracheal mucociliary transport in patients with cystic fibrosis and its stimulation by terbutaline. *Am. Rev. Respir. Dis. 111*, 733–738

Discussion

Reid: What do you find in the 500 μm thick section, and in the dog how deep does this go?

Nadel: We dissect off the muscle from the posterior membrane of the trachea. Although we do not study the areas containing cartilage, the preparations contain glands.

Reid: That is one of the regions where there are a lot of glands.

Nadel: The main problem is that if cartilage is present we cannot dissect off the airway epithelium and cannot maintain viability of the whole membrane. In smaller airways (e.g. in the rabbit), we have demonstrated prolonged viability of preparations that include cartilage.

Reid: Have you tried to remove less and make the layer much thinner so that you really do get just the surface epithelium? Which cells and which levels of the structures we have talked about might be responsible for what you have told us?

Nadel: Certainly one does not need substantial numbers of glands to have an electrical potential difference (p.d.) or short-circuit current (I_{SC}), since rabbits (a species with few glands) have p.d. and I_{SC} values similar to dogs.

Jeffery: You need a little histology after your experiment to see what you have actually been looking at.

Nadel: We have studied anatomical sections of the airways in our preparations. The surface layer will be difficult to dissect away from all glandular tissue. I believe that dissecting the gland away from the duct will be easier. If the gland can be removed without contaminating surface cells, we will be able to study isolated cell function. In addition, our approach *in vivo* is to look at the subunit of the gland and gland duct system with micropipettes.

Silberberg: Are the cilia still beating?

Nadel: Yes.

Silberberg: Then why isn't there transport when you put powder on the surface?

Nadel: The purpose of the tantalum is to bind the surface, so we 'pack' the surface with particles.

Donald: When you stimulate with acetylcholine, are there hillocks of mucus from the gland?

Nadel: The mucus emanates from the gland duct openings.

Donald: So why do you have to dust if you see it come up?

Nadel: We now have three methods available for identifying the duct opening. One is to use the tantalum technique; the second is to put in Neutral red, a vital dye that stains the ducts; and the third is to replace the Krebs–Henseleit solution with a fluorocarbon that has a different refractive index so that we can see the secretions directly.

Guz: The extraordinarily small coefficient of variation of your potential difference is impressive. Can you remind us of Ussing's classical preparation and tell us what there is in the toad bladder besides the epithelium, and what sort of coefficient of variation do you find with the p.d.?

Nadel: The coefficient of variation varies from tissue to tissue and depends, for example, on the thickness of the membrane and how rigorously the oxygenation and temperature are maintained.

Guz: Was there much submucosa in the toad bladder?

Nadel: How many cells thick is the toad bladder?

Jeffery: The layers are quite thick and there are about 10 cell layers. The toad bladder is quite elastic and there is a transitional epithelium so it is rather different from the system in the respiratory tract.

Nadel: Very few of the systems studied are single cell systems. Other techniques are required to identify the exact functions of specific subunits and cells. For example our tantalum and micropuncture studies indicate that most of the fluid secreted during stimulation of the vagus is derived from glands.

Godfrey: Could this p.d. be picked up by a suitable electrodc passed into the bronchial tree via a fibre-optic bronchoscope?

Nadel: No, because if you do that you have to flood the airway.

Godfrey: Transmucosal potential differences have been measured successfully in the stomach and rectum; you might add support to your concept of ion-exchange pump dysfunction by measuring potentials in the bronchi.

Nadel: The gut is normally filled with liquid. The lung is normally filled with air. This difference makes *in vivo* measurement of p.d. difficult in humans.

Cumming: I was interested in your hypothesis that ion pump failure might explain some of the problems in cystic fibrosis. In some of our experiments (to be published) we have shown that in the normal human there is a flux of water and heat from the upper airways during inspiration and expiration which extends down five or six orders of bronchi. If the amount of water available is diminished the flux may be altered and therefore the flux in people with cystic fibrosis would be different from the flux in normal humans. Our measurements show no difference whatever but there still may be enough water available from a defective ion pump.

Nadel: This gives me the opportunity to comment on certain implications of drugs. For example, if furosemide were given to a patient with chronic lung disease, what would it do to mucociliary clearance? That is something that can be studied. Secondly, there is the question of the availability of these various 'pumps' and glands and subunits to the drugs that we use. Terbutaline put into the airway lumen may have little or no effect on ion transport compared to the effect when it is given intravenously. Similarly, what are the implications of delivering water aerosol into the airway versus intravenous fluids?

J. G. Jones: In the clinical description of mucoviscidosis the cutaneous loss of sodium is striking and very large, but it seems to be inappropriate to the water loss in that the water loss seems to be normal. Is this also true of the internal membranes or is this peculiar to skin? Does your work explain the observations of cutaneous sodium loss and possible mechanisms inside mucous glands in mucoviscidosis?

Davis: The absorption of electrolytes and water in sweat gland ducts produces a hypotonic secretion. Mangos (1973) found that if sweat from patients with cystic fibrosis was placed in normal glands *in vitro* it inhibited sodium reabsorption and was excreted with increased salinity. The control of secretion in the airway glands is probably different since most mucous secretions in cystic fibrosis are hypertonic (Dearborn 1976).

Nadel: There is clearly a difference in the ability to concentrate sweat; this is an active transport process and involves the pump in the sweat gland.

J. G. Jones: So sweat is related to the problem?

Nadel: We suggest that ion transport may be defective in cystic fibrosis and that this defect prevents adequate production of the sol layer in the airway lumen, so preventing normal ciliary motion and clearance. The chloride pump in the airway is not surprising: these cells derive from the primitive foregut, a locus known for the presence of chloride pumps.

Guz: I was going to raise the question of the massive use of furosemide in clinical medicine and whether it does any harm or good. Have you tried to see whether furosemide in doses that almost completely block renal tubular absorption affect the 'dryness' of the airway? Could one do that in animals by using Dr Cumming's sampling system with a mass spectrometer probe for H_2O vapour?

Nadel: What you can do is to find out whether, in any circumstances of health or disease, furosemide impairs clearance.

Godfrey: As a physician I have never heard a patient complain of difficulties with sputum, and there are plenty of patients being treated with furosemide.

Nadel: I believe the problem needs to be studied in a controlled fashion.

Cumming: In two or three patients with chronic bronchitis who were being treated with furosemide because of dependent oedema from their lung disease, the flux of water in the upper airways was no different from normal. But this was a small series and it may not be relevant.

Nadel: We are now talking about the difference between the vapour phase and the liquid phase in the airway.

Proctor: I believe that there is a wide range in these functions in both experimental animals and in man, and I will say something about that later (p. 226). A good way to test this question of furosemide would be in something like our dog preparation, where we are collecting secretions at the same time as we measure clearance. We can look for clearance of surface particles as well as clearance of periciliary fluid. I suspect we could detect a change if furosemide resulted in a change in airway secretions. When I get home we shall try it.

Richardson: Dr Nadel, you speculated that the hypertrophy of the mucous gland in bronchitis may be due to an increased activity of secretomotor nerves. Brody *et al.* (1972) found that when they denervated one lung of a dog, the mucous glands on the denervated side atrophied. That lends some support to your speculation. It is not very surprising if the muscle hypertrophies in asthmatics more than in bronchitics and if there is more hypertrophy of the mucous glands in bronchitics than in asthmatics, because the nerves controlling the glands seem to be quite distinct from those controlling bronchial muscles. Widdicombe (1966) described two sets of nerves to the airways, group III which probably innervate bronchial glands and group I which constrict bronchial muscles. They seemed to be controlled independently.

Widdicombe: That the so-called group III nerves were going to the glands was an assumption based mainly on elimination of other possibilities. We found these nerves in both the sympathetic and the parasympathetic nervous systems, so the idea that there may be a double innervation is entirely consistent with these results (Widdicombe 1966).

Nadel: Which sensory stimuli are most potent in the bronchosecretory system?

Richardson: One that causes tracheal secretion in the cat is stimulation of the nasopharynx. At the same time as causing bronchial secretion (mainly through the parasympathetic nervous system) it will switch off the parasympathetic nervous system to the bronchial muscle, so when the nasopharynx is rubbed the bronchi dilate because of a lessening of the parasympathetic nerve tone (Tomori & Widdicombe 1969). At the same time there will be tracheal secretion from increased parasympathetic activity, probably in the group III nerves (Phipps & Richardson 1976).

Nadel: Isn't that a sympathetic nervous response?

Richardson: Probably part of it is sympathetic but the major part is parasympathetic. Most of the effect disappears if the vagus nerves are cut.

Widdicombe: Another example is that an increase in blood pressure, probably working through the carotid sinuses, will cause both a reflex bronchodilatation and a reflex increase in activity in secretomotor fibres simply going to the airways (Nadel & Widdicombe 1962; Salvato 1968). So again there is a difference in the reflex autonomic output with the same afferent input.

Silberberg: Have you combined your two approaches and studied whether secretion occurs when a potential is applied across the mucosa and whether and how an applied external potential influences the secretory process?

Widdicombe: I think you are asking what would happen to mucus secretion if a potential was applied across the epithelium. Tantalum might be a wonderful preparation for testing this because it is a highly conducting medium and lies like a kind of plate-electrode on one side of the airway wall. If you put a potential difference across the epithelium with a tantalum sheet as one electrode would you produce a hillock, Dr Nadel?

Nadel: An interesting idea!

Richardson: Kim Balfre (personal communication) working in my laboratory has been studying the relationship between the potential and secretion of mucin in the chicken trachea. She has found so far that any stimulus which augments mucin secretion also increases the potential across the trachea. However one or two things she has tested increase the p.d. without increasing the mucin secretion, so she would say that the potential doesn't cause the mucin secretion. Whether it causes water secretion is doubtful.

Nadel: The number of cells from which you can choose is limited. I think one of the major questions has to do with regulation of the gland. It is another way of looking at the difference between the gland and all the surface cells.

I am inclined to believe—although no one has proved it yet—that much of the water secretion of the pump occurs outside the glandular secretion, and that is why I was asking about the microvilli. These surface cells themselves, I believe, are reasonable candidates for pumping ions.

Allison: I wouldn't mind betting that the microvilli are good ion pumpers.

References

BRODY, J. S., KLEMPFNER, G., STAUM, M. M., VIDYASAGAR, D., KUHL, D. E. & WALDHAUSEN, J. A. (1972) Mucociliary clearance after lung denervation and bronchial transection. *J. Appl. Physiol. 32*, 160–164

DEARBORN, D. G. (1976) Water and electrolytes of exocrine secretions, in *Cystic Fibrosis: Projections into the Future* (Mangos, J. A. & Talamo, R. C., eds.), p. 179, Stratton Intercontinental Medical Book Corp., New York

MANGOS, J. A. (1973) Microperfusion study of the sweat gland abnormality in cystic fibrosis. *Tex. Rep. Biol. Med. 31*, 651–663

NADEL, J. A. & WIDDICOMBE, J. G. (1962) Effect of changes in blood gas tensions and carotid sinus pressure on tracheal volume and total lung resistance to airflow. *J. Physiol. (Lond.) 163*, 13–33

PHIPPS, R. J. & RICHARDSON, P. S. (1976) The effects of irritation at various levels of the airway upon tracheal mucus secretion in the cat. *J. Physiol. (Lond.) 261*, 563–581

SALVATO, G. (1968) Some histological changes in chronic bronchitis and asthma. *Thorax 23*, 168–172

TOMORI, Z. & WIDDICOMBE, J. G. (1969) Muscular, bronchomotor and cardiovascular reflexes elicited by mechanical stimulation of the respiratory tract. *J. Physiol. (Lond.) 200*, 25–49

WIDDICOMBE, J. G. (1966) Action potentials in parasympathetic and sympathetic efferent fibres to the trachea and lungs of dogs and cats. *J. Physiol. (Lond.) 186*, 56–88

General discussion II

Allison: When we discussed the biochemical control of mucin production we were dealing with short-term events. Longer-term events—over a period of days or longer—were alluded to but I understand that there is no information at the biochemical level about long-term changes in the quantity and quality of mucin produced. There is morphological evidence of the increase in the number of mucus-secreting cells, but nothing on the biochemistry. Is that a fair statement?

Phelps: I would say so. My only fear is of stresses arising if we go much beyond the 6 hours which has been the absolute maximum running time for our system.

Allison: I wasn't suggesting that experimental approach but the question is interesting. If the stimulus were applied *in vivo* for a relatively long time one could look at the associated biochemistry and find out whether there were differences in enzyme levels and so on.

Phelps: Yes, I think that is a good idea.

Nadel: I have suggested that chronic vagal reflux overstimulation of glandular secretion (secondary to epithelial damage in the airway) may be the cause of glandular hypertrophy in disease. We are attempting to show that chronic vagal stimulation causes gland hypertrophy.

Reid: Isn't this the sort of classical experiment that was done some decades ago—stimulating, chronically, nerves to salivary glands by filing down the teeth and watching the salivary glands hypertrophy?

Nadel: You are correct! Salivary gland hypertrophy has been shown after vagal reflux stimulation. It was from this model that I got the idea that airway gland hypertrophy could be vagal in origin. Two 'models' of gland hypertrophy used in your laboratory involve cigarette smoke and sulphur dioxide. We have shown that the bronchomotor responses to these stimuli result from vagal reflexes (Nadel & Widdicombe 1963). Similarly, I now propose that the gland hypertrophy is also due to reflex cholinergic stimulation.

Allison: Considering the control of enzyme activity, the effects of changes in nucleotide composition were revealing but there is little information about changes in the nucleotide concentrations in intact cells.

Phelps: We have tried but it is almost impossible to rock the nucleotide sugar pool. So there is a very high level of homeostasis.

Allison: It is tightly controlled. It might be possible to determine NAD/NADH levels in intact cells by spectrophotometry.

Phelps: I think one could make an approximation just from the lactate: pyruvate levels. But the point is that, at the substrate level, the fluxes are so small compared with what is going on in the catabolic nature of things that we are always looking at a 1% margin of economic effort whilst 99% is going to the profit of glycolysis and the energy production inherent in that.

Allison: So the concentration of enzymes concerned with mucin synthesis is rather small compared with the concentration of those catalysing glycolysis, and the activities of the former are further restricted by nucleotide levels. Here it is doubtful whether greatly increased enzyme levels would be needed to step up mucin synthesis, although it would be interesting to know whether these can be induced by chronic stimulation.

Nadel: I have a minor point which has to do with 5HT. In dogs, when the vagus nerves are cut and stimulated there is a potent interaction between 5HT and vagal stimulation. Low concentrations of 5HT which have no effect on the muscle itself markedly increase the cholinergic effect on the contraction of the muscle induced by low levels of vagal stimulation. Thus, 5HT released by cells could 'modulate' vagal effects (Hahn *et al.* 1976).

Richardson: I didn't know that, but I shall try it.

Douglas: Is the cholinergic stimulation through the nerves or by applied acetylcholine?

Nadel: The interaction with 5HT exists in the absence of central connections, but one must stimulate the nerves. If acetylcholine is put into the airway the interaction with 5HT does not occur. If you put in histamine rather than 5HT you do not get the interaction. It is quite specific to 5HT; the exact site in the efferent vagal system is not known.

Widdicombe: Should we add a 12th epithelial cell to Dr Jeffery's list—the mast cell, which has been described in the epithelium, certainly for human asthmatics and for some non-asthmatic animals? Would Dr Jeffery or Dr Thurlbeck like to comment on whether epithelial mast cells might be important in releasing mediators which in turn will affect these mucus-secreting mechanisms?

Thurlbeck: Guerzon *et al.* (1977) certainly think it is important and they have recently completed a quantitative survey of mast cells in the monkey, *Macaca fasicularis*. They found a small but significant number of mast cells in the epithelium. This is of considerable importance because it looks as though the initial reaction may be mediated at the surface of the epithelium rather than the submucosa. Their idea is that the release of mediators may initiate the attack of asthma and then make the epithelium permeable to antigens, and that the initial reaction would then be amplified. Mast cells are abundant in the airways of man and guinea pig (Connell 1971; Trotter & Orr 1973).

Widdicombe: We have looked for mast cells in guinea-pig epithelium, but they are very infrequent.

Thurlbeck: They are more commonly found in the submucosa than outside the wall, or in the epithelium.

Proctor: We find mast cells in the surface fluid in our dog preparation and also in human nasal secretions, and they seem to be viable and functional.

Godfrey: I think it is true that they have been seen actually lying in the epithelial layer in asthmatics who have died in attacks.

Widdicombe: Does anybody know whether slow-reacting substance A (SRS-A) has an action on mucus secretion? This mediator would be released when mast cells break down.

Guz: We have heard a lot about glands being stimulated to enlarge by chronic cholinergic mechanisms. Does anyone know anything about the glands and their secretion in a disease like acromegaly where, at least in the skin, there are very large sweat glands which produce a lot of sweat? Do we know whether the glands are very large in the airways of acromegalics and whether they secrete a lot? That would be a system without involvement of nerves. If we don't know the answer, presumably if one gave growth hormone to newborn animals one could create the appropriate experimental situation.

Reid: Brody has studied animals treated with excessive amounts of growth hormone (Brody *et al.* 1976). But nobody has looked at the mucus glands; obviously it could be studied.

Thurlbeck: I am surprised that people accept John Widdicombe's statement, or implied statement, that we know very precisely the cholinergic distribution of nerves within the human lung. It appears that the bronchial mucous glands are primarily served by the submucous plexus, which in turn comes primarily from the plexus around the bronchial arteries. This plexus in turn comes primarily from the cholinergic peribronchial plexus which is also the source of the nerves of the airway muscle. There is a complex electrical connection between the glands and the bronchial muscle. The major difference between the gland and muscle may be the inhibitory nervous system. J. B. Richardson (Richardson & Bouchard 1975; Richardson & Beland 1976) has shown that the inhibitory nervous system to the smooth muscle of the lung is not the adrenergic nervous system; it is Burnstock's non-adrenergic inhibitory nervous system or 'purinergic' system. Puig *et al.* (1977) have shown that there may be inhibitory opiate receptors in the gut. Conceivably, endorphins may be mediators in the gut and thus airways as well. There are a lot of interesting implications in the management of asthma if this is true.

Widdicombe: Let me put the record straight. What I said was that there has been a fair amount of work studying the patterns of activity in nerves going into the lungs, but where the nerves end up nobody knows.

Davis: I have a comment about the interpretation of experiments in which a radioactive precursor is incorporated into mucin in a cell, and is used to measure the rate of mucin secretion. Since there is a store of mucins in the tissue, the radioactive precursor may not be distributed among all the stored mucins during baseline measurements. The rate at which the precursor is taken up by the mucins may be different during the control and the experimental periods. Thus, varying amounts of radiolabel can be excreted without any change in the rate of mucus secretion. If the tissue was stimulated maximally in the presence of the precursor the unlabelled stored mucus could be expelled before the baseline secretion rate was measured. It is also important to determine the effect of the experimental conditions on the incorporation of the precursor into the mucin.

Phelps: I support that. We have had examples here of people who have used, and clearly had to use, glucose as a label instead of glucosamine and that is a perfect example of somebody penalizing himself, unless there is a trivial reason why glucosamine didn't get into the system. The difference in the selectivity of incorporation of glucosamine over something like glucose should be very great.

Jeffery: In our experiments the concentration of the glucosamine given was higher than that of the glucose, yet glucosamine was not taken up though we had good uptake of glucose. I think perhaps we should repeat the experiments.

Phelps: The transport systems are identical.

Jeffery: I agree. I was most surprised to find that glucosamine wasn't a good marker for glycoprotein.

Richardson: You said that there were many different sorts of glucosamine. Perhaps we were just using the wrong sort (D-glucosamine).

Phelps: That is possible. There might be a case for clever exploitation of other materials, for instance 2-deoxyglucose. It should not be taken up into the glycogen side but might bamboozle the systems which lead to polymer production or perturb the pool of precursors in some way. Or there are 6-fluoroglucose and *N*-fluoracetamidoglucosamines. What we really need is a specific additive which would find universal favour in not being subject to the heavy 'metabolic' dilution from which glucose suffers but which is specifically incorporated into the polymers that we are interested in.

Reid: With glucose, isn't it possible to trace it into a number of other amino sugars and thus get a higher concentration than with glucosamine? We can get glucosamine to go into our organ culture system but on the whole we get higher concentrations of glucose.

Phelps: I think there is both a kinetic and a partitioning answer to your question. Kinetically, if the fluxes are as they have been shown, so little is going into polymer and so much into other things that one really is penalizing oneself by using glucose as a specific label to look at the pathway of synthesis. On the other hand, if one is interested in the partition of label and where it is going at various times under different stimuli, that is different.

Allison: There seems to be a message from the biochemists to the histochemists as to the most appropriate label. In the organ culture system one could simply raise the specific activity of the label but that might be more difficult to achieve *in vivo*.

References

BRODY, J. S., MANALO, A., KAGAN, H. & GONNERMAN, W. A. (1976) Lysil oxidase: regional concentration during normal and hypoxia induced lung growth. *Am. Rev. Respir. Dis. 113*, 261

CONNELL, J. T. (1971) Asthmatic deaths: role of the mast cell. *J. Am. Med. Assoc. 215*, 769

GUERZON, G., PARE, P. D. & HOGG, J. C. (1977) The distribution of mast cells and eosinophils in monkey lungs. *Clin. Res. 24*, 691

HAHN, H. L., GRAF, P. D. & NADEL, J. A. (1976) Serotonin-induced bronchoconstriction in dogs: interaction with the cholinergic nervous system. *Clin. Res. 24*, 465A

NADEL, J. A. & WIDDICOMBE, J. G. (1963) Reflex control of airway size. *Ann. N.Y. Acad. Sci. 109*, 712–722

PUIG, M. M., GASCON, T., CRAVISCO, G. L. & MUSACCHIO, J. M. (1977) Endogenous opiate receptor ligand: electrically induced release in the guinea pig ileum. *Science (Wash. D.C.) 195*, 419–420

RICHARDSON, J. B. & BELAND, J. (1976) Demonstration of non-adrenergic inhibitor system in human airways. *J. Appl. Physiol. 41*, 764

RICHARDSON, J. B. & BOUCHARD, T. (1975) Demonstration of the non-adrenergic inhibitory system in the trachea of guinea pigs. *J. Allergy Clin. Immunol. 56*, 473

TROTTER, C. M. & ORR, T. S. C. (1973) A fine structure study of some cellular components of allergic reaction. *Clin. Allergy 3*, 411

Chemical aspects of tracheal glycoproteins

P. W. KENT

Glycoprotein Research Unit, Durham University

Abstract The chemical characteristics of tracheal mucus obtained directly from the epithelial surface of the trachea indicate that the mucus from each animal source consists of a group of sulphated sialic acid-containing glycoproteins. Fractionation of the native glycoprotein from the cat by gel chromatography in the presence of urea and dithiothreitol suggests a value of about 3×10^6 for the molecular weights. The chief monosaccharide constituents are *N*-acetylneuraminic acid, *N*-acetylglucosamine, *N*-acetylgalactosamine, fucose and galactose. In the goose tracheal mucin, mannose is present (serum proteins being absent).

Doubly labelled cat mucus, obtained by giving $Na_2{}^{35}SO_4$ and [^{3}H]glucose simultaneously into the lumen of the trachea, is massively released by parasympathetic agents, e.g. pilocarpine. The resulting mucus has a high content of ^{35}S and is derived largely from submucosal gland cells. Subsequent exposure to an irritant, ammonia, releases a low sulphation fraction, highly labelled with ^{3}H, arising from goblet cells. Evidence supports the view that the overall mucus is composed of mixed secretions, chemically distinct, from different cellular synthesizing sites. Differential nervous stimulation of the various sites may cause far-reaching changes in the chemical and physical properties of the mucus by selective action on the secretion of one or more of the contributing glycoproteins.

In the trachea, mucus constitutes a viscous mobile barrier protecting the ciliated surface from dust, bacteria and viruses. It also provides the surface with an appropriately buffered, aqueous micro-environment, affording it some protection against chemical irritants. In each individual, mucus, both in 'insoluble' and soluble forms, appears to comprise a series of glycoproteins present in differing amounts which interact to form the characteristic highly viscous gross secretion. Evidence has been obtained, supplementary to the histological results, that different contributing cells synthesize distinctive glycoproteins, and that these cells may be under separate nervous control. In these terms, investigations have been concerned with the basis of the changes in the chemical composition of tracheal mucus.

Early investigations of the chemical composition of tracheal mucus preparations from a variety of sources showed that these were composed chiefly of glycoproteins in which *N*-acetylglucosamine, *N*-acetylgalactosamine, fucose and galactose (mannose) accounted for the neutral hexose constituents. The characteristic acidic property of mucus arose from the presence of sialic acid, particularly *N*-acetylneuraminic acid in humans, but with *N*-glycolyl- and other *O*-acetylated sialic acids in other mammals. Ester sulphate residues, usually between 2 and 3%, also contributed to the acidic function. Close investigation, however, has been made more difficult because of the high viscosity of the material which makes it unsuitable for most fractionation techniques, and because of the difficulty of obtaining fractions sufficiently large for detailed analysis. Frequently, tracheal mucus has been obtained from sputum and it became increasingly apparent that such material was subject to gross contamination by saliva and secretions of the upper airways as well as by bacteria and their products. The presence of bacterial polysaccharides and DNA is not unusual.

Successful isolation of bronchial glycoproteins has been achieved by fractionation after reduction or proteolysis of the fibrillar network in sputum (Biserte *et al.* 1963; Havez *et al.* 1967). In a recent study, Roussel *et al.* (1972, 1975) have obtained by these means a series of glycoproteins from the sputum of a child suffering from cystic fibrosis. The principal constituent was a sulphated glycoprotein (2.1% ester sulphate) possessing blood group H activity. A range of oligosaccharide side chains composed of fucose (16.6%), galactose (29.0%), *N*-acetylglucosamine (24.6%), *N*-acetylgalactosamine (8.9%) and *N*-acetylneuraminic acid (3.4%) were present. These could be cleaved from the peptide by sodium hydroxide and the presence of sodium borohydride was consistent with *O*-seryl and *O*-threonyl linkages existing between the peptide and the carbohydrate. The amino acid composition was typical of mammalian glycoproteins, being rich in threonine, serine, proline, alanine and glycine. The cysteine and aromatic amino acid contents were low. Some 14 different oligosaccharides were separated and analysed, four of which were non-sulphated.

Overall, the chain length of these oligosaccharide side chains ranged from five to twenty monosaccharide residues. It is assumed that these different chains were associated with a single type of glycoprotein and thus illustrate the extensive variations in chemical structure which can occur. Though the initial glycoprotein fraction possessed some evidence of purity, it is clear that its carbohydrate chains have a wide heterogeneity at least with regard to acidity and molecular size.

High molecular weight glycoproteins have been obtained by fractionation of sputum of patients suffering from bronchorrhoea (Roberts 1974). The carbohydrate content (58% to 69%) was composed of fucose, galactose, glucosamine, galactosamine and *N*-acetylneuraminic acid and was present as *O*-glycosidic side chains of the protein core. As in the case of cystic sputum, sulphate ester groups and sialic acid residues were present together in most chains. Separate fuco-, sialo- and sulpho-glycoproteins were not obtained. The larger oligosaccharides appear to have the greater sulphate content, whereas the sialic acid content was highest in the smaller oligosaccharides.

Extensive fractionation analyses have been made in a number of laboratories of human tracheal glycoproteins obtained from other sources than sputum, e.g. by bronchoscopy (Potter *et al.* 1963; Chernick & Barbero 1959, 1963). While these methods obviate some sources of contamination, the effects of pathological agents present in the trachea remain (Potter *et al.* 1963).

Recent investigations (E. A. Davidson, personal communication 1977) have been made of human lung glycoproteins obtained from bronchial washings. The major component was a glycoprotein fraction separable by chromatography on Sephadex 4B with a molecular weight of the order of 2.5×10^6, though higher aggregates may also have been present. The materials appear not to be dissociated into subunits by dithiothreitol. As Roussel *et al.* (1975) found, the sugar constituents were galactose, *N*-acetylglucosamine, *N*-acetylgalactosamine, fucose and *N*-acetylneuraminic acid (in the ratio 3:2:1:3:1 respectively). Again the carbohydrate peptide linkage was of the *O*-glycosidic type through seryl and threonyl residues, cleaved by alkaline borohydride. A range of oligosaccharides was found, from the disaccharide (Gal-GalNAcitol) to octa- and nonasaccharides. It will be of much interest to know about the distribution of sialic acids among these various side chains and whether ester sulphate groups are also involved.

It is apparent that despite the fact that these glycoproteins behave as single components on sedimentation and gel fractionation, a high degree of internal inhomogeneity nevertheless persists. It is a matter for speculation and for further investigation whether the oligosaccharide variants are attached as a group to a single peptide or whether several glycoproteins are present, each with its own distinctive pattern of oligosaccharide structure. The origins of microheterogeneity (Gottschalk 1969) have been frequently considered in terms of variations of specificity, rates and distributions of enzymes within a single type of glycoprotein-synthesizing cell. When the biosynthetic system has been a cultured cell line or bacterial culture, this hypothesis may be valid, though it cannot be held with certainty, since carbohydrate synthetic activity may well be related to cell age (passage number) (Mora 1973). The possibility has to be envisaged that variations in glycoprotein structures may reflect enzymic differences between individual cells.

Epithelial tissues, including those of mammalian trachea, are furnished with a series of glycoprotein-synthesizing cells which have been well identified histologically and by radioautography. In human, cat, and other trachea, these include goblet cells and subepithelial glands, both serous and mucous. Elsewhere, as for example in the goose (Phipps *et al.* 1977), only goblet cells are present, as is discussed by Dr Jeffery (this volume, pp. 5–20). An abundance of histological and radiographical evidence, to which Professor Lynne Reid (this volume, pp. 297–304) has contributed notably, had correlated glycoprotein biosynthesis in these various biosynthetic sites with the formation of mucin components. The evidence points strongly to biochemical specialization at these sites, each seeming capable of producing structurally distinctive glycoproteins (Lamb 1975). The proportion of the various glycoprotein-synthesizing cells is not constant but is found to vary significantly with age, as well as in response to irritants and to pathogenic viruses (Falk *et al.* 1963). It is important to explore in further detail the extent to which individual biosynthetic sites contribute to the chemistry and to the physical properties as well as to the rate of production of the overall mucus.

STIMULATION OF GLYCOPROTEIN SECRETION IN THE TRACHEA

In 1962, Dische *et al.* observed that in series of glycoprotein preparations the sialic acid content varied inversely with the fucose content. In particular, this was demonstrated in samples from urine, duodenal mucus and bovine cervical mucus. It was further shown (Dische 1963) that the sialic acid/fucose ratio of glycoproteins of the submaxillary gland was decreased on electrical stimulation of the parasympathetic nerve chorda tympani or after intravenous injection of pilocarpine. Further investigations (Winzler 1973; Lombart & Winzler 1974) of that organ showed that the ester sulphate content of the mucin was also sensitive to stimulation. No differences were detected in the amino acid composition of glycoproteins isolated from the gland after electrical stimulation or after early and late pilocarpine administration. Alkaline borohydride reduction of the normal mucus gave two identifiable tetrasaccharides; one contained sialic acid and the other a sulphate ester (attached to $C_{(3)}$ of *N*-acetylglucosamine), as mentioned by Professor Phelps (Phelps & Stevens, this volume, pp. 91–107).

An interpretation of these findings has been made assuming homocellular

TABLE 1

Carbohydrate composition of principal tracheal glycoproteins (fractionated on DEAE-Cellulose DE-52)

	Rabbit[a]		*Dog*[a]	*Cat*[b]	*Goose*[b]
	Soluble	*Insoluble*	*Soluble*	*Soluble*	*Soluble*
Fucose	0.37	0.23	0.84	0.65	1.56
Galactose	1.03	0.92	1.60	1.30	1.00
N-Acetylglucosamine	1.00	1.00	1.00	1.00	1.00
N-Acetylgalactosamine	1.83	1.00	0.74	1.25	0.94
Sialic acid[c]	0.93	0.77	0.28	0.36	0.40
Sulphate	++	++	++	++	++

[a] from organ culture [b] from tracheal perfusion [c] as *N*-acetylneuraminic acid

secretions, i.e. secretions arising from a population of identical cells acting by closely similar mechanisms. The stimulating agents are thus envisaged as influencing synthetic enzyme steps or enzyme organization.

Glycoprotein secretion in the respiratory tract (as in the digestive tract) has long been known to respond to parasympathomimetic and sympathetic agents. The trachea is a particularly favourable organ in which to trace the nervous supply and from which to isolate epithelial glycoprotein specimens. Two principal techniques have been employed, trachea perfusion in acute experiments in cats (Gallagher *et al.* 1975) and in geese (Phipps *et al.* 1977) and tracheal organ cultures (Gallagher & Kent 1975; Ellis & Stahl 1973). The carbohydrate composition of a number of epithelial glycoproteins is shown in Table 1. In the cat, tracheal glycoproteins are synthesized by goblet cells and by submucosal glands (both serous and mucous) and experiments were designed to test the hypothesis that these sites can be separately stimulated with a consequent change in their contribution to the final mucus and thus to its analytical composition. This process may be designated heterocellular mucus secretion.

Tracheal mucus was doubly labelled in cat experiments by introduction of [^{35}S]sulphate and D-[1-^{3}H]glucose into the lumen. After one hour, the precursors were washed out and mucus was collected at intervals, using the system described by Richardson *et al.* (this volume, pp. 111–126). Parasympathetic stimulation was invoked by giving pilocarpine (6.5 μg/ml) into the tracheal lumen for four separate periods of 15 min. After an interval of 30 min, four further exposures to pilocarpine were given. Then after a further interval of 15 min, two exposures, each of 15 min, were given to ammonia vapour

(1:100) in air. After each exposure to stimulant, the secreted mucus was washed out of the trachea and fractionated, and the ^{35}S and ^{3}H levels were determined (Gallagher *et al.* 1977).

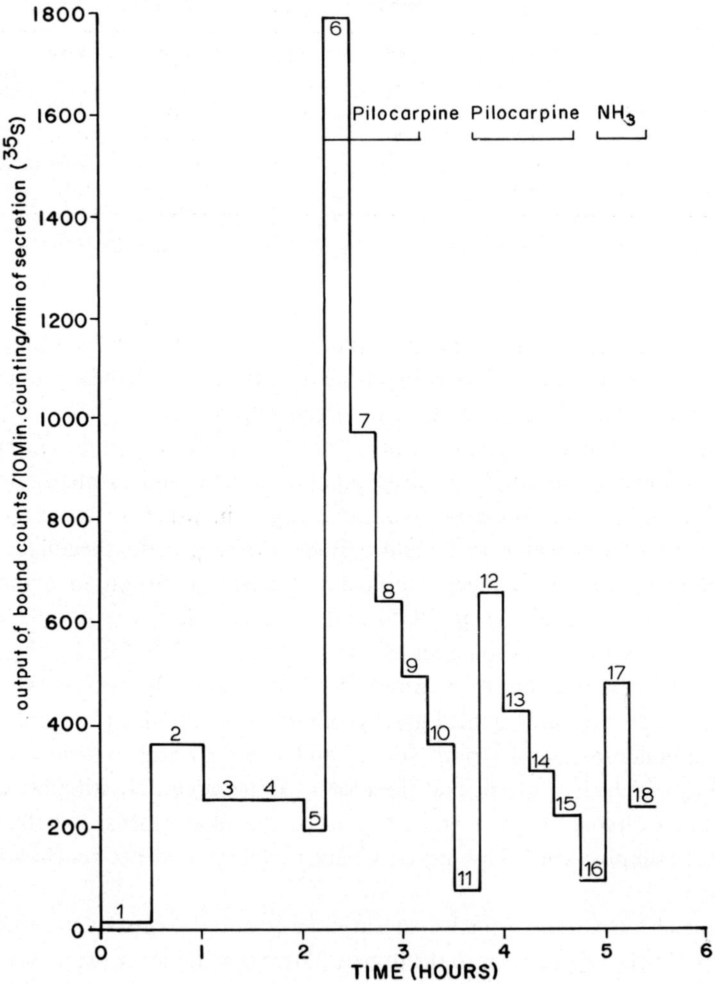

FIGS. 1 and 2. The histograms show the level of bound radioactivity from [^{35}S]sulphate and [^{3}H]glucose in secreted cat tracheal mucins. The first five samples collected over the first 2.25 h (four 30-minute collections and one of 15 minutes) were pooled to give the control (nos. 1–5) samples with which subsequent secretions evoked by pilocarpine and ammonia are compared. Samples were usually pooled as follows: controls (nos. 1–5), pilocarpine (no. 6), pilocarpine (nos. 7, 8 and 9), pilocarpine (nos. 12–15), controls (nos. 10, 11 and 16) and ammonia (nos. 17 and 18).

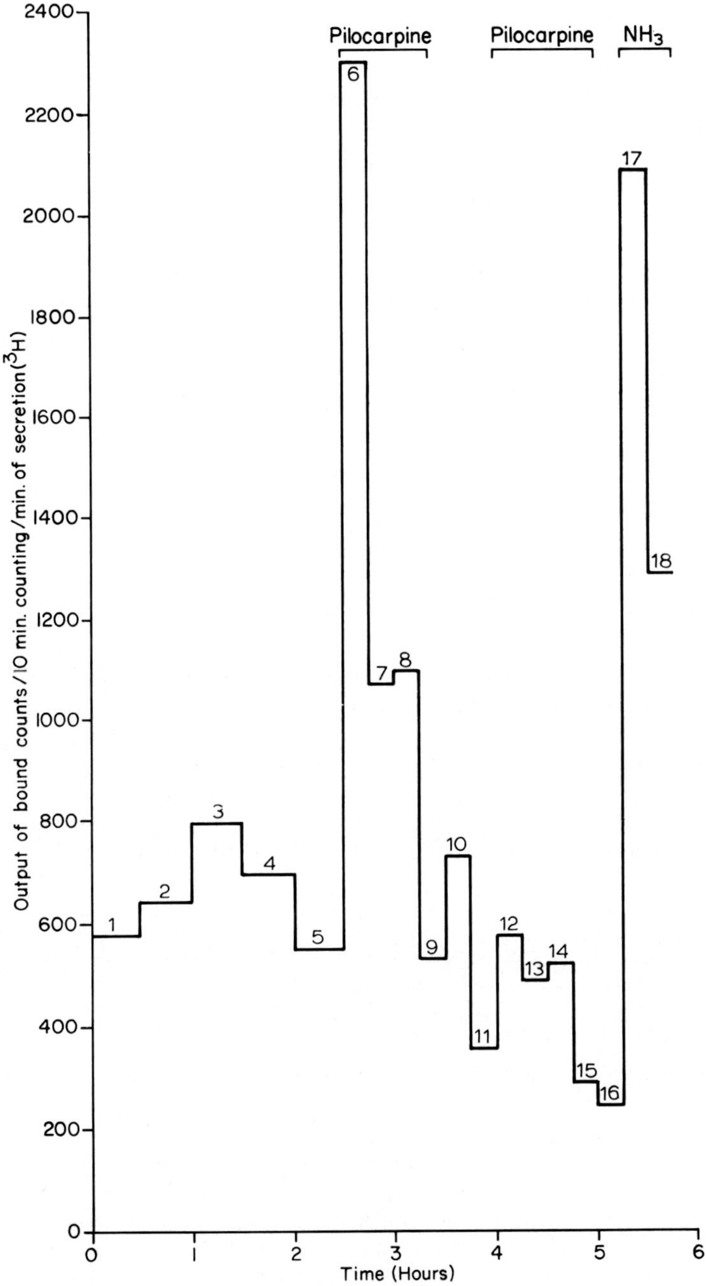
Pilocarpine
Pilocarpine
NH_3
Output of bound counts/10 min. counting/min. of secretion (^3H)
Time (Hours)
0
200
400
600
800
1000
1200
1400
1600
1800
2000
2200
2400
1
2
3
4
5
6
7
8
9
10
11
12
13
14
15
16
17
18

FIG. 2

FRACTIONATION AND ANALYSIS OF GLYCOPROTEINS FORMED UNDER STIMULATED SECRETION

Two modified chromatographic techniques have been developed to fractionate native viscous mucus. In the first method, labelled mucins were fractionated on a column of Sepharose CL-4B using a dissociating sodium phosphate buffer system (10 mM, pH 7.2) containing 6M-urea and dithiothreitol (10 mM). In the second method, native samples were fractionated by ion-exchange chromatography on DEAE-cellulose (DEAE-DE52) using a starting buffer of sodium phosphate (10 mM, pH 7.2), 6M-urea and 10 mM-sodium chloride. A linear sodium chloride gradient, 10 mM to 0.4 M, was then applied in buffer–urea.

After administration of $Na_2{}^{35}SO_4$ and D-[1-^{3}H]glucose into the lumen of the cat trachea, the mucus became labelled with both isotopes at a steady rate within the first two hours (Fig. 1, Fig. 2—samples 1 to 5). The first pilocarpine exposure caused the usual massive and immediate release of mucus labelled both with ^{35}S (Fig. 1, sample 6) and ^{3}H (Fig. 2, sample 6). Subsequent stimulations with pilocarpine also promoted release of mucus but with decreasing amounts of labels (Figs. 1 and 2). Between pilocarpine stimulation the labelling of mucus returned to the control value. In contrast, ammonia vapour given after secretion appeared to have become exhausted and gave a large release of ^{3}H-labelled glycoprotein (Fig. 1, Fig. 2, sample 17). The

TABLE 2

Mean percentage changes (%) in output of mucin-bound ^{35}S- and ^{3}H-radioactivity

	1st pilocarpine run (Sample 6)		*2nd pilocarpine run (Sample 12)*		*NH_3 vapour (Sample 17)*	
	^{35}S	*^3H*	*^{35}S*	*^3H*	*^{35}S*	*^3H*
%	+583	+144	+235	+86	+415	+1009
± S.E. (%)	117	35	104	32	130	244
n	7	7	7	7	7	7
P	0.005	0.005	0.005	0.005	0.005	0.005

The above changes refer to a comparison of the radioactivity in the 15-min control sample taken immediately before application of either pilocarpine or ammonia, and the first 15-min collection of mucus after the stimulus was given. For example, in the column headed '1st pilocarpine run' the data refer to a comparison of radioactivity in sample no. 6 – the first pilocarpine sample – with that in sample no. 5, the last control sample taken before administering the pilocarpine (see also Figs. 1 and 2).

TABLE 3

Ratio of ^{35}S-sulphate- and ^{3}H-glucose-derived radioactivity in cat tracheal mucins before and after administration of irritants

Irritant	*Collection*	*Ratio ^{3}H:^{35}S*
Controls	(1–5)	6.23
Pilocarpine	(6)	2.07
Pilocarpine	(7)	3.19
Pilocarpine	(8, 9)	3.73
Pilocarpine	(12–15)	4.46
Controls	(10. 11. 16)	5.03
Ammonia	(17, 18)	11.11

Separate mucin collections were pooled as indicated. Controls 1–5 represent the first five collections of radioactive mucin before addition of pilocarpine. Three fractions, Collections 7, (8 + 9) and (12 to 15) were examined after pilocarpine treatment. Controls nos. 10, 11 and 16 represent mucin samples taken before and after the second phase of pilocarpine stimulation (nos. 12–15). Pooled fraction (17 + 18) was taken after ammonia treatment.

TABLE 4

Comparison of sugars in cat mucins

Molar ratios (GlcNAc = 1)			
Sugar	*Pilocarpine (No. 6)*	*Control (1–5)*	*Ammonia (17–18)*
Fucose	1.51	1.25	0.12
Galactose	1.64	1.45	1.15
N-acetylgalactosamine	0.70	0.80	0.65
N-acetylglucosamine	1.00	1.00	1.00
Sialic acid	0.62	0.55	1.15

The above data were obtained by gas liquid chromatographic analysis of tracheal mucins after fractionation by DEAE-DE52 ion-exchange chromatography.

increases in amounts of radioactivity released into the lumen under these conditions are given in Table 2. The ratios ^{35}S/^{3}H of the labels in the respective fractions suggest that pilocarpine stimulates secretion (or biosynthesis) of the sulphated component(s) while ammonia stimulates preferentially release (or biosynthesis) of the glycoprotein derived from the [^{3}H]glucose (Table 3). It

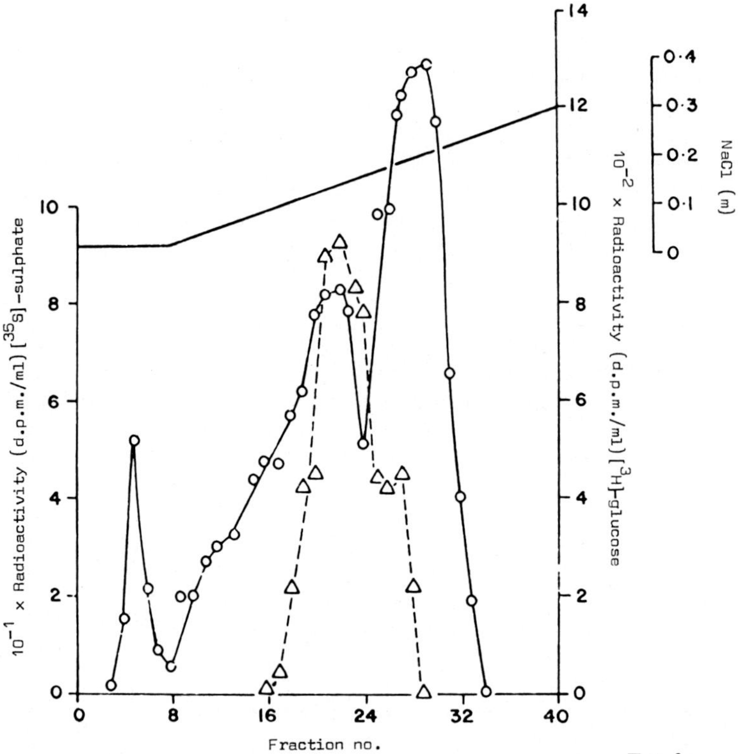

FIG. 3a

FIG. 3. Control mucins (nos. 1–5) (Fig. 3*a*) and the first pilocarpine mucin (no. 6) (Fig. 3*b*) were dialysed against starting buffer (6 M-urea, 10 mM-phosphate, pH 7.2, 10 mM-NaCl) and then applied to the ion-exchange column. The mucins were then eluted by a linear gradient of NaCl from 10 mM → 0.4 M-NaCl. Fractions of 3–4 ml were collected and 200 μl aliquots taken for radioactivity determinations. The flow rate was 6 ml/h. ○——○ = [^{3}H]glucose; △---△ = [^{35}S]sulphate; —— = NaCl.

is necessary to recall that ammonia has toxic properties and in low concentrations may provoke metabolic disturbances.

The question is whether these stimulatory effects are achieved by release of macromolecular material not present normally. Ion-exchange chromatography in the buffer–urea–NaCl system, described above, showed that both control mucin (Fig. 3*a*, samples 1 to 5) and pilocarpine-stimulated mucin (Fig. 3*b*; sample 6) contained a neutral sulphate-free component. The effect of pilocarpine is clearly to increase the sulphate labelling of the main fraction (Fig. 3*b*), while ammonia causes release tentatively from another cellular site of a different

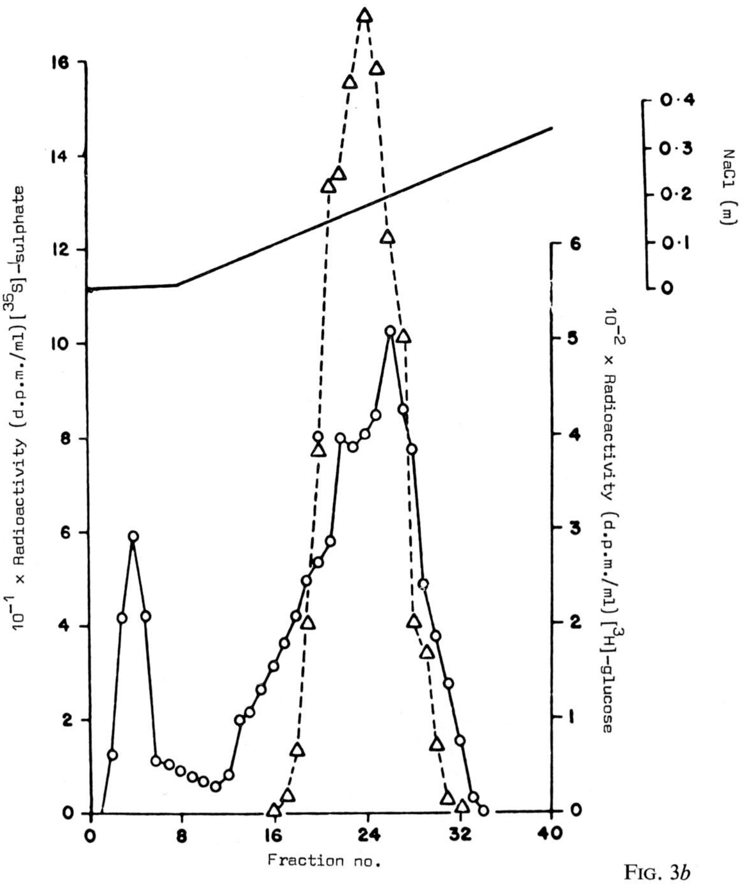

FIG. 3*b*

glycoprotein characteristically highly labelled from [^{3}H]glucose (Fig. 3*a*). Repeated ion-exchange chromatography of the principal labelled peaks (Fig. 4) shows a small but significantly stronger retention of the pilocarpine-stimulated material in comparison with control or ammonia-stimulated mucin. Significant differences exist, especially in the sialic acid content of both mucins (Table 4).

Gel filtration of these control fractions in buffer–urea–dithiothreitol (Fig. 5) indicated that the molecular weight was in excess of 3×10^{6}. All other fractions obtained under conditions of stimulation had similar profiles and as yet no major structural differences have been detected. However, as a function of the molecular size, the $^{35}S/^{3}H$ ratio (Fig. 6) indicates that a higher degree of sulphation is present in the lower molecular weight fractions of the pilocarpine-

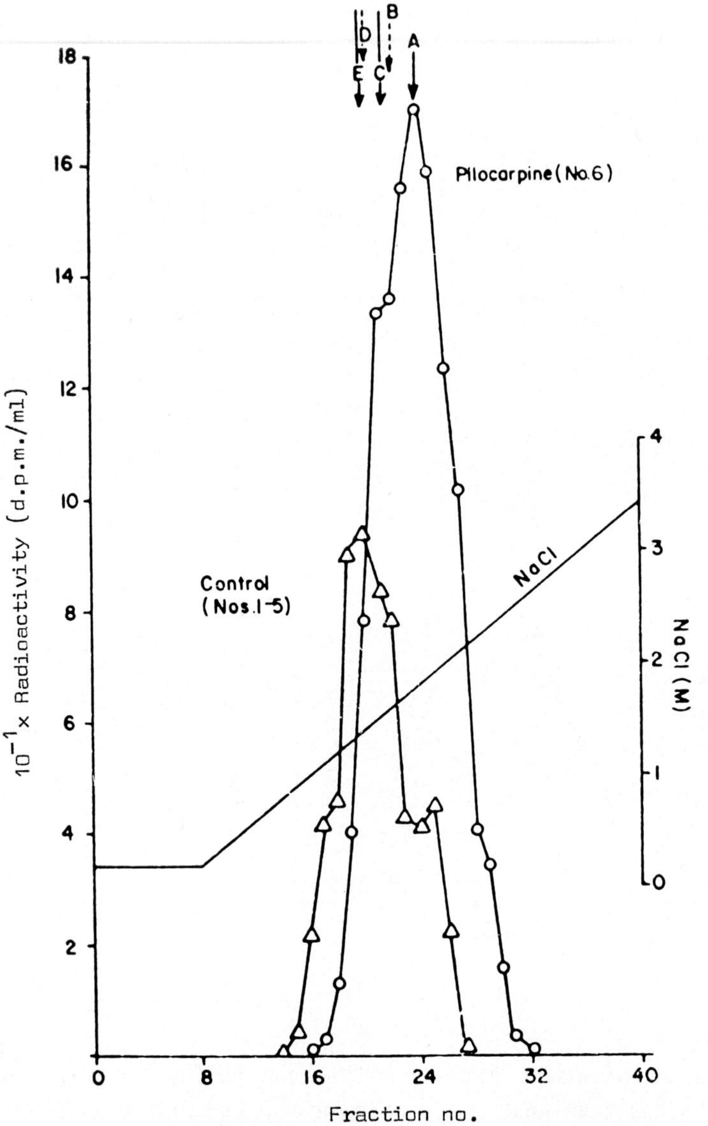

ARROWS ^{35}S-PEAKS
A = Pil. No. 6
B = NH_3 17–18
C = Pil. Nos. 7, 8, 9
D = Pil. Nol. 12–15
E = Control 1–5

FIG. 4. All mucin fractions collected and pooled as described in Figs. 1 and 2 were fractionated by ion-exchange chromatography under conditions described for Fig. 3. The graph shows a comparison of the elution of the peak for [^{35}S]sulphate in controls (nos. 1–5) and pilocarpine (no. 6) mucins and the arrows indicate the apex of the [^{35}S]sulphate peak for all other mucins collected. Controls (nos. 10, 11 & 16) are not shown but their elution peak corresponds to controls (nos. 1–5) indicated by arrow 'E'. With the exception of controls (nos. 1–5) the [^{35}S]sulphate and [^{3}H]glucose peaks coincided. It is noteworthy that the main [^{3}H]glucose peak in controls (nos. 1–5) – see Fig. 3 – corresponded, in terms of the NaCl concentration required to elute it from the column, to the [^{3}H]glucose/[^{35}S]sulphate peak in ammonia mucins – arrow 'B' in this figure.

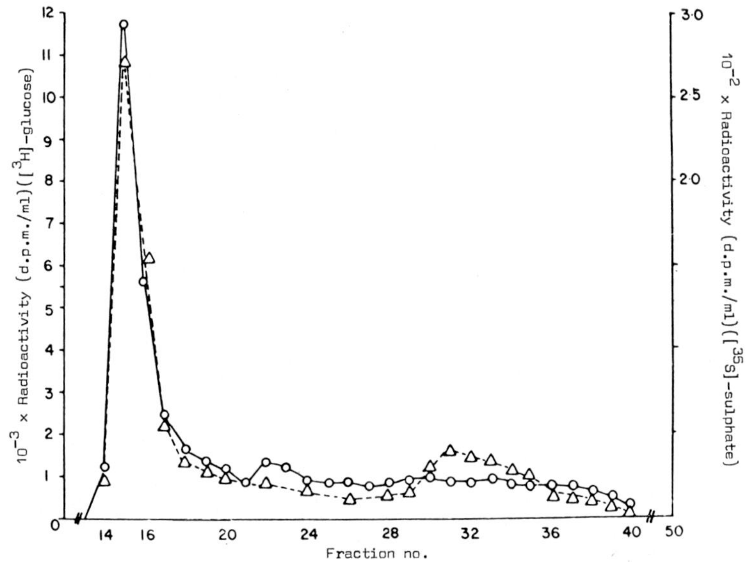

FIG. 5. Mucins were equilibrated by dialysis with the eluting buffer (6 M-urea, 10 mM-DTT, 10 mM-phosphate, pH 7.2) before application to the Sepharose CL-4B column. Elution was carried out at a flow rate of 6 ml/h, and 4 ml/h fractions were collected. Column void volume (V_o) was 60 ml (fraction 15) and the total included volume (V_i) was 180 ml (fraction 45). ○——○ = [^{3}H]glucose; △---△ = [^{35}S]sulphate.

TABLE 5

Carbohydrate composition of various preparations of goose tracheal mucins

Molar ratios of monosaccharides present (N-acetylglucosamine = 1.00) in various fractions						
Monosaccharide	*A*	*B*	*C*	*D1*	*D2*	*E*
Galactose	1.37	0.87	++	2.14	2.05	1.39
N-Acetylgalactosamine	1.60	1.18	1.19	1.01	0.53	0.67
N-Acetylglucosamine	1.00	1.00	1.00	1.00	1.00	1.00
Sialic acid	1.97	1.08	0.64	0.57	0.20	0.87
Mannose	0.19	0.17	0.05	0.53	0.95	0.24

Fractions A–E represent mucin samples obtained from different geese and fractionated by various methods. A, void volume (V_o) peak from Sephadex G-200; B, from Sepharose 2B; C, V_o peak from Ultrogel AcA22; D1; DEAE-ion exchange chromatography, fraction one; D2, DEAE-ion exchange chromatography, fraction two; E, unfractionated sample.

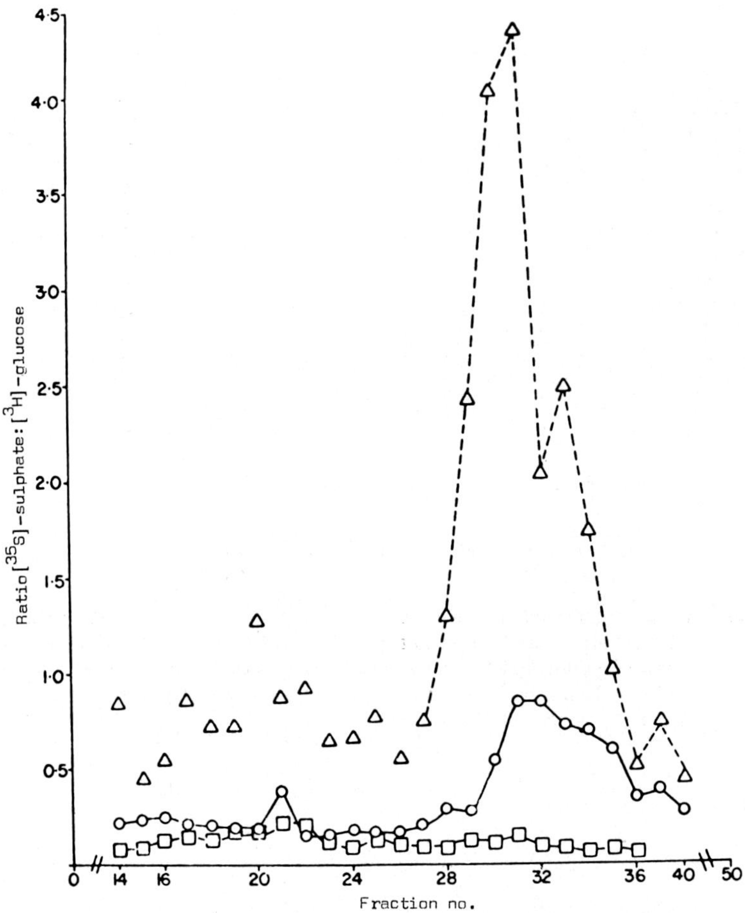

FIG. 6. The graph shows a comparison of the ratio of ^{35}S:^{3}H-radioactivity in each 4 ml fraction of control (nos. 1–5), pilocarpine (no. 6) and ammonia (nos. 17–18) mucins fractionated on Sepharose CL-4B as described in Fig. 5. ○——○ = control mucin; △---△ = pilocarpine mucin; □——□ = ammonia mucin.

stimulated mucin. The results imply that there is probably no metabolic or structural precursor product relationship between the high and low molecular weight fractions (Gallagher *et al.* 1977).

The histological and radioautographic studies which form an important part of the study (Jeffery, this volume, pp. 5–20) strongly support the view that pilocarpine selectively stimulates the secretion of highly sulphated material from submucosal gland cells but with little effect on goblet cell secretion. By contrast, the irritant action of ammonia is exerted on goblet cells.

In the goose, tracheal mucus arises solely from goblet cells since there are no mucous or serous glands. The glycoprotein, isolated by perfusion and subsequently fractionated by various methods, has distinctive properties (Table 5). Fucose is absent and sialic acid content is relatively high compared with cat or dog mucins. Mannose was consistently present, care having been taken to exclude the possibility of serum contamination.

CONCLUSIONS

A growing body of evidence suggests that consideration of the properties and composition of overall mucus secretions, both of surface epithelia and of glands, must take into account the nature and variety of cell types from which the mucin component arises. Compositional changes in the final mucus can be achieved through selective stimulation or inhibition of the formation of one of the contributing glycoproteins. There is also evidence, however, that within one cell differences may exist between secretory granules, and that these differences may contribute to microheterogeneity. Biochemical as well as histological evidence supports the view that different contributing cells synthesize chemically distinct glycoproteins. The macromolecular interactions which lead to the characteristically high viscosity may thus be in part extracellular. This property may also be significantly influenced by the cationic composition of the secretions as well as by concentration effects arising from water transport by the tissue.

It is of interest to investigate further the chemical structures of goblet cells and mucous gland glycoproteins, the factors which govern their rates of secretion, and the extent to which extracellular interactions influence mechanical properties.

ACKNOWLEDGEMENTS

The contributions of Dr J. T. Gallagher, Dr A. Corfield, Mr D. J. Mortimer, Ms C. Anderson, Mrs B. Chorley and Mrs S. Jobling in these studies are gratefully acknowledged. The investigations are supported by grants from the Cystic Fibrosis Research Trust and the Wellcome Trust.

References

BISERTE, G., HAVEZ, R. & CUVELUR, R. (1963) Les glycoprotéides des secrétions bronchiques. *Expo. Annu. Biochim. Med. 24*, 85–120

CHERNICK, W. S. & BARBERO, G. J. (1959) Composition of tracheobronchial secretions in cystic fibrosis of the pancreas and in bronchiectasis. *Pediatrics 24*, 739

CHERNICK, W. S. & BARBERO, G. J. (1963) Studies on human tracheobronchial and submaxillary secretions in normal and pathophysiological conditions. *Ann. N.Y. Acad. Sci. 106*, 698–708

DISCHE, Z. (1963) Reciprocal relation between fucose and sialic acid in mammalian glycoproteins. *Ann. N.Y. Acad. Sci. 106*, 259–270

DISCHE, Z., PALLAVICINI, C., KAWASAKI, H., SMIRNOW, N., CIZEK, L. J. & CHIEN, S. (1962) Influence of the nature of the secretory stimulus on the composition of the carbohydrate moiety of glycoproteins of the sub-maxillary saliva. *Arch. Biochem. Biophys. 97*, 459–469

ELLIS, D. B. & STAHL, G. H. (1973) Biosynthesis of respiratory-tract mucins. *Biochem. J. 136*, 837–844

FALK, H. L., KOTIN, P. & ROWLETTE, W. (1963) The response of mucus-secreting epithelium and mucus to irritants. *Ann. N.Y. Acad. Sci. 106*, 583–608

GALLAGHER, J. T. & KENT, P. W. (1975) Structure and metabolism of glycoproteins and glycosaminoglycans in organ cultures of rabbit trachea. *Biochem. J. 148*, 187–196

GALLAGHER, J. T., KENT, P. W., PASSATORE, M., PHIPPS, R. J. & RICHARDSON, P. S. (1975) The composition of tracheal mucus and the nervous control of its secretion in the cat. *Proc. R. Soc. Lond. B Biol. Sci. 192*, 49–76

GALLAGHER, J. T., KENT, P. W., PHIPPS, R. J. & RICHARDSON, P. S. (1977) Influence of pilocarpine and ammonia vapour on the secretion and structure of cat tracheal mucins: differentiation of goblet and submucosal gland cell secretions, in *Mucus in Health and Disease* (Elstein, M. & Parke, D. V., eds.), Plenum Press, London

GOTTSCHALK, A. (1969) Biosynthesis of glycoproteins and its relationship to heterogeneity. *Nature (Lond.) 222*, 452–454

HAVEZ, R., ROUSSEL, P., DEGAND, P. & BISERTE, G. (1967) Etude des structures fibrillaires de la secrétion bronchique humaine. *Clin. Chim. Acta 17*, 281–295

JEFFERY, P. K. (1978) Structure and function of mucus-secreting cells of cat and goose airway epithelium, in this volume, pp. 5–20

LOMBART, C. G. & WINZLER, R. J. (1974) Isolation and characterization of oligosaccharides from canine submaxillary mucin. *Eur. J. Biochem. 49*, 77–86

LAMB, D. (1975) appendix, see Gallagher, J. T. *et al.* (1975)

MORA, P. T. (1973) Cell growth regulation; cell selection and the function of membrane glycolipids, in *Membrane Mediated Information* (Kent, P. W., ed.), vol. 1, pp. 64–84, Medical and Technical Publishing, Lancaster

PHELPS, C. F. & STEVENS, A. M. (1978) Studies on the control of mucin production, in this volume, pp. 91–107

PHIPPS, R. J., RICHARDSON, P. S., CORFIELD, A., GALLAGHER, J. T., JEFFERY, P. K., KENT, P. W. & PASSATORE, M. (1977) A physiological, biochemical and histological study of goose tracheal mucin and its secretions. *Philos. Trans. R. Soc. Lond. B Biol. Sci. 279*, 513–543

POTTER, J. L., MATTHEWS, L. W., LEMM, J. & SPECTOR, S. (1963) Human pulmonary secretions in health and disease. *Ann. N.Y. Acad. Sci. 106*, 692–697

RICHARDSON, P. S., PHIPPS, R. J., BALFRE, K. & HALL, R. L. (1978) The roles of mediators, irritants and allergens in causing mucin secretion from the trachea, in this volume, pp. 111–126

REID, L. (1978) Animal models in clinical disease, in this volume, pp. 297–307

ROBERTS, G. P. (1974) Isolation and characterization of glycoproteins from sputum. *Eur. J. Biochem. 50*, 265–280

ROUSSEL, P., LAMBLIN, G., DEGAND, P. & HAVEZ, R. (1972) Isolement des mucines bronchiques sécrétées au cours de la mucoviscidose. *Clin. Chim. Acta 36*, 315–328

ROUSSEL, P., LAMBLIN, G., DEGAND, P., WALKER-NASIRE, E. & JEANLOZ, R. W. (1975) Heterogeneity of the carbohydrate chains of sulphated bronchial glycoproteins isolated from a patient suffering from cystic fibrosis. *J. Biol. Chem. 250*, 2114–2122

WINZLER, R. J. (1973) A model for control of oligosaccharide structure in membrane glycoproteins, in *Membrane Mediated Information* (Kent, P. W., ed.), vol. 1, pp. 3–19, Medical and Technical Publishing, Lancaster

Discussion

Richardson: We originally did these experiments to try to separate goblet cell secretions from those of gland cells. After the submucosal glands had been virtually exhausted by repeated doses of pilocarpine, ammonia vapour put into the tracheal segment yielded a secretion which was very heavily labelled with tritiated glucose. We expected, therefore, that autoradiographs would reveal that the goblet cells were heavily labelled with [^{3}H]glucose, but this was not so. What was labelled in the autoradiographs was the luminal edge of the ciliated cells, so the labelled glycoprotein that ammonia released was from the luminal edge of the ciliated cells and probably not from the goblet cells. There must have been goblet cell secretion there but it wasn't heavily labelled.

Kent: Luminal edge secretion has been observed before and could be deposition of glycoprotein on the epithelial surface concentrated by water reabsorption—a precipitation phenomenon. If the chemical composition is markedly different from submucosal gland secretion, its origin must be more complicated than that. We do know that in the glycoproteins resulting from goblet cell stimulation the sugars are contained as oligosaccharides split off by sodium hydroxide and borohydride and that sialic acid and sulphate are present in the same unit.

Silberberg: I was a little surprised that you could not reduce these washings with dithiothreitol (DTT). We have managed to dissolve lung mucus with DTT and find units of a molecular weight of about 500 000 after the reduction. It is interesting, however, that the disulphide bonds of bovine cervical mucin were not fully reduced when DTT was used. Only after performic acid reaction did the resulting mucin come down to the same size as the unit that we found with other mucins. There are cases therefore where the reagent does not produce total disulphide splitting.

Kent: The mechanism of reduction is complex and the existence of disulphide bridges is probably not the only factor involved. If hydrogen-bond-breaking reagents are also included, the cleavage of S-S bonds will probably be facilitated. There are very considerable differences between viscous mucins. But we do not yet know accurately the total number of cysteine residues in our glycoprotein, nor the extent to which they are reduced. The cysteine contents are very small indeed.

Reid: Roberts (1976) found that there are only a handful of disulphide bonds and this fits with Allen's work (Snary *et al.* 1971) in relation to gut mucus. Either it has already been split or there is some species difference. The question of SH bonds is an extremely important aspect of the macromolecule. Where are these formed within the cell? In the stomach and in human airway epithelium there is evidence that there are five to six disulphide bonds in the macromolecule.

Phelps: Would you see this as a means of hybridizing different molecules by way of their disulphide bridges to make a matrix outside, tailor-made to the physical conditions?

Reid: I see the matrix coming earlier, somewhere within cells and perhaps disulphide bridges could condense outside the cell rather than within. They might even be added outside the cell?

Phelps: I see no reason why they can't be 'zipped' outside the cell. The requirements within the cell are to make a concentrated bulk of material which will be exported from the cell with minimum collateral nuisance. Thereafter a different set of conditions must operate on the material—it has to become a vast property occupier.

Kent: It is a very attractive hypothesis in that the final viscous molecular state involves extracellular hybridization or zipping, at least in part, and at present one sees no evidence to rule that out.

Allison: Masson (1973) makes the point that the polypeptide chains are relatively short (about 30 000 daltons), so that several are present in the macromolecule (over 500 000 daltons). Would you accept that evidence, which is based on N-terminal and recent C-terminal studies?

Kent: Yes.

Allison: So if there is a large molecule of this size there must be cross-bonding of one sort or another. Disulphide bonding represents one possibility; another is that sugar chains might link polypeptide chains. This is the concept of transglycolysation which began by being unorthodox but is now accepted by several authorities. Roth (1973) believes that apposed cells can be covalently linked together by carbohydrate units and that there are specific enzymes which catalyse the process.

Kent: I think that is possible. If there are to be intercalary carbohydrate chains, one has to postulate some new forms of carbohydrate-peptide linkage involving a non-glycosidic attachment (*O*-ether). One still has to make quite certain that it is not hydrogen bonding and hydrophobic interactions which predominate.

Silberberg: It is our impression that neither of these secondary bond types is important. We find no change in the rate of molecular degradation whether mucus is heat-solubilized in saline or in such media as 6M-guanidine hydrochloride or sodium dodecyl sulphate.

Allison: I was referring not only to the molecular weight but also to the molecular properties which relate to their viscous structure.

Reid: We need to be clear what aspect we are talking about. It is sputum if it is above the larynx and bronchial liquid if it is below. If we take either of these from man, viscosity can certainly be reduced by urea. If you refer to purified glycoprotein, I agree.

Guz: Are there any data on how many disulphide bonds there are?

Reid: Allen & Snary (1972) have good data that in gastric mucosa there are something like four or five bonds per macromolecule of, say, 1 or 2 million daltons, and Roberts (1976) reports five to seven bonds in purified respiratory glycoprotein.

Silberberg: The 30 000 mol.wt. unit that Bushana Rao & Masson (1977) find contains two cysteine residues, which is what we find in bovine cervical mucin. It agrees also with data of Roussel *et al.* (1972) for human bronchial glycoprotein.

Allison: So the total number of disulphide bonds in the macromolecule (1–2 million daltons) is about 50.

Silberberg: But the majority, if they are in one molecule, would probably not be used for intermolecular connections but rather for intramolecular bonding, the creation of a specifically shaped structural entity. The tempting thing about the 30 000 unit on the other hand is that two cysteines are just the minimum number needed to build up chains.

Allison: Do we accept that disulphide bonding is the most likely mechanism by which the subunits are held together?

Kent: It is one of the mechanisms.

Reid: Hydrogen bonding doesn't seem to be so important for purified glycoprotein, at least not in the sense that Dr Allison was referring to.

Kent: On the other hand there are examples known of gel formation and molecular aggregation which are not dependent on SH interactions, for example gel formation in the Tamm & Horsfall urinary glycoprotein which is a very rapid process and is closely calcium-dependent.

Silberberg: The cysteine bonds certainly do not form the gel. They are only the device by which a large specially shaped unit is built up, perhaps from smaller subunits.

Allison: How do you start from a relatively small polypeptide unit to build up a macromolecule by covalent bonding?

Silberberg: The covalently linked unit probably has a molecular weight of the order of 0.5×10^6. This, however, does not tell us anything about the number, or the lengths, of the peptide chains involved with it. Even if there are many very short peptide chains linked by carbohydrate to carbohydrate links, this still makes up a single covalently linked structure. In this case the carbohydrate-to-carbohydrate links must be parallel to the cysteine linkages, since breaking the latter does not produce a marked change in molecular weight. Nobody has yet found a 30 000 mol.wt. unit by any physicochemical technique. Bushana Rao & Masson (1977) on their own preparation find a molecular weight of 500 000, and they put forward a possible explanation to account for it—aggregation by hydrophobic bonding. We do not believe, however, that hydrophobic bonding can be involved, because the unit, when suspended in a hydrophobic-bond-breaking medium such as sodium dodecyl sulphate, does not change in molecular weight. If build-up from a 30 000 molecular weight unit is involved we therefore tend to favour carbohydrate linkages. The evidence for the 30 000 mol.wt. unit comes from N- and C-terminal determinations. If the analyses are in error and there are fewer linkages, the protein chain would be longer and one wouldn't have to stipulate the carbohydrate-to-carbohydrate links.

Allison: If, on the other hand, the carbohydrate chains were screening the terminal groups, one would expect to find fewer and not more terminal groups. Hence it is unlikely that the number of terminal groups is over-estimated. The observations do pose the problem of how such small polypeptide chains are covalently bonded together to form the macromolecule.

References

ALLEN, A. & SNARY, D. (1972) The structure and function of gastric mucus. *Gut 13*, 666–672

BUSHANA RAO, K. S. P. & MASSON, P. L. (1977) A tentative model for the structure of bovine oestrus cervical mucin, in *Mucus in Health and Disease* (Elstein, M. & Parke, D. V., eds.), Plenum Press, London

MASSON, P. L. (1973) Carbohydrate component of cervical mucus, in *Cervical Mucus in Human Reproduction* (Elstein, M. *et al.*, eds.), p. 82, Scriptor, Copenhagen

ROBERTS, G. P. (1976) The role of disulfide bonds in maintaining the gel structure of bronchial mucus. *Arch. Biochem. Biophys. 173*, 528–537

ROTH, S. (1973) A molecular model for cell interactions. *Q. Rev. Biol. 48*, 541–563

ROUSSEL, P., LAMBLIN, G., DEGAND, P. & HAVEZ, R. (1972) Isolement des mucines bronchiques sécrétées au cours de la mucoviscidose. *Clin. Chim. Acta 36*, 315–328

SNARY, D., ALLEN, A. & PLAIN, R. H. (1971) The structure of pig gastric mucus. *Eur. J. Biochem. 24*, 183–189

The glycoproteins of secretory cells in airway epithelium

ROSEMARY JONES

Harvard Medical School, The Children's Hospital Medical Center, Boston, Massachusetts and Department of Experimental Pathology, Brompton Hospital, London

Abstract Quantitative histochemical methods demonstrate a variety of glycoproteins within mucus-secreting cells of airway epithelium. A single cell may synthesize one or a combination of four major types—(*i*) neutral glycoprotein, (*ii*) and (*iii*) sialylated glycoprotein either sensitive or resistant to sialidase and (*iv*) sulphated. In human airway disease, or in experimental response to inhalation of an irritant, there is mucus cell hyperplasia and change in the proportion of cells synthesizing the various types. Experimental studies show how speedily these changes occur. In rats exposed to tobacco smoke changes are found within 20 h of the first exposure. Only in the extrapulmonary epithelium is there discharge of the secretions, with an apparent fall in cell number. Modification of glycoprotein may occur with an unchanged or increased cell number, suggesting that it occurs in existing and newly appearing secretory cells. Modification of the contents of the granule occurs toward the cell apex. Modification of glycoprotein synthesis towards the normal is also the most sensitive and earliest sign of recovery.

This paper describes both the range of glycoproteins identified within secretory cells of the airway surface and submucosal gland, and the results of experimental studies that illustrate that, within the airway surface, the epithelial cells are a labile population and may transform from one cell type to another. This change may be induced in response to irritation (Lamb & Reid 1968; Jones *et al.* 1973) or drugs (Sturgess & Reid 1973; Baskerville 1976; Kleinerman *et al.* 1976). More recently it has also been shown that such a change may be induced in response to elastase (EC 3.4.21.11) (Christensen *et al.* 1977).

The secretory cell populations of the airways include the cells of the submucosal gland and of the airway surface. Within the gland two secretory cell types are present, both mucous and serous cells (Meyrick & Reid 1970). Within the airway surface three secretory cell types are now recognized—the Clara, serous and mucous (also known as the 'goblet') cells (Jeffery & Reid

1975). The morphology of the secretory granules of the goblet cell as demonstrated by electron microscopy resembles that of the mucous cell of the gland. Each of these cell types synthesizes glycoproteins that are packaged within granules within the cell.

It is now known that the mucus glycoprotein identified from bronchial secretion (Degand *et al.* 1973) and from sputum (Reid 1977; J. M. Creeth *et al.* unpublished work) is a large macromolecule that seems unlikely to be secreted from one granule of a secretory cell but may rather be formed from the contents of several granules. Little is known, however, of the structural arrangement of the content of a granule or its molecular size. Recent chemical studies have shown that the glycoprotein present in both the sol and the gel phase of sputum is similar, although within the sol phase the concentration of the total glycoprotein is lower and that of sialic acid higher (I. Das *et al.* unpublished work). Both phases nevertheless are secreted by the cell populations of the airways that produce glycoproteins. Histochemical analysis of glycoproteins is concerned with their intracellular demonstration.

HISTOCHEMICAL ANALYSIS OF EPITHELIAL GLYCOPROTEINS

In some secretory cells of the airways, as in other epithelial tissue sites (Eversole 1972; Fletcher *et al.* 1976), acid groups may be identified by histochemical stains, while in other cells containing glycoprotein they cannot (Jones *et al.* 1973, 1975), this form of cell product being termed neutral (Fig. 1). The acid groups include the carboxyl group of sialic acid, either sensitive or resistant to removal from the glycoprotein structure by sialidase (neuraminidase: EC 3.2.1.18), or ester sulphate. After histochemical staining the secretory

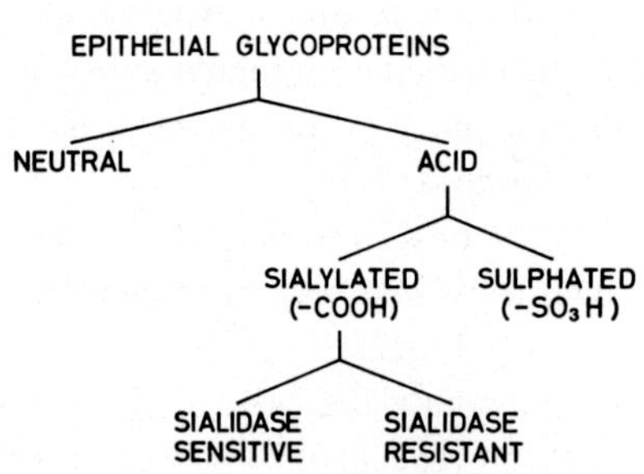

FIG. 1. When stained by histochemical techniques, epithelial glycoproteins may (acid) or may not (neutral) demonstrate acid groups. When present, the acid groups may be sialic acid, either sensitive or resistant to sialidase digestion, or ester sulphate.

TABLE 1

Identification of epithelial glycoproteins in consecutive tissue sections each stained with a variation of the AB–PAS technique.

Section	*Stain*	*Group identified*
1	AB–pH 2.6–PAS	All acid glycoprotein stains blue
2	Sialidase AB–pH 2.6–PAS	Sialylated glycoprotein resistant to sialidase and sulphated glycoprotein stain blue
3	AB–pH 1.0–PAS	Sulphated glycoprotein stains blue

cells of the airways display specific staining properties but the type of acid group(s), or neutral glycoprotein, that may be present within a cell cannot be identified by a single histochemical method. A combination of the Alcian blue and periodic acid Schiff (AB–PAS) techniques, each used on a consecutive tissue section, has proved a useful way of identifying these glycoproteins (Table 1). With Alcian blue at pH 2.6 all acid glycoprotein stains blue. After sialidase treatment and similar staining with AB at pH 2.6 only sialidase-resistant and sulphated glycoprotein retain their blue staining; with AB at pH 1.0 only sulphated glycoprotein stains blue. By this sequence of techniques, the neutral form of glycoprotein and acid groups that fail to stain with AB stains with PAS (Jones & Reid 1973). Analysis of the different glycoproteins within cells of the airway surface is by counting various types of secretory cell, identified by their glycoprotein content (see section below), while for the gland a method of point-counting is used (see Lamb & Reid 1972*a*). It cannot be too strongly emphasized that, to establish the glycoproteins present within a cell population, it is necessary to analyse quantitatively the staining response to the above group of AB–PAS techniques.

RANGE OF GLYCOPROTEINS WITHIN AIRWAY SECRETORY CELLS

Histochemical analysis has demonstrated a range of glycoproteins in secretory cells of the airways, both of the gland and of the surface epithelium (Lamb & Reid 1969, 1970; Jones & Reid 1973; Jones *et al.* 1973, 1975). Each species has a particular pattern of glycoprotein synthesis (Table 2). Even within a single species, secretory cell types vary within a single tissue site; for example, in the submucosal gland the mucous and serous cell populations each have different patterns of synthesis for both the type and amount of glycoprotein

TABLE 2

Species variation in glycoprotein type within mucous and serous cells of the submucosal gland

Species	*Cell type*	*NGP*	*AGP*		
			Sialylated		*Sulphated*
			Sensitive	*Resistant*	
Rat	Mucous	±	—	+	+
(Sprague-Dawley)	Serous	+	+	+	+
Mouse	Mucous	+	+	—	—
Cat	Mucous	±	—	+	+
	Serous	+	—	+	+
Dog	Mucous	+	—	+	+
	Serous	+	—	—	—
Pig	Mucous	+	+	+	+
	Serous	+	—	+	+

NGP: neutral glycoprotein
AGP: acid glycoprotein

present. The difference between species is illustrated in Table 2, where it can be seen that while neutral glycoprotein is present in the mucous cells of the gland in mouse, dog and pig, it is rarely found in the rat or cat. In the rat the acid group within the mucous cells is sulphated (at least in Sprague-Dawley animals). In the mouse the only acid group is sialidase-sensitive sialylated glycoprotein (McCarthy & Reid 1964*a*) while in the cat (Gallagher *et al.* 1975) and dog (Spicer *et al.* 1971) there is again a mixture of sulphated and sialidase-resistant sialylated glycoprotein. The glycoproteins within mucous cells of the pig submucosal gland most closely resemble those of man, although here also there is a species difference in that proportionally more neutral glycoprotein is synthesized in the pig than in man (Jones *et al.* 1975).

In man, while each of the four types of glycoprotein is present in the mucous cells of the adult gland (Lamb & Reid 1969), this is not so at birth. There is a pattern of maturation such as there is in the gut, although in gut the pattern is the reverse—from mostly sialylated glycoprotein in the fetal gut (Lev 1968) to sulphated glycoprotein in the adult large intestine (Filipe & Branfoot 1974). In mucous cells of the human fetal airway gland, only sulphated glycoprotein is present. This then decreases in amount while sialylated glycoprotein appeasr after birth and increases during childhood (Lamb & Reid 1972*b*) to reach

TABLE 3

Range of acid glycoproteins within secretory cells of rat airway epithelium

Type of acid glycoprotein	*Individual cell type*				
	I	*II*	*III*	*IV*	*V*
Sialylated glycoprotein					
Sialidase-sensitive	+	+			
Sialidase-resistant		+	+	+	
Sulphated glycoprotein				+	+

the adult pattern of both the sialidase-sensitive and resistant forms. In the adult, one or a range of acid groups may be present within a single mucous cell although they are present only in certain combinations (Lamb & Reid 1972*a*). Despite the wide range of glycoproteins that may be present within mucous and serous cells of the submucosal gland (Lamb & Reid 1969, 1970), their variation is less within the bronchial tree of one individual than between one individual and another (Lamb & Reid 1972*a*), and this is reflected in the analysis of glycoproteins from sputum from different individuals (Lopez-Vidriero 1976). Recent studies (Jones 1976) have shown that even within secretory cells of the airway surface population there is a similar range of intracellular combinations of glycoproteins (Table 3). Sialidase-sensitive sialylated glycoprotein may be present alone within a cell or in combination with the resistant form. The latter may also be present alone, as may sulphated glycoprotein, or these two may be present in combination. This has been demonstrated in airway epithelium in the rat, which is the species included in the experimental studies discussed below.

CHANGE IN GLYCOPROTEIN SYNTHESIS IN HUMAN AIRWAY DISEASE

In addition to analysis of the secretory glycoproteins present within cell populations of normal airway epithelium, histochemical analysis has provided information on the changes occurring in disease. In human airway disease secretory cell hyperplasia is accompanied by a shift in the proportion of cells synthesizing a particular acid glycoprotein. In chronic bronchitis there is within mucous cells of the gland an increase in sialidase-resistant sialylated glycoprotein relative to the sensitive form and an increase in sulphated glycoprotein (McCarthy & Reid 1964*b*; deHaller & Reid 1965; Lamb 1968).

There is also an increase in sulphation within cells of the airway surface (Lamb 1969). Similar changes in the glycoprotein occur after inhalation of an irritant (Lamb & Reid 1968; Jones *et al.* 1973) but until recently little has been known of the speed or the pattern of development of these changes.

The results that follow are from experimental studies that illustrate three aspects of the changes that occur within the cells of the surface epithelium of the airways in response to irritation—the speed of the appearance of new secretory cells, the pattern of modification to glycoprotein synthesis that accompanies or precedes the increase, and the reversibility of these changes.

EXPERIMENTAL STUDIES OF SECRETORY CELL HYPERPLASIA

Distribution of secretory cell types in normal rat airway epithelium

When stained with AB-pH 2.6-PAS the secretory cells of rat airway epithelium are characterized both by the type of glycoprotein and its amount (Jones *et al.* 1973). A cell may synthesize a single type of granule that contains glycoprotein that is acid and stains blue (AB +ve), or one that is neutral and stains red (PAS +ve) or a combination of granules of either type (AB–PAS +ve). A cell may contain a large (L) number of granules that extend throughout the cell or only a small (S) number that are present in the apical region. Thus six secretory cell types are characterized within the surface epithelium of the rat by their glycoprotein content: L.AB, S.AB, L.AB–PAS, S.AB–PAS, L.PAS and S.PAS.

The results of the study presented here are for one extrapulmonary and one intrapulmonary airway region—the lower trachea and main bronchi and upper part of the main axial pathway respectively. In both these regions most secretory cells in the normal airway epithelium contain only a small number of granules of glycoprotein but each synthesize different amounts of each type, as judged by the numbers of the various cell types present. In the lower trachea and main bronchi, the distribution for AB, AB–PAS and PAS cell types is 48, 32 and 20% while in the upper axial pathway it is 5, 30 and 65% respectively. In this way the effect of irritation on different baseline secretory cell populations within the airways can be studied.

Change in the distribution of secretory cell types in rat airway epithelium induced by irritation

Rats were exposed to the tobacco smoke of 25 cigarettes a day for 1, 2, 3, 7 or 14 days. These animals were killed 20 hours after their last exposure period;

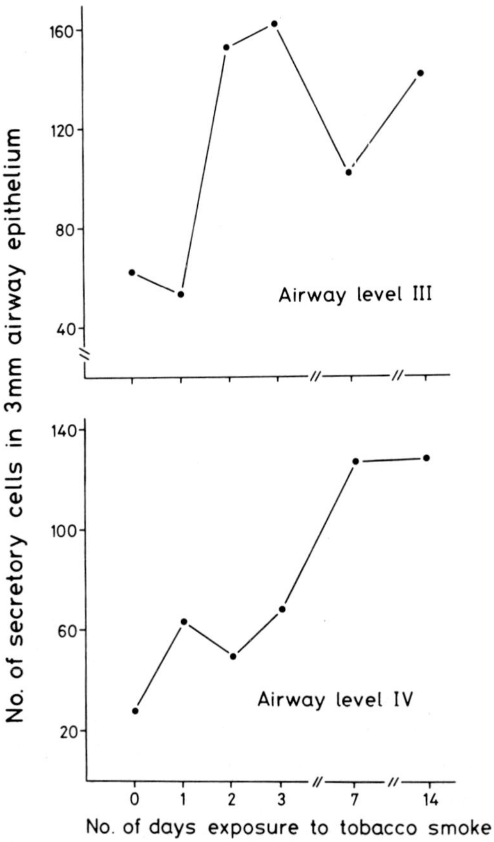

FIG. 2. Number of secretory cells in 3 mm airway epithelium of control rats (Day 0) and rats exposed to tobacco smoke for periods up to 14 days: airways levels III – lower trachea and main bronchi – and IV – upper part of the axial pathway (along the medial wall).

control animals were killed at the beginning or at the end of the exposure period of 14 days and the results for these animals were taken together.

The numbers of secretory cells in the lower trachea and main bronchus (Airway level III) and in the upper axial pathway (Airway level IV) of control rats and rats exposed to tobacco smoke are illustrated in Fig. 2. The pattern of change in secretory cell number after exposures to smoke is different in the two airway regions in that only in the lower trachea and main bronchus did the exposures produce a substantial fall in the secretory cell number. The fall after the first exposure is followed by an increase in the cell number that is significantly above the control value by day 3 ($P < 0.001$) when the maximum number of secretory cells is seen. The number then falls again after 7 days of exposure and a further increase is seen after 14 days. Within the lung there is a pattern of overall increase, with the maximum number of secretory cells present after the longest period of exposures.

The apparent fall in secretory cell number is due to discharge of secretory product from cells within the population. Although there was a delay of 20 h between the end of exposure and the killing of an animal, many of the secretory cells were still empty. The discharge effect occurred only at certain times: that is, after the first exposure to the irritant and after the seventh, when the pattern mimicked that of the first day. The animals killed after seven days' exposure had received six consecutive days of exposure to the smoke, one day's rest and a single further exposure, so that a period of rest preceded the final exposure. Animals killed after 14 days' exposure also had received a day's rest, but this was two days before the final exposure; here the pattern mimics that of day 2 and an increase above the control level is seen, although it is not as great as that of the early period.

It seems that tolerance to a stimulus develops within airway epithelium between 20 and 44 h after a single exposure to tobacco smoke and that there is then stabilization against overwhelming discharge despite continued exposure to the irritant. A balance is again achieved between the rates of synthesis and discharge within cells of the stimulated epithelium. Tolerance to the dose, however, is then lost by removal of the stimulus for 44 h and empty cells are again present, with a corresponding reduction in the apparent secretory cell population.

It is interesting that the pattern of cell division closely resembles that of discharge. In rats from the same experiment, it was shown that the increase in mitotic index (number of nuclei in division per 1000/24 h) after exposure to the irritant was greater after the first and after the seventh day of exposure (Bolduc 1976). This effect is more pronounced in the extrapulmonary airways where there is a greater basal cell population since these are the cells that are stimulated to divide. The stimulus to discharge for the superficial secretory cell and to mitosis for the basal cell has the same timing and suggests some relationship but whether it is causal is not clear.

In both the extrapulmonary and intrapulmonary regions the contribution by individual secretory cell types to the overall increase in total secretory cell number in response to irritation is mainly by cells containing a small number of granules of glycoprotein that are either acid and neutral in combination (S.AB–PAS) or acid glycoprotein alone (S.AB) (Jones 1976). Cells containing any number of granules that are only neutral glycoprotein (S.PAS and L.PAS) are rarely seen within the airway epithelium after exposure to tobacco smoke.

A few cells containing a large number of granules that include the acid form —acid and neutral glycoprotein (L.AB–PAS) or acid glycoprotein alone (L.AB)—are present but these contribute less to the increase than cells containing similar glycoprotein present in a smaller amount.

When the proportional increase in each cell type is related to the total number of secretory cells the glycoprotein in the population is modified in both airway regions despite differences in the baseline secretory cell population (Jones 1976). This occurs when the total number of secretory cells remains the same or is increased and suggests that modification to synthesis occurs both in existing and in the newly appearing secretory cells. Modification of glycoprotein synthesis implies an even more rapid modification of enzyme systems within the cell that is apparent within 20 h of stimulation. This occurs not only in previously secreting cells but also in previously non-secreting cells where there is a switch to glycoprotein synthesis.

Intracellular location of granules (number and type)

Further information on the way changes occur is obtained by considering the granules within a cell. In cells of the normal airway granules are present in the cell apex. This intracellular distribution represents the balance between synthesis and discharge. In the early stage of irritation, that is, after 14 days of exposure to tobacco smoke as illustrated by our experiments, this balance is maintained, although organ culture studies in our Department have shown an increase in synthesis and discharge at this time. After six weeks of exposure to tobacco smoke, however, the balance has changed and many cells now contain granules that extend throughout the cell (Jones *et al.* 1973). It has not yet been established from organ culture what the rates of synthesis and discharge are at this time. It seems that the rate of synthesis may be increased and that of discharge normal or reduced, or that the rate of synthesis is normal and that of discharge decreased. This suggests that in the secretory cell populations of the airway epithelium the two are independent.

When both acid and neutral glycoprotein are present together, the granules of acid glycoprotein are apical to the neutral glycoprotein within the cell. Quantitative analysis and assessment of the results for the number of secretory cells of each type within the airway epithelium of the rat by the χ^2 test (Jones 1976) has shown that granules containing either type of sialylated or sulphated glycoprotein are present alone within a cell either at the cell apex or throughout the cell. And when both forms of sialylated glycoprotein are present within a cell, the resistant form is apical to the sensitive form. When sialylated and sulphated glycoproteins are present together the sulphated form is apical. The basis for this intracellular location of granules containing different glycoproteins is not clear, but it may be that enzymes present on the granule membrane continue to modify the contents of the granule during migration to the cell apex before discharge. Since the granule membrane is derived largely from the Golgi lamellae (Jamieson & Palade 1971), it might be expected to have a similar complement of enzymes.

Conversion of cell types

Analysis of the results of the early changes after exposure to tobacco smoke (illustrated above) and of those from the more long-term exposure for six weeks (Jones *et al.* 1973) shows a pattern of change first in type and then in amount. There is a reduction in the number of cells with a small number of granules that stain with PAS, through a population of cells with both AB and PAS granules, to the cell with AB granules; and cells with only a small number of granules eventually change to ones stuffed with granules (Fig. 3). Our studies of the changes in the cell populations of the airway surface after exposure to tobacco smoke have been extended to the ultrastructural level

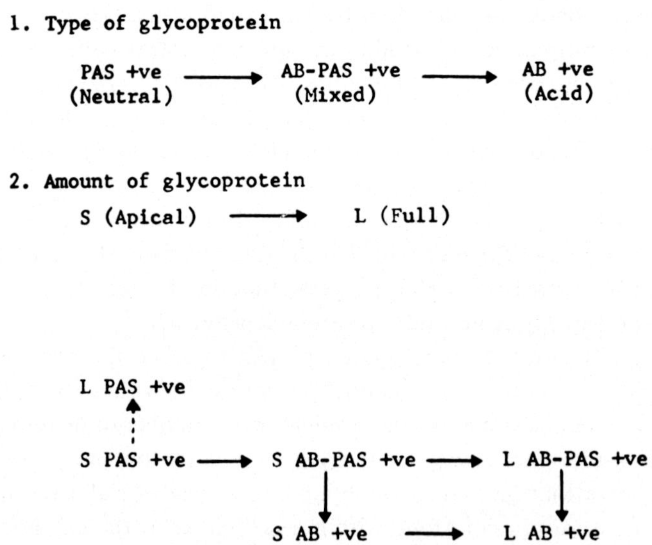

FIG. 3. Pattern of modification in type and amount of intracellular glycoprotein in secretory cells of rat airway epithelium after irritation, and suggested flow chart whereby one secretory cell type is converted to another.

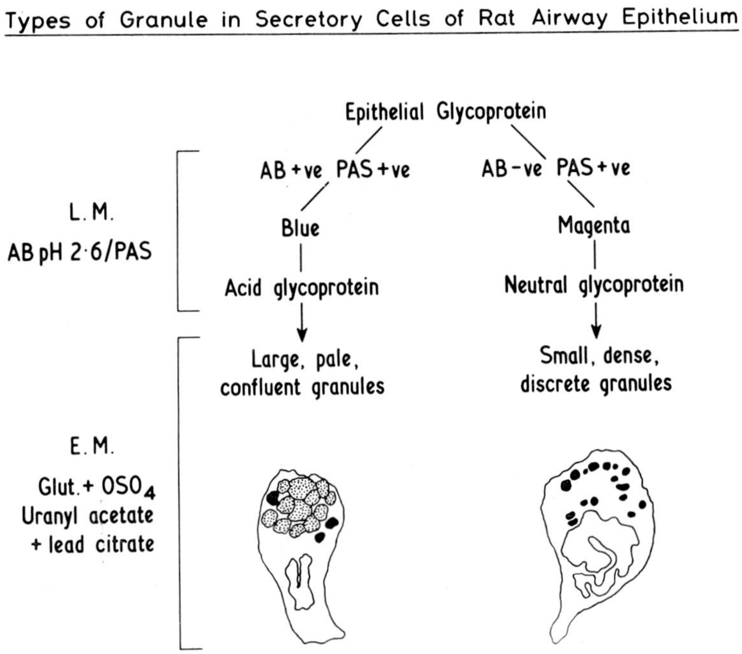

FIG. 4. In secretory cells of rat airway epithelium granules staining with AB contain acid glycoprotein and correspond to the large, pale and confluent granules seen in the cell at the ultrastructural level. Those staining with PAS contain neutral glycoprotein and correspond to the small, dense and discrete granule.

by Dr Jeffery. There is evidence that granules containing acid glycoprotein that stain with AB at the light microscope level are those which, at the ultrastructural level, are large, electron-lucent and confluent (Fig. 4), and those granules containing neutral glycoprotein that stain with PAS are those that are small, discrete and electron-dense. In both cell types seen at both the light and ultrastructural levels, some cells contain granules of both types. There is a correlation in the pattern of transformation between secretory cell types in response to irritation when studied at both the light and electron microscope levels (Jones 1976; Jeffery 1973).

From the ultrastructural studies it would seem that there is transformation within the lung from the Clara to the serous cell and, throughout the airways, from the serous to the goblet cell (Jeffery 1973). It is the non-ciliated cell without granules—the intermediate cell—that is believed to transform to a secretory cell type.

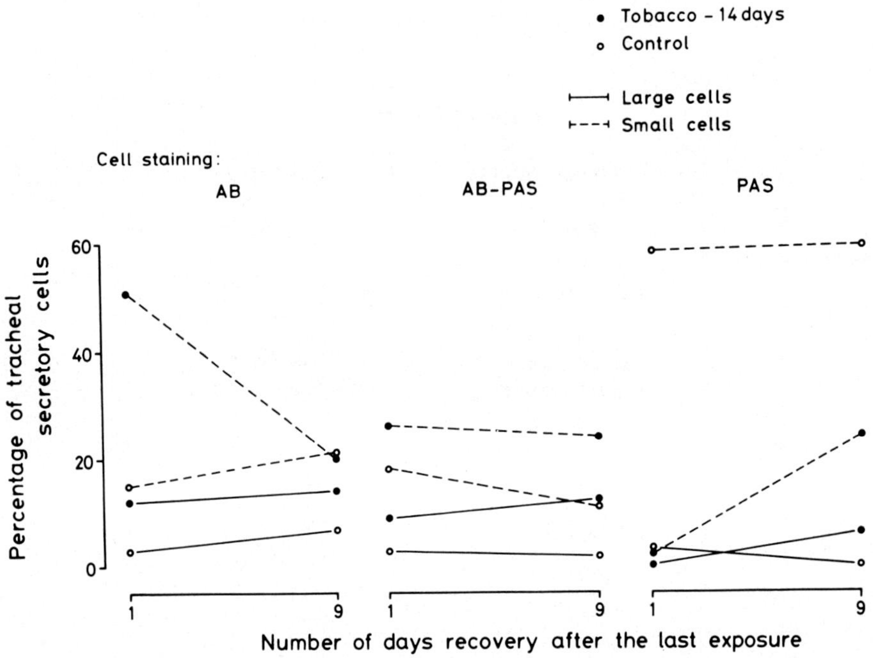

FIG. 5. Percentage of tracheal secretory cells staining with AB, AB–PAS or PAS in control rats and in rats 1 and 9 days after removal from tobacco smoke, after exposure for 14 days.

Although our studies have been concerned mainly with producing and following the pattern of change after stimulation, the question of reversal is of clinical interest. It is the reversal of the pattern of glycoprotein synthesis that is proving the most sensitive sign of recovery. Nine days after removal from the stimulus, the earliest time studied to date, the total number of secretory cells is increased but many cells have changed their pattern of glycoprotein synthesis. The proportion of cells synthesizing only acid glycoprotein (AB) is reduced (Fig. 5) while that synthesizing only the neutral (PAS) is increasing towards the control value.

The results of our combined studies have shown that, in terms of glycoprotein synthesis, the cells of the airway surface are labile. In response to irritation they are able to transform the population to one containing increased numbers of secretory cells and, after removal of the irritant, to transform it back again. It seems likely that this happens in human airways also, at least before the chronic stage of disease when secretory cells appear but do not regress. The epithelial cell population is labile to a degree we had not previously recognized.

ACKNOWLEDGEMENTS

The work reported here has in the past been supported by the Tobacco Research Council of Great Britain and currently by the Council for Tobacco Research USA.

References

BASKERVILLE, A. (1976) The development and persistence of bronchial gland hypertrophy and goblet cell hyperplasia in the pig after injection of isoprenaline. *J. Pathol. 119*, 35–47

BOLDUC, P. (1976) *Cell Turnover of the Bronchial and Alveolar Lining in the Rat Lung in Various Types of Hypertrophy*. Ph.D. Thesis, University of London

CHRISTENSEN, T. G., KORTHY, A. L., SNIDER, G. L. & HAYES, J. A. (1977) Irreversible bronchial goblet cell metaplasia in hamsters with elastase-induced panacinar emphysema. *J. Clin. Invest. 59*, 397–407

DEGAND, P., ROUSSEL, P. & LAMBLIN, G. (1973) Purification et étude des mucines de kystes bronchogéniques. *Biochim. Biophys. Acta 320*, 318–330

DEHALLER, R. & REID, L. (1965) Adult chronic bronchitis, morphology, histochemistry and vascularisation of the bronchial mucous glands. *Med. Thorac. 22*, 549–567

EVERSOLE, L. R. (1972) The histochemistry of mucosubstances in human minor salivary glands. *Arch. Oral Biol. 17*, 1225–1239

FILIPE, M. I. & BRANFOOT, A. C. (1974) Abnormal patterns of mucus secretion in apparently normal mucosa of large intestine with carcinoma. *Cancer 34*, 282–290

FLETCHER, T., JONES, R. & REID, L. (1976) Identification of glycoproteins in goblet cells of epidermis and gill of plaice (*Pleuronectes platessa* L.), flounder (*Platichthys flesus* (L.)) and rainbow trout *(Salmo gairdneri Richardson)*. *Histochem. J. 8*, 597–608

GALLAGHER, J. T., KENT, P. W., PASSATORE, M., PHIPPS, R. J., RICHARDSON, P. S. & LAMB, D. (1975) The composition of tracheal mucus and the nervous control of its secretion in the cat. *Proc. R. Soc. Lond. B Biol. Sci. 192*, 49–76

JAMIESON, J. D. & PALADE, G. E. (1971) Synthesis, intracellular transport and discharge of secretory proteins in stimulated pancreatic exocrine cells. *J. Cell Biol. 50*, 135–158

JEFFERY, P. K. (1973) *Goblet Cell Increase in Rat Bronchial Epithelium arising from Irritation or Drug Administration – an Experimental and Electron Microscopic Study*. Ph.D. thesis, University of London

JEFFERY, P. K. & REID, L. (1975) New observations of rat airway epithelium: a quantitative and electron microscopic study. *J. Anat. 120*, 295–320

JONES, R. (1976) *A Quantitative Analysis of the Effect of Tobacco Smoke and Phenylmethyloxadiazole on Rat Airway Epithelium*. M. Phil. thesis, University of London

JONES, R. & REID, L. (1973) The effect of pH on Alcian blue staining of epithelial acid glycoproteins II. Human bronchial submucosal gland. *Histochem. J. 5*, 19–27

JONES, R., BOLDUC, P. & REID, L. (1973) Goblet cell glycoproteins and tracheal gland hypertrophy in rat airways: the effect of tobacco smoke with or without the anti-inflammatory agent phenylmethyloxadiazole. *Br. J. Exp. Pathol. 54*, 229–239

JONES, R., BASKERVILLE, A. & REID, L. (1975) Histochemical identification of glycoproteins in pig bronchial epithelium: (a) normal and (b) hypertrophied from enzootic pneumonia. *J. Pathol. 116*, 1–11

KLEINERMAN, J., SORENSEN, J. & RYNBRANDT, D. (1976) Chronic bronchitis in the cat produced by chronic methacholine administration. *Am. J. Pathol. 82*, 45A

LAMB, D. (1968) Mucous secretion in hypersecretory states. *Bronches 18*, 453–465

LAMB, D. (1969) *Intracellular Development and Secretion of Mucus in the Normal and Morbid Bronchial Tree*. Ph.D. thesis, University of London

LAMB, D. & REID, L. (1968) Mitotic rates, goblet cell increase and histochemical changes in mucus in rat bronchial epithelium during exposure to sulphur dioxide. *J. Pathol. Bacteriol. 96*, 97–111
LAMB, D. & REID, L. (1969) Histochemical types of acidic glycoprotein produced by mucous cells of the tracheobronchial glands in man. *J. Pathol. 98*, 213–229
LAMB, D. & REID, L. (1970) Histochemical and autoradiographic investigations of the serous cells of the human bronchial glands. *J. Pathol. 100*, 127–138
LAMB, D. & REID, L. (1972*a*) Quantitative distribution of various types of acid glycoprotein in mucous cells of human bronchi. *Histochem. J. 4*, 91–102
LAMB, D. & REID, L. (1972*b*) Acidic glycoproteins produced by the mucous cells of the bronchial submucosal glands in the fetus and child: a histochemical autoradiographic study. *Br. J. Dis. Chest 66*, 248–253
LEV, R. (1968) A histochemical study of glycogen and mucin in developing human foetal epithelia. *Histochem. J. 1*, 152–165
LOPEZ-VIDRIERO, M. T. (1976) *Neuroaminic Acid, Fucose and Sulphate Content of Sputum in Disease and during Treatment*. Ph. D. thesis, University of London
MCCARTHY, C. & REID, L. (1964*a*) Acid mucopolysaccharide in the bronchial tree in the mouse and rat (sialomucin and sulphomucin). *Q. J. Exp. Physiol. 49*, 81–84
MCCARTHY, C. & REID, L. (1964*b*) Intracellular mucopolysaccharides in the normal human bronchial tree. *Q. J. Exp. Physiol. 49*, 85–94
MEYRICK, B. & REID, L. (1970) Ultrastructure of cells in the human bronchial submucosal glands. *J. Anat. 107*, 281–299
REID, L. (1977) Secretory cells. *Fed. Proc.*, in press
SPICER, S. S., CHAKRIN, L. W., WARDELL, J. R. & KENDRICK, W. (1971) Histochemistry of mucosubstances in the canine and human respiratory tract. *Lab. Invest. 25*, 483–490
STURGESS, J. & REID, L. (1973) The effect of isoprenaline and pilocarpine on (a) bronchial mucus-secreting tissue and (b) pancreas, salivary glands, heart, thymus, liver and spleen. *Br. J. Exp. Pathol. 54*, 388–403

Discussion

Thurlbeck: You said that the cells that multiplied were the basal cells? Was this at all levels in the airway?

R. Jones: In the rat, the basal cell population is present predominantly in the extrapulmonary airways. There are a few basal cells in the proximal parts of the lung but they are virtually absent in the peripheral regions, where it is a single-cell cuboidal epithelium. Other cells do divide; even secretory cells may divide in response to irritation (Jeffery 1973). But in the irritated airway it is essentially the normal pattern that one sees and most of the cells in division are basal.

Thurlbeck: Do you think the cell division is producing one particular form of cell?

R. Jones: Dr Jeffery's studies (Jeffery 1973) have shown that there is an increase in the mean cell concentration: that is, an increase in the total number of cells per unit length of epithelium, in the extrapulmonary airways of rats exposed to tobacco smoke for 1 to 2 weeks. This implies that more than one cell type is increased in number since both basal and superficially situated cells increase. A first burst of mitosis occurs on day 1 and is mainly in the basal cell population. By day 2 there is an increase in the percentage of basal cells within the total and this level is maintained with continued exposures to smoke; presumably some of these are daughter cells. We do not know the pattern of development of new superficial cells but later the secretory cells increase both their absolute and percentage number within the population and so do the ciliated cells.

Thurlbeck: So in addition to the increase in overall cell number there is a change in cell type—metaplasia—towards a particular form of mucus-secreting cell?

R. Jones: There are two processes in operation. One is the stimulation of the basal cell population to produce daughter cells, which in turn give rise to new secretory cells. The other is transformation within the existing cell population; the non-secretory intermediate cell is converted to a secretory cell; and secretory cells of one type are converted to another, with the production of forms of glycoprotein other than those present in the normal airway. The Clara cell is thought to become the serous cell and the serous the 'goblet' cell (Jeffery 1973).

Guz: What is the evidence for the second process? How do you differentiate between them?

R. Jones: If tobacco smoke is used with an anti-inflammatory agent, the secretory cell population can be held stable; it does not increase in number but the secretory cell type present is changed. With the light microscope there is a change from cells containing neutral glycoprotein (PAS +ve) to cells containing acid (AB +ve) (Jones *et al.* 1973). In the electron microscope there is a change from cells with dense granules to ones in which the granules have a dense core and lucent halo and finally to cells with purely lucent granules.

Guz: You are implying that Clara cells could transform. What is the evidence for that?

R. Jones: In light microscopy studies, most of the secretory cells within the lung, in control animals, produce acid glycoprotein but in one peripheral airway region the population produces the neutral form. These cells have the typical caps containing granules that stain with PAS. I think that it is now accepted that the granules of the Clara cell stain with PAS. In response to irritation this secretory cell population is changed to one in which there are more granules within the cell and these have changed to acid glycoprotein.

Jeffery: I have looked at this at two airway levels in the electron microscope: at the proximal airway level (i.e. in the main bronchus) and at the distal airway level which is less than 0.4 mm in diameter and where there are mainly Clara cells. Proximally after exposure to tobacco smoke we found a decrease in the number of serous cells and an increase in the number of goblet cells. Distally after sulphur dioxide we found a decrease in the number of Clara cells and an increase in goblet cells. In each case we found intermediate cells—i.e. cells with features of both serous and goblet and of both Clara and goblet cells in response to the respective irritants. From single pictures of these cells one can build up a hypothetical sequence of events of the change from a serous to a goblet and a Clara to a goblet cell, but we now need to put in a radioactive tag, say of [^{3}H]thymidine, to see whether the proposed sequence is indeed correct. The evidence from electron microscopy, though somewhat circumstantial, supports a transformation of both the serous and the Clara cell into a goblet cell.

Thurlbeck: It depends on the level of airway you are looking at. Evans *et al.* (1976) were describing peripheral airways and found that only non-ciliated (Clara) cells multiply, which in turn, after cell division, produced ciliated cells, presumably 'goblet' cells.

Jeffery: After sulphur dioxide the mitotic index is not significantly increased in a distal airway and yet goblet cells appear where there were none before (Lamb & Reid 1968), so there must be a transformation of existing cell types.

Allison: We need to define what we mean by transformation. The term 'transformation' is used in so many senses—for malignant change, blast formation by lymphocytes and so on. This sounds like metaplasia but that term is also used in different senses.

Jeffery: If used here it is a very narrow definition of metaplasia because we presume that the Clara cell is a secretory cell anyway, so it is only changing its type of secretion.

Proctor: Was there an increase in both types of cells? The epithelial surface is normally rather crowded, so where do these other cells go? How can there be an increase in total number of cells on the surface without an elongation of the airway? It seems more logical to assume that one cell population increases at the expense of the other.

Jeffery: To quantify this, there are about 200 cells in a high-power field (i.e. 0.18 mm length of epithelium) in the normal animal and this increases to 300 cells in the exposed animal. The epithelium becomes hypertrophied (i.e. thickened) and this is not due to stratification of cells but mainly to a change in cell shape, although there is an element of cell hypertrophy as well.

Proctor: It is difficult to visualize the change in the shape of a ciliated cell since the surface is so crowded with cilia to begin with.

Jeffery: Not if you look down a microscope. It is very obvious—they become thin and elongated (along the axis base to lumen) but the concentration of cilia doesn't change.

R. Jones: There is cell crowding. And this fits with the earlier statement made by Dr Jeffery that after irritation the microvilli are more prominent on the secretory cell surface. This is known to occur when the secretory cell surface is less distended.

Silberberg: Are you saying that the number of nuclei per unit area of epithelium is increasing?

Jeffery: Within each cell the area occupied by the nucleus stays the same but the area of the cell occupied by cytoplasm is increasing. The number of nuclei per unit *length* of epithelium is increased, because the cells are elongated.

Kramer: In the gastric mucosa the cells move from the bottom upwards along the pits in the gastric surface as they grow older. It takes six days in the rat and after one or two days these cells stop incorporating sulphate. The loss of the capacity to incorporate sulphate might be a signal that cells are becoming older. So when you talk about a higher index of mitotic activity it is possible that your cells are younger than usual when they are shed from the epithelium and do not reach the point of losing the capacity to incorporate sulphate or sugar. As a result the amount of sugars or sulphate incorporated in the cell could show differences. Are the cells older or younger?

R. Jones: The pattern of development of secretory cells within the airway is quite different from what one sees in gut, where there is maturation as the cell migrates up the villus and, as you say, there is incorporation of sulphate until the cell reaches a stage after which there is no more incorporation and finally the cell is shed.

Kramer: You are speaking about gut. I am speaking about stomach and all cells along these pits have the same appearance, with no differences in their function at all.

R. Jones: But is there a pattern of maturation?

Kramer: There is a point where incorporation of sulphate stops while galactose incorporation, for instance, continues.

R. Jones: Little is known of the lifespan of secretory cells in the respiratory tract. But it does not seem that differences in glycoprotein reflect the age of cells. In the main bronchus, where the replacement of the cell population as a whole is relatively fast (Bolduc & Reid 1976), neutral glycoprotein predominates within the cell population and the same glycoprotein is produced in the most peripheral part of the airway within the lung where replacement is relatively slow.

Kramer: With cigarette smoke does the amount of sulphate in cells increase?

R. Jones: It is not sulphate; it is the sialic acid which is resistant to sialidase.

Cumming: I am prejudiced in favour of believing that there is a dynamism of the cell population. In the graphs you showed of exposure of rats to tobacco smoke, how precise are your measurements of different levels of airways?

R. Jones: We compared the total number of secretory cells and their type of glycoprotein in carefully measured regions of the airways in control and exposed rats (Jones 1976). The level of significance between the control and exposed animals was < 0.001.

Iravani: Is it an increase in the number of the ciliated cells or an increase in turnover of these cells?

R. Jones: They are increased in number.

Iravani: Do you see more younger ciliated cells with fewer cilia and a vast number of microvilli?

R. Jones: We have not done counts.

Jeffery: There are more cells which show evidence of ciliogenesis, i.e. fibro-granular accumulations, but we haven't counted the percentage of those cells as a distinct unit.

Kent: In your stimulated situation where new secretory cells are arising, is it known whether these are producing more glycoproteins and are the secretory granules expelled more rapidly or retained?

R. Jones: In the extrapulmonary airways there is rapid discharge initially. By 20 hours after the first stimulus this is stabilized, but during the first two weeks of exposure the rates of both glycoprotein synthesis and discharge are increased. Later, after six weeks of exposure the cells are stuffed with granules but we do not know what the rates of synthesis and discharge are at this time.

Kent: It is interesting to speculate whether secreted glycoprotein retained in a cell undergoes postsynthetic modification—whether the addition of more acidic function goes on after the main structure has been completed.

R. Jones: The intracellular location of granules containing neutral or acid glycoprotein, and different types of acid, suggests modification of the granule before discharge.

Kent: You suggested that the sialic acid residues and the sulphate residues can reside in the same structures. Do you feel that your distinction between sialomucins and fucomucins is reasonable when what we may have, in fact, is a range of species in which different ratios of sialic acid and sulphate are present in the same basic molecule?

Jones: In the light microscope studies it does seem that individual granules produce individual types of glycoprotein that may be either neutral glycoprotein or acid and, if acid, then either sialic or sulphate.

Reid: Some of the granules contain both sialic acid and sulphate within the same cell.

Allison: Then the mixed species must come from these mixed granules.

Kent: This has many implications on the biochemical side if it can be correlated with molecular structure.

Jeffery: Staley & Trier (1965) looked at Paneth cells in the gut and found on electron microscopy that this cell has a two-tone appearance, i.e. an electron-dense core with an electron-lucent halo. They made some very thin (2 μm) sections for light microscopy and stained them with combined Alcian blue and periodic acid-Schiff. They found that the central core stained with periodic acid-Schiff, indicating a neutral mucin, and the halo stained with Alcian blue, indicating an acidic mucin, so there is some evidence for a correlation between electron-density and periodic acid-Schiff reactivity and electron-lucency and 'alcianophilia', at least in the alimentary and respiratory tracts.

References

Bolduc, P. & Reid, L. (1976) Mitotic index of the bronchial and alveolar lining of the normal rat lung. *Am. Rev. Respir. Dis. 114*, 1121–1128

Evans, M. J., Johnson, L. V., Stephens, R. J. & Freeman, G. (1976) Renewal of terminal bronchiolar epithelium in the rat following exposure to $NO_2 + O_3$. *Lab. Invest. 35*, 246–257

Jeffery, P. K. (1973) *Goblet Cell Increase in Rat Epithelium Arising from Irritation or Drug Administration – an Experimental and Electron Microscopic Study*. Ph. D. thesis, University of London

Jones, R. (1976) *A Quantitative Analysis of the Effect of Tobacco Smoke and Phenylmethyl-Oxadiazole on Rat Airway Epithelium*. M. Phil. thesis, University of London

Jones, R., Bolduc, P. & Reid, L. (1973) Goblet cell glycoprotein and tracheal gland hypertrophy in rat airways: the effect of tobacco smoke with and without the anti-inflammatory agent phenylmethyloxadiazole. *Br. J. Exp. Pathol. 54*, 229–239

Lamb, D. & Reid, L. (1968) Mitotic rates, goblet cell increase and histochemical changes in mucus in rat bronchial epithelium during exposure to SO_2. *J. Pathol. Bacteriol. 96*, 97–111

Staley, M. W. & Trier, J. S. (1965) Morphologic heterogeneity of mouse Paneth cell granules before and after secretory stimulation. *Am. J. Anat. 117*, 365–384

General discussion III

Nadel: We have been saying that we have cells containing granules that move up, fuse with the surface and then somehow come out. And depending on the milieu of the granule, its covering and the external milieu—at some point it is modified, perhaps picks up water, explodes or whatever we like to call it. Now somewhere inside the cell there is a membrane which keeps this process separate from the rest of the milieu of the cell. Are there materials in that membrane, say ATPases, that actively transport materials out and maintain the milieu of the cell? If it is not known, can it be tested?

Allison: It is not known. To test it one can perform electron microscope histochemistry which gives some information, but obviously the best way would be to isolate the granules. Is this possible?

Nadel: Isolation of the granule raises the question of what is maintaining the intact granule.

Douglas: All sorts of manoeuvres have proved successful, but one of the problems is that granules in many cells seem to become confluent within the cell, so that it becomes difficult to isolate them. But certainly in pancreatic or salivary cells one can isolate beautiful granules.

Silberberg: What do you mean by confluent? With membranes still separating them?

Douglas: No, I mean where several granule cores come to lie within a single limiting membrane. That is where granules have fused and ruptured amongst themselves.

Jeffery: The membrane of the secretory granule fuses with that of the cell.

Allison: And the granule membranes fuse with one another.

Reid: You can imagine the cell like a tube of toothpaste. In a mucous cell secretion is 'squeezed' out almost without any loss of membrane, but not from the serous cell.

Allison: That is what the older histologists meant by an apocrine secretion.

Kent: Biochemically, the question is whether the granule inside the cell is being maintained at a high and, as it were, abnormal concentration. If it is being compacted and held in some concentrated form, there must be some mechanism to maintain it so. Is there an ATPase in the granule membrane which is pumping out water and keeping it folded?

Kramer: There is no direct evidence for any ATP-dependent transport system. There is only an indirect argument against it from work with the Golgi system of pancreas (Jamieson & Palade 1971). There, vacuoles with rather loose contents become free and are called condensing vacuoles, still with loose contents. Then they change into granules that are very compact. To find out what causes withdrawal of water and ions, Jamieson & Palade did experiments with blockers of energy production but found no change in this transformation. They suggested that the condensing process is not energy-dependent, so there would be no pumps. This was in serous cells of guinea-pig pancreas, not in glycoprotein-secreting cells.

Phelps: Of course, we are dealing with highly charged components. They must have a counter-ion present and the problem is how to control the counter-ion behaviour.

Silberberg: I don't think this is very important, at physiological ionic strengths, for this level of charging. Meyer *et al.* (1975) have removed sialic acid without seriously affecting the structure of the material, as evidenced by the absence of a change in rheological properties or in the dimensions of the isolated mucin molecule.

Allison: It would be easier to package this material if the acidic groups were counteracted in some way, and the most obvious possibility is divalent ions. Is there a relatively high concentration of calcium or magnesium in these granules?

Kent: We really do not know the concentration of glycoprotein in the granules, do we?

Phelps: That is right, and, with all respect to the electron microscopists, looking at something that is electron-lucent and electron-dense does not necessarily mean that there is any change in the concentration of the components.

Kramer: Berg & Young (1971) have found that even in serous cells like those in the guinea-pig pancreas there is a certain degree of sulphate binding in the Golgi system. Regio & Palade (1976) are now looking for sulphated proteins within the granule fraction. Salt binding may decrease the number of active molecules within such a granule and make it possible for the water to flow from low molarity to high molarity by degrees. The sulphate esters should help in the binding.

Allison: Let us get back to the question of how we should try to isolate the granules.

Douglas: I would look for a more abundant source of mucus such as a tumour. Before one can talk sensibly about packaging mechanisms one needs to have the isolated granule and study its composition. We have excellent information about chromaffin and other granules which can be relatively easily isolated. But one needs a good source. Surely there must be a tumour around which is appropriate.

Reid: You could use a mucus-secreting tumour of lung.

Kramer: Parotid glands have been used but they have a more serous type of glycoprotein-containing granule; these granules do not swell and they do not fuse with each other in unstimulated conditions.

Richardson: Would it be possible to get a cell culture going of either mucous cells or serous cells?

Davis: Wissig & Satir (1976) have used *Tetrahymena pyriformis* to study the role of divalent cations in the regulation of mucocyst secretion. Large quantities of these organisms can be harvested from cultures.

Kent: I believe there are cell lines from tumour-bearing cells in the colon which produce vast amounts of mucus from goblet cells.

Allison: Plasmacytomas have given us an enormous amount of information about how immunoglobulins are synthesized, for example, and I think it would be a good beginning to have a uniform population of mucus-secreting tumour cells.

I said earlier that in some circumstances divalent ions help to stabilize membranes. In these circumstances you probably wouldn't want calcium ions because they are likely to promote fusion. So the main point in isolating the granules would be careful attention to osmolarity and perhaps also having magnesium ions present.

Douglas: One would certainly want to remove the calcium and that is done fairly routinely, with EGTA for example. I am not sure how important the addition of magnesium would be.

Allison: Magnesium helps to stabilize and re-seal plasma membrane vesicular preparations, so it may be useful for preserving granule integrity.

Kent: There is a good deal of circumstantial evidence that cation modifiers like ouabain and chlorpromazine seem to influence the pattern of granule release.

Reid: We have evidence that, in the human bronchial gland for both serous and mucous cells, it is possible to dissociate uptake, synthesis and discharge by varying the pulse label and the use of toxic and pharmacologically active agents.

Allison: In a number of cell types microtubules are important in establishing polarity, particularly after cell division when cells are essentially symmetrical. Is there any information about the possible role of microtubules in the determination of polarity in mucus-secreting cells? When you are stimulating development, does colchicine in organ cultures disturb normal differentiation?

Reid: Colchicine has been used in growing lung to show how important the tubules are in dividing epithelium but I don't know anything about the adult.

Allison: Another example is the Kartagener syndrome: the association of chronic bronchitis and bronchiectasis with situs inversus and ciliary immobility (Afzelius 1976). There you have an inherited defect of dynein sidearms of microtubules, abnormal ciliary movement and abnormal embryonic development giving rise to situs inversus which is associated with an increased predisposition to chronic obstructive pulmonary disease.

Silberberg: What is it that actually produces secretion from the cell—mechanically? Professor Reid spoke of the cell as being like a tube of toothpaste, but something has to squeeze the tube. Are microtubules or microfilaments involved in this?

Douglas: We should ask whether we are dealing here with an artifact. I am not sure whether there is such a thing as intracellular fusion of granules before secretion. Dr Kramer has shown us that in a preparation where there seemed to be intracellular fusion of granules, a different fixation procedure caused this to disappear and a more conventional picture then emerged. In my view the granules are not being squeezed out of the cell, but rather there is compound exocytosis of the sort I illustrated for mast cells and the 'cell surface' is coming to the granules.

Silberberg: But what brings the granule up to the cell membrane?

Douglas: The mast cells are so crammed with granules that they are almost touching the plasma membrane and each other. No migration is needed to expose the granule cores by compound exocytosis which involves a progressive inward fusion and fission of granule membranes.

Allison: We really know nothing about how these granules move to the upper surface of the cell where they accumulate. There may be active translocation or diffusion, and the granules may be guided by microtubules or even propelled by them.

Silberberg: These things are waiting for the opportunity to secrete so there is a stimulus but evidently we don't know what it is.

Allison: Once membrane fusion occurs, surface tension effects come in and gradually the membrane will be smoothed out and the granules will be released. We just don't know what event on the cell surface triggers off secretion. It could be depolarization, or it could be calcium ion accumulation by another mechanism.

Douglas: I doubt if it is depolarization in this exocrine gland; none of the other mammalian exocrine glands respond to depolarization.

Jeffery: It has been suggested that ammonia causes goblet cells on the surface epithelium to secrete. We have studies to indicate that, in the cat, these cells are not under neural control though there seems to be a species difference here. What actually causes that goblet cell to release its secretion?

Douglas: Calcium, of course! All effective physiological stimuli I believe introduce calcium into the cell or mobilize cellular calcium. You might find that ammonia does one or the other. I would like to learn what is known of the energetics of secretion of this cell and the involvement of calcium.

Allison: I should like to see the very simple experiment of just adding ionophores to some of these systems for a start. I don't think it has ever been done.

Silberberg: I cannot accept the idea that it is surface tension. We are dealing with a lipid bilayer of given area. The only way in which that could compress is by expelling membrane material. What must be happening is a sideward squeeze on the cell that causes it to elongate, thereby inverting the sac which has been formed and spurting out the contents. Later on vesicle formation may occur which interiorizes some of the lipid and restores lost cell volume. Alternatively there might be a sudden influx of water into the cell. This again would expel the contents of the sac without a decrease in bilayer area.

Allison: That is a perfectly good notion but it would be associated with changes in membrane permeability. Have you found any indication that this happens—perhaps by dilution of cytoplasmic contents?

Reid: You lose the top half of the cell. In organ culture you can tell the cells that have secreted by their height. They don't fill up and stay big pale cells; they become small cells.

Allison: A third possibility is that some active contractile system is involved and it would be interesting to see whether there is any effect from cytochalasin D, which unlike cytochalasin B does not block transport of sugars and amino sugars across the plasma membrane.

Richardson: You asked whether ionophores caused secretion in these mucous cells. Kim Balfre (personal communication) has put a calcium ionophore, A 23187, into a segment of hen trachea suspended in the organ bath and has found that it does cause secretion.

Allison: This may be similar to Professor Douglas's situation where decreasing the extracellular free calcium level tends to make the plasma membrane permeable, or it could arise from an intracellular source of calcium or something like that. Professor Douglas, how would you set about finding out what it is that triggers secretion in these cells? We have heard about the ionophore experiments and the EGTA experiments; what would you do next?

Douglas: The most obvious gambit is to look at the energetics of the situation to see whether, as in other cells, this is a secretory process which requires ATP. I am still disturbed by the suggestion that the cell is getting smaller after secretion. If the compound exocytotic mechanism were operating in the cell, the cell surface should be enormously increased. I am trying to fit this cell into a general pattern with which I am familiar.

Jeffery: The answer is the difference between merocrine secretion and apocrine secretion. In the cells that Professor Reid was referring to it was obviously an apocrine secretion. There was a massive discharge involving both membrane and cell content and this is why the cell was getting smaller.

Douglas: What is the conventional thinking now on apocrine secretion? How does the cell surface re-form?

Jeffery: I don't know.

Reid: I don't think we know but one idea which comes from freeze–fracture work is that in the mucous cell not every granule on the surface pops; perhaps only one of them does. If that is so, there may literally be a collapse from the lateral walls inwards into space which is left; the whole of the cell top is not opening up and bursting out. A lot of the contents are lost but what I am suggesting is that thanks to your compound exocytosis the secretion gets out through what is now a continuous tube. And as that happens the cell collapses inwards.

Allison: The trouble with the toothpaste model is that it leaves so much membrane unaccounted for. I believe that a kind of waist forms at the middle of the cell where there is fusion of apposed plasma membranes. The surface part is shed while the lower part is retained. There must be fusion.

Reid: The cell doesn't die; that is the first thing to be clear about. It used to be said that the goblet cell died when it discharged—it doesn't.

Douglas: I couldn't be happy with this explanation until I had evidence that the cell was losing cytoplasm. You say it is, and the morphologists used to say that it occurred, but what is the chemical evidence? What cytoplasmic material is being lost? Without evidence of such loss I can't subscribe to apocrine secretion.

References

AFZELIUS, B. A. (1976) A human syndrome caused by immotile cilia. *Science (Wash. D.C.) 193*, 317–318

BERG, N. B. & YOUNG, R. W. (1971) Sulfate metabolism in pancreatic acinar cells. *J. Cell Biol. 50*, 469–483

JAMIESON, J. D. & PALADE, G. E. (1971) Condensing vacuole conversion and zymogen granule discharge in pancreatic exocrine cells. Metabolic studies. *J. Cell Biol. 48*, 503–522

MEYER, F. A., KING, M. & GELMAN, R. A. (1975) On the role of sialic acid in the rheological properties of mucus. *Biochim. Biophys. Acta 392*, 223–232

REGIO, H. & PALADE, G. E. (1976) Sulfated compounds in the secretion and zymogen granule content of the guinea pig pancreas. *J. Cell Biol. 70*, 360A

WISSIG, S. L. & SATIR, B. (1976) Ionophore-induced secretion in *Tetrahymena*. *J. Cell Biol. 70*, 172A

Structure and function of mucus

F. A. MEYER and A. SILBERBERG

Weizmann Institute of Science, Rehovot, Israel

Abstract A glycoprotein building block is common to mammalian mucins. This structure is composed of several protein chains having the same sequence. The carbohydrate side chains, which constitute over three-quarters of the weight, coat only some two-thirds of the backbone chain. The bare protein chains are linked by disulphide bridges and can be digested away with trypsin. Either procedure rapidly solubilizes mucus and results in a structural unit of about 500 000 molecular weight. Mucus solubilizes spontaneously. The first size unit which reaches solution is about 15×10^6 molecular weight but continues to break down further. Mechanical agitation considerably speeds up this process. The gel-like character which is an essential feature of mucus—which cannot otherwise act as transport coupler—is thus a transient phenomenon. The problem of how such a structure can arise from the building blocks known to be available is discussed.

Most secretory mucociliary epithelia play an important role in the transport of material over their surface. Most such epithelia, moreover, are very similar in structure. It is reasonable to assume therefore that this similarity is strong and fundamental enough for studies and information obtained on one system to be applied to other mucosae.

The means to test this research approach was provided by Sadé *et al.* (1970). It was demonstrated, using detached frog's palate, that the depletion of mucus from the epithelium prevented transport of particle loads over the mucosa even though cilia continued to beat actively. Restoration of the mucus to the epithelium by mechanically replacing it restored the ability of the epithelium to effect transport. Moreover, recovery of transport velocity was complete, with the particles moving as fast as on the freshly excised palate. Other epithelia, for example excised trachea, could be shown to act similarly. A depleted frog's palate was thus a means of testing whether a given system could replace mucus (and to what extent) in its role as mechanical coupler.

Sadé *et al.* (1970) then established, in confirmation of the basic working hypothesis, that mucus samples from different epithelia all restored transport although not necessarily to the same velocity. Moreover, King *et al.* (1974) could show that aqueous systems, based on completely synthetic macromolecules, would also function as mechanical couplers provided that the macromolecular species was capable of cross-linking and was present in sufficiently high concentration to give an incipient gel.

While the special rheological properties of mucus were thus not necessarily linked to the glycoprotein character of its biopolymeric component—not, at least, the property of mucus for acting as a mechanical coupler in transport—biochemical evidence accumulated, again in keeping with and in confirmation of our basic working hypothesis, that the composition and size of the characteristic glycoprotein from various mammalian sources was common to many mucociliary secretions (Meyer *et al.* 1973; Meyer 1976, 1977). It also became clear that while mucus is secreted in a form which gives it the needed gel-like properties, this structural arrangement is not its equilibrium character (Meyer 1976), but is a consequence of the way it was synthesized and/or secreted by the cell. Mucus, left to itself, will in time spontaneously lose its gel character and go into solution, and then relax into a form in which it no longer acts as a mechanical coupler (Meyer 1976; Silberberg *et al.* 1977). Mechanical agitation can also disperse normal mucus without breakage of covalent bonds (Robson *et al.* 1975).

Some of the things that mucus does and is are thus relatively well understood (Gilboa & Silberberg 1976). Many of the most important details, however, still escape us. It is the purpose of this paper to try to assess what is known. In this we shall continue to take the view that epithelial mucins from mammalian sources are very similar and that epithelial secretions which are mucus-like in character have similar properties and are based on similar structural units.

THE GLYCOPROTEIN OF MUCUS AND MUCUS STRUCTURE

It is today fairly well established that there is one dominant glycoprotein species which gives mucus its special character (Meyer *et al.* 1973, 1977; Hatcher & Jeanloz 1974*a*; Allen *et al.* 1976; Gibbons & Glover 1959; Roberts 1974; Bushana Rao & Masson 1977; Litt *et al.* 1974). It seems, moreover, that the composition and structure of this material is rather similar when isolated from different mucociliary secretions. Characteristically, mucociliary glycoproteins are made up of a protein backbone with short sugar side chains linked to serine and threonine (Meyer *et al.* 1977; Hatcher & Jeanloz 1974*a*; Degand *et al.* 1973; Roberts 1974). The sugar side chain distribution over the protein core is such as to give rise to a sugar-rich and a sugar-poor section (Gelman & Vered 1976; Masson 1973; Hatcher & Jeanloz 1974*b*; Scawen & Allen 1975; Roberts 1976). For bovine cervical mucin, for example, the sugar side chains seem to involve some nine monosaccharide residues with average composition: sialic acid, 1; fucose, 1; galactose, 3; *N*-acetylglucosamine, 2; *N*-acetylgalactosamine 2, with sialic acid and fucose as terminal units (Meyer *et al.* 1977).

Various studies in our laboratory (Meyer 1976; Silberberg *et al.* 1977) and elsewhere (Allen *et al.* 1976; Bushana Rao & Masson 1977; Hatcher & Jeanloz 1974*a*) show that a fundamental glycoprotein building block is involved. The molecular weight of this glycoprotein has been reported to be about 2 million (Allen *et al.* 1976). This molecular entity is thought to be composed of several glycoprotein molecules of about 500 000 mol. wt. held together by disulphide bridges. Solubilization of mucus by disulphide bond breakage is thus due to a 'crumbling' of the fundamental structural unit rather than a breakdown of a true covalently bonded network.

Treatment with dithiothreitol (DTT) followed by carboxymethylation gave a soluble stable glycoprotein material which could be separated from proteins by CsCl density gradient centrifugation. Materials from several sources were tested, including mucus from the middle ear. It was found that good separations were obtained for all mammalian source materials by gradients derived from an initial density of 1.42 g/ml. For subsequent analysis material recovered between 1.43 and 1.57 g/ml was used (Meyer 1976, 1977).

Bovine cervical mucin so prepared still contained some unreduced disulphide bonds which could, however, be cleaved when the material was treated with performic acid. Table 1 compares the sedimentation coefficients of materials so obtained with those treated with DTT only (Meyer 1977).

The banding of these preparations on a CsCl gradient results in a distribution

TABLE 1

Effect of total cleavage of disulphide bonds

Mucin	*Sedimentation coefficient* ($s^{0}_{20,w}$)	
	After DTT only	*After DTT and performic acid*
Bovine cervix (oestrus)	26.0	12.3
Human ear	11.8	12.5
Human lung	10.7	11.1

which is practically identical for all mammalian glycoproteins. The glycoproteins moreover have similar amino acid and carbohydrate compositions.

The sugar side chains however are unevenly distributed over the protein core. This can be shown in several ways, for example by analysing the cyanogen bromide peptides from cervical mucin. One of the peptides so obtained has a particularly low sugar content (Hatcher & Jeanloz 1974*b*); Gelman & Vered 1976). It turns out, moreover, that trypsin solubilizes mucus (Gibbons & Mattner 1967), leaving mainly a glycoprotein of molecular weight very similar to that of the reduced fundamental unit obtained by total disulphide cleavage (Allen *et al.* 1976). For example, we find that, with bovine cervical mucin after trypsin digestion, the sedimentation coefficient is 13.8S (compare Table 1) and is unaltered if the trypsin digest is further treated with DTT. Bushana Rao & Masson (1977), who have been working on the same mucin, have determined amino acid composition and terminal (N and C) amino acid placements, and have partially sequenced the two trypsin peptides obtained. It turns out that the heavy peptide contains practically all the carbohydrate and the small peptide practically all the cysteine. There is only one N-terminal amino acid (Ala) which suggests a unique protein sequence and a single chain type. From the number of N-terminal groups found, this chain is apparently only 68 amino acid residues long and has a molecular weight of 30 000, close to 80% of which is carbohydrate. After trypsin digestion, the part of the protein backbone to which the carbohydrate attaches is reduced to some 42 amino acids. The peptide which has been detached is almost free of carbohydrate and represents only 8% of the total molecular weight.

It will be noted that there is a large discrepancy between a molecular weight of 30 000 and the value of 500 000 which is found by physical chemical characterization. Since Bushana Rao & Masson (1977) also find a unit of 500 000 by equilibrium centrifugation they suggest that this is an aggregate made up of the 30 000 molecular weight units. However, it seems unlikely that this is a consequence of hydrophobic bonding, as they suggest, since we do not find a change in the physical properties when the measurements are made in strong dissociating agents such as 6M-guanidinium HCl or 1% sodium dodecyl sulphate (Meyer 1976; Meyer *et al.* 1977). Their suggestion that bonds between the sugar side chains could hold the structure together is most interesting.

A basic chemical unit of some 70 amino acids has some very interesting features. It would contain one methionine, one tyrosine and one lysine residue. It is thus the minimal, unique chain length which can be constructed. It contains two cysteine residues, both in the region not covered by carbohydrate side chains, which again is the minimum number required to tie the chains together by interchain disulphide bonds. On the other hand, one may question the need for disulphide bridges when the structure is in any case already tied together. It is therefore of interest to discuss mucus structure from another point of view—that of the gel-like network which characterizes the freshly secreted system.

PHYSICOCHEMICAL CHARACTERIZATION OF THE MOLECULAR ENTITIES WHICH CONSTITUTE MUCUS

As already described, mucus, in the form secreted, possesses a gel-like character but not as a result of a macroscopic, three-dimensional network of covalent bonds. The glycoprotein moiety which is held together by disulphide bonds is large and very effectively entangled. These entanglements are hard to break and even at 40 °C we find that it takes more than one day to obtain a soluble product. At lower temperatures much longer times are required for the disentanglement process and at close to 0 °C mucus can be stored for long periods without a noticeable change in properties. The process can be speeded up considerably by raising the temperature to, say, 60 °C, or by stirring. The first molecular entity into solution obtained by stirring does not seem to differ from that obtained by thermal degradation alone, judging by sedimentation coefficient and intrinsic viscosity. Moreover, subsequent treatment with DTT and performic acid leads to the same product, which has a molecular weight of about 500 000. From the angular dependence of light scattering, the radius of gyration of this product is 57 ± 10 nm and it seems to be rather rod-like in character. This is in reasonable agreement with figures for a rod-like model where the intrinsic viscosity corresponds to a radius of gyration of about 49 nm and the sedimentation coefficient to a radius of 46 nm.

The molecular weight of the first molecularly disperse unit into which the system disentangles is about 15×10^6 (from light scattering and from sedimentation and viscosity: Meyer 1976; Silberberg *et al.* 1977). The angular dependence of light scattering corresponds to a radius of gyration of about 210 nm and the structure is that of an extended coil. This is confirmed by interpreting the intrinsic viscosity and sedimentation coefficient as either a coil or a rod. The estimates so obtained lie either side of the value of 210 nm. It is most interesting that a molecular weight of some 15×10^6 is also the estimate for the size of the structural unit derived from the value of the elastic modulus. This result agrees extremely well moreover with the result, 10×10^6, calculated by Lee *et al.* (1977) from their analysis of bovine cervical mucus by laser light scattering spectroscopy.

The breakdown of this unit can be monitored by following the changes in specific viscosity as a function of time and temperature. An activation energy of some 30 kcal/mol (126 kJ/mol) is obtained for the process. The kinetics of breakdown do not change when the study is performed in 6M-guanidinium hydrochloride or in sodium dodecyl sulphate (SDS). Hence it is very unlikely that secondary bonds are being broken in the process. It also makes it most unlikely that an enzymic process is involved. Most proteins denature in this kind of environment and so presumably would an enzyme had one been involved. The intrinsic viscosity study can, moreover, be extended to 60 °C with no change in activation energy and the same kinetics. Few enzymes would withstand such high temperatures without denaturation. All the evidence points to a very complex macromolecular unit which is capable of particularly effective entanglement. Dissolution of mucus by breaking disulphide bonds is thus an indirect attack on the structural network in that this action destroys the aggregates from which it is built.

RHEOLOGICAL REQUIREMENTS FOR MUCUS

We have already indicated that non-mucus systems as well as mucus systems are capable of restoring transport on the depleted frog palate. Several non-mucus systems were tested and the ratio of the velocity to which transport was restored by the system to the velocity of normal transport was evaluated. With guaran, a plant galactomannan, we did a systematic study and measured this ratio as a function of guaran concentration. No effect is observed below the gel point, but almost complete restoration of transport is obtained over a range of concentrations just above the gelation point. If the consistency of the gel is increased beyond that range, however, the added 'mucus' acts less and less as a mechanical coupler and becomes more and more the load. Hence in a given system, including mucus itself, there exists an optimum for transport function; if mucus flows too thinly or is too highly consistent, clearance will suffer (King *et al.* 1974; Sadé *et al.* 1975).

We have investigated this question by testing bovine cervical mucus on the frog's palate after introducing additional cross-links using glutaraldehyde. At the same time the rheological properties, notably the dynamic storage modulus G′, were measured at a frequency of about 1 Hz. Whereas the unmodified mucus restored transport to about 30%, an optimum of 70% could be attained by increased cross-linking. This corresponded to a G′ value of about 2 dynes/cm^2 (2×10^{-5} N/cm^2) (Silberberg *et al.* 1977) as compared with 1 dyne/cm^2 (1×10^{-5} N/cm^2) for unmodified mucus (Eliezer 1974). The optimum velocity ratio attained is thus still below that given by frog's mucus, showing that mucus function is presumably dictated not only by an increase in number of cross-links but also by the manner in which they are introduced and arranged.

Rheologically speaking, this implies that a system which functions as mucus must possess a significant number of relaxation mechanisms with very long time constants. In practical terms, these are time constants at least 10 times larger than the period of the ciliary beat. A material having such characteristics would store energy elastically during its contact with the beating cilium, whereas it would be capable of relaxation and flow given longer periods of time. On the other hand, if we take into consideration that mucus has to be secreted and spread over the surface of the epithelium, this would be impossible were it a fully developed gel with an 'infinite' network involving 'infinite' relaxation times.

The structure of mucus is changing all the time, probably from the moment of secretion. There is first a building up and then a gradual loss of gel-like properties. Hence the questions of major interest are how mucus, which is stored in granules in the cell, is converted into a transient gel in the course of secretion, and how the covalently linked units, which may be of about 2×10^6 molecular weight and are most likely only entangled, nevertheless undergo such a very slow structural relaxation. How can we make these requirements consistent with what we now know about the chemical structure? Finally, can we understand what function this structure serves in addition to those already recognized?

DISCUSSION

It seems almost certain that the transient mucus structure will be found to possess unusual features. The building blocks must be elongated in order to form a gel at a low (1 mg/ml) glycoprotein concentration. These requirements are not unreasonable for the 500 000 molecular weight fundamental unit if it is considered as one chain, but some special assumptions are needed if the unit is only of 30 000 molecular weight. In whatever way the unit is constituted, it is not unreasonable to think that the bare protein portion, which contains the cysteine, is folded into a special conformation by intramolecular disulphide bonds to constitute a mechanical structure which has the ability to create the long-lived links.

Specifically this could be a ring structure, or a loop, in which other entities, particularly the sugar-rich portions, are caught. These could be envisaged as barbed structures whose release by thermal agitation would be a very slow process. Opening up the ring or loop by breaking the disulphide bonds or digesting the entire ring or loop away by trypsin would, however, give a very fast response.

Clearly, these are speculations. Even if they are in accord with the features of the system as we have come to know them, our information in this area is far too poor as yet to take it any further. Compared with the state of affairs of only a few years ago, however, enormous strides have been made.

ACKNOWLEDGEMENT

The results quoted derive in part from work supported by Grant No. NS 10048 from the National Institutes of Health, USA.

References

ALLEN, A., PAIN, R. H. & ROBSON, T. R. (1976) Model for the structure of the gastric mucus gel. *Nature (Lond.) 264*, 88

BUSHANA RAO, K. S. P. & MASSON, P. L. (1977) A tentative model for the structure of bovine oestrus cervical mucin, in *Mucus in Health and Disease* (Elstein, M. & Parke, D., eds.), Plenum Press, London

DEGAND, R., ROUSSEL, P., LAMBLIN, G., DURAND, G. & HAVEZ, R. (1973) Données biochimiques et rhéologiques dans l'expectoration. *Bull. Physio-Pathol. Respir. 9*, 199

ELIEZER, N. (1974) Viscoelastic properties of mucus. *Biorheology 11*, 61

GELMAN, R. A. & VERED, J. (1976) Cyanogen bromide fragments of bovine cervical mucus. *Biochim. Biophys. Acta 427*, 627

GIBBONS, R. A. & GLOVER, F. A. (1959) The physicochemical properties of two mucoids from bovine cervical mucin. *Biochem. J. 73*, 217

GIBBONS, R. A. & MATTNER, P. (1967) Some aspects of the chemistry of cervical mucus, in *Fertility and Sterility*, Proceedings of the Fifth World Congress, Stockholm 1966 (Eds. B. Westin and N. Wiqvist). ICS no. 133, p. 695, Excerpta Medica, Amsterdam

GILBOA, A. & SILBERBERG, A. (1976) Characterization of epithelial mucus and its function in clearance by ciliary propulsion, in *Air Pollution and The Lung* (Aharonson, E. F. *et al.*, eds.), p. 49, Wiley, New York

HATCHER, V. B. & JEANLOZ, R. W. (1974*a*) The use of glycosidases in the structure elucidation of the carbohydrate chain of alpha-acid glycoprotein from *Macacca radiata*, in *Methodologie de la Structure et du Métabolisme des Glyconjugés*. Centre National de la Recherche Scientifique No. 221, p. 329, Paris

HATCHER, V. B. & JEANLOZ, R. W. (1974*b*) Studies on cyanogen bromide fragments from monkey cervical glycoprotein, in *Methodologie de la Structure et du Métabolisme des Glyconjugés*, Centre National de la Recherche Scientifique No. 221, p. 381, Paris

KING, M., GILBOA, A., MEYER, F. A. & SILBERBERG, A. (1974) On the transport of mucus and its rheological simulants in systems. *Am. Rev. Respir. Dis. 110*, 740

LEE, W. I., VERDUGO, P., BLANDAU, R. J. & GADDUM-ROSSE, P. (1977) Molecular arrangement of cervical mucus: a re-evaluation based on laser light-scattering spectroscopy. (Personal communication.)

LITT, M., KHAN, M. A., CHAKRIN, L. W., WARDELL, J. R. & CHRISTIAN, P. (1974) The viscoelasticity of fractionated canine tracheal mucus. *Biorheology 11*, 111

MASSON, P. L. (1973) Carbohydrate component of cervical mucus, in *Cervical Mucus in Human Reproduction* (Elstein, M. *et al.*, eds.), p. 82, Scriptor, Copenhagen

MEYER, F. A. (1976) Mucus structure, relation to biological transport function. *Biorheology 13*, 49

MEYER, F. A. (1977) Comparison of structural glycoproteins from mucus of different sources. *Biochim. Biophys. Acta*, in press

MEYER, F. A., ELIEZER, N., SILBERBERG, A., VERED, J., SHARON, N. & SADÉ, J. (1973) An approach to the biochemical basis for the transport function of epithelial mucus. *Bull. Physio-Pathol. Respir. 9*, 259

MEYER, F. A., VERED, J. & SHARON, N. (1977) Studies of glycoproteins from mammalian mucociliary secretions, in *Mucus in Health and Disease* (Elstein, M. & Parke, D., eds.), Plenum Press, London

ROBERTS, G. P. (1974) Isolation and characterization of glycoproteins from sputum. *Eur. J. Biochem. 50*, 265

ROBERTS, G. P. (1976) The role of disulfide bonds in maintaining the gel structure of bronchial mucus. *Arch. Biochem. Biophys. 173*, 528

ROBSON, T., ALLEN, A. & PAIN, R. H. (1975) Non-covalent forces hold glycoprotein molecules together in mucus gel. *Biochem. Soc. Trans. 3*, 1105

SADÉ, J., ELIEZER, N., SILBERBERG, A. & NEVO, A. C. (1970) The role of mucus in transport by cilia. *Am. Rev. Respir. Dis. 102*, 48

SADÉ, J., MEYER, F. A., KING, M. & SILBERBERG, A. (1975) Clearance of middle ear effusions by the mucociliary system. *Acta Oto-Laryngol. 79*, 277

SCAWEN, M. & ALLEN, A. (1975) The digestion of the glycoprotein from pig gastric mucus with pepsin and other proteolytic enzymes. *Biochem. Soc. Trans. 3*, 1107

SILBERBERG, A., MEYER, F. A., GILBOA, A. & GELMAN, R. A. (1977) Function and properties of epithelial mucus, in *Mucus in Health and Disease* (Elstein, M. & Parke, D., eds.), Plenum Press, London

Discussion

Phelps: Are the properties of your system fully dependent on having four pairs of disulphide bonds? Is it an all-or-nothing type of phenomenon which functions best in a high state of 'orderedness'?

Silberberg: No, not at all! It can be done with zero interchain disulphide bonds as well. What is needed is an interaction, an entanglement, between the covalently intact structural units which requires no bonding but will take a very long time to come apart. This interaction must, moreover, be such that on disulphide bond breakage or trypsin digestion the constraint is removed and the interaction is almost instantly broken.

Let us assume for a moment that the 500 000 molecular weight unit contains only a single peptide chain. Its structure could then be something like Fig. 1 (below). The carbohydrate-rich region constitutes some two-thirds of the chain, but the bare protein part contains practically all the cysteine. It could, therefore, form the ring shown by intramolecular disulphide bridges. A network could be built up if the bristly carbohydrate-rich region were threaded through one, two or more rings. Threading one ring over a carbohydrate-rich region gives only an elongation of the chain but threading two or more rings constitutes a branch or a cross-link (see Fig. 1b). If the covalently linked structural unit is larger than 500 000 molecular weight, being composed, say, of four of

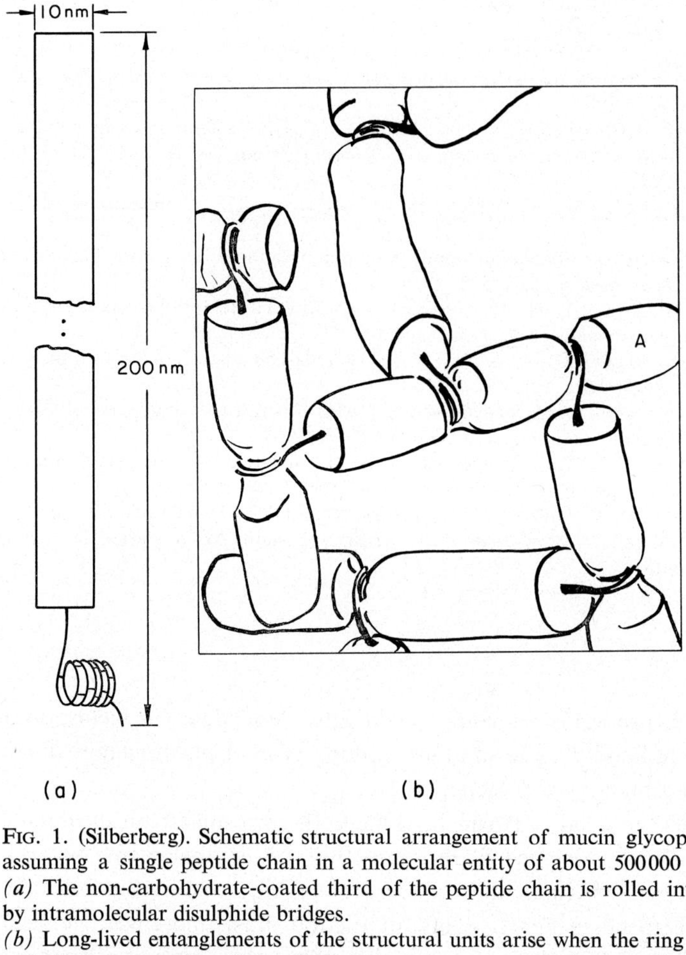

(a) (b)

FIG. 1. (Silberberg). Schematic structural arrangement of mucin glycoprotein (speculative, assuming a single peptide chain in a molecular entity of about 500000 molecular weight).
(a) The non-carbohydrate-coated third of the peptide chain is rolled into a ring stabilized by intramolecular disulphide bridges.
(b) Long-lived entanglements of the structural units arise when the ring is slipped over the carbohydrate-coated section. Cross-links arise, as at A, when two rings are slipped over the same chain.

the chains in Fig. 1a, the four carbohydrate-bare regions could be combined by disulphide bonds into one ring. This would give a unit of about 2×10^6 molecular weight as proposed by Scawen & Allen (1975). The same threading process could build up networks in this case as well.

I would like to stress however that I would not like Fig. 1 to be taken too seriously. It should be regarded as a pure speculation but as one which possesses the required features. Unthreading would indeed be a very slow process. Each sugar side chain would have to undergo a rather specific conformational collapse before the ring could move up or down the chain by one unit. On the other hand, breakage of disulphide bonds would, as required, rapidly open the rings. Trypsin digestion would, similarly, cut them off near the start of the carbohydrate-rich region. In either case there would be an almost instant resolution of the entanglement and release of the subunit.

Kent: How far is it essential to this interpretation that all the carbohydrate lies in one block, as indicated by your diagram?

Silberberg: This would obviously not be necessary but it is a fairly well established fact which was incorporated into the model.

Kent: Is there just one polysaccharide, not a series of oligosaccharides?

Silberberg: There seems to be only one important protein backbone chain. There could be and most likely is microheterogeneity in the length and composition of the sugar side chain. In bovine cervical mucin, however—and here I am quoting Bushana Rao & Masson (1977)—there is only one N-terminal and one C-terminal amino acid: alanine and leucine, respectively. The numbers of both these terminal amino acids tend to indicate that the molecular weight associated with each peptide chain is about 30 000, corresponding to some 68 amino acids. On the assumption of a single unique amino acid sequence this corresponds to one methionine, one tyrosine, one phenylalanine and one lysine per chain. A chain of some 70 amino acids is thus the shortest unique sequence which could be constructed, given the amino acid composition.

Kent: So it is a carbohydrate-enriched part of the peptide chain, as Masson showed. It must be a polyanion of considerable magnitude, and interaction between these will be a feature of the cooperativity of the molecule.

Silberberg: The glycoprotein is indeed a polyanion but it is not this feature of its structure which seems to be important. The difficulty which we have with this molecule is concerned with the number of peptide chains which constitute one covalently linked molecular entity. Even after total disulphide bond cleavage the molecular weight of the glycoprotein in solution is about 500 000. This is not only our finding but is also what Bushana Rao & Masson (1977) and everyone else so far has obtained. There would be no difficulty with this result if the peptide chain and its carbohydrate side chains looked like Fig. 1a, but according to Bushana Rao & Masson (1977) it looks like Fig. 2a (below). Some 20 of these units must therefore be linked together, say, as in Fig. 2b. Disulphide bridges are, as indicated in Fig. 2b, involved in this structure but disulphide bridges (reaction at points 1 in Fig. 2a) cannot be the only internal cross-links which exist. If this were the case dissolution of the disulphide bonds would result in the liberation of the 30 000 molecular weight moiety (Fig. 2a), which is not what is found. We must assume therefore that there are other interactions, say, the carbohydrate-to-carbohydrate linkages

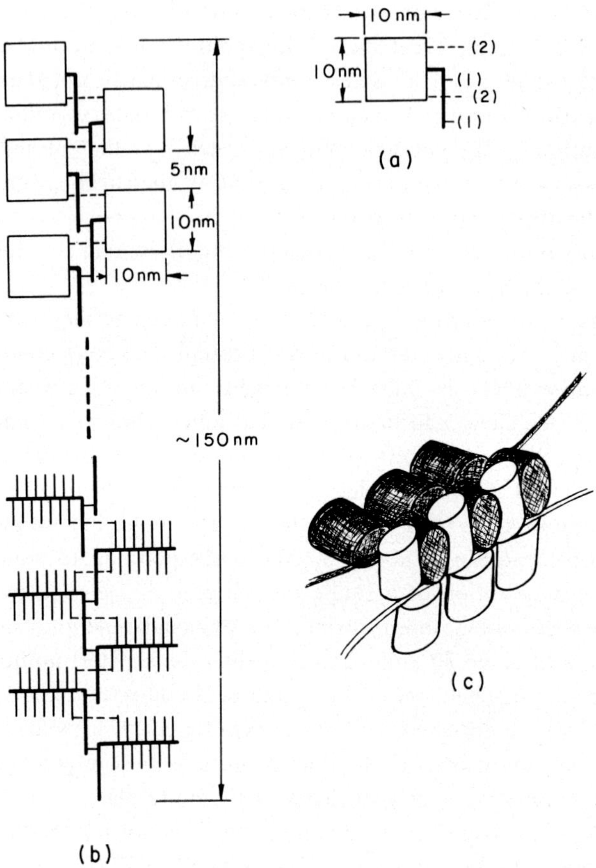

FIG. 2. (Silberberg). Schematic structural arrangement of mucin glycoprotein (speculative, assuming that each peptide chain is associated with a molecular weight of 30 000).
(a) The structure associated with each peptide chain. Two disulphide bridges can arise at points (1). Carbohydrate-to-carbohydrate linkages arise at (2).
(b) Proposed assembly of a 500 000 molecular weight unit using both disulphide bridges and carbohydrate-to-carbohydrate linkages. It is assumed that a fairly stiff backbone is formed and that free spaces arise between the tufts of carbohydrate-coated side structures.
(c) 'Zipping' together two chains such as (b) produces long-lived entanglement cross-links.

mentioned by Dr Allison, which occur at points such as (2) in Fig. 2a. These would have to parallel the disulphide bridges. Bushana Rao & Masson (1977) have suggested that hydrophobic bonding is involved. We find, however, that working in 6M-guanidinium-HCl, or in 1% sodium dodecyl sulphate, has no effect on the stability of the glycoprotein. Hence we favour the carbohydrate-to-carbohydrate bonds. Moreover there must be some structural involvement of the disulphide bonds. Their presence as shown in Fig. 2b would considerably stiffen the assembly and one might then conceive of the 'zipper'-like engagement (shown in Fig. 2c) as being the mechanism by which the units (Fig. 2b) would interact and entangle. Disulphide bond breakage, or trypsin digestion, would in this case produce a 'floppy' chain, held together by the carbohydrate-to-carbohydrate bonds only. Interactions of the type in Fig. 2c would therefore be broken. Again it is important to stress that we have no direct evidence that a structure like Fig. 2b really exists or that interactions of the type in Fig. 2c occur. This model is only intended to set out ideas and illustrate what kind of situation might satisfy the known facts.

Kent: Certainly it is an extremely important proposition. In the general properties and the spontaneous loss, how much variation is there between one preparation and another?

Silberberg: I presume that your question refers to variability between the properties of various mucus secretions. If there is indeed one structural unit common to most mammalian mucins, as Meyer (1977) suggests, are the properties of the secretions also comparable? There is some evidence that they are. We (Silberberg *et al.* 1977) have looked at the dynamic shear modulus of bovine cervical mucus. Litt (1977) has done similar work on respiratory mucus. Under similar test conditions we both find a result of about 0.1 N/m^2 (1 $dyne/cm^2$). We have both tried to modify the mucus and increase the number of cross-links. We have both tested these preparations for their ability to restore velocity of conveyance on the depleted frog palate and correlated this effect with changes in dynamic shear modulus. We both agree that the point of best transport lies at about 0.2 N/m^2. On the other hand frog mucus itself does better; we have looked at the rheological characteristics on the epithelium of the frog *in situ*, but have yet to do the dynamic test. Frog mucus has a much more gel-like character than the other secretions which we have looked at (Gilboa & Silberberg 1976); it also has a different composition (Meyer 1977). Perhaps only mammalian sources give mucus secretions that are very similar, and amphibian mucus may be different—it has far less sialic acid, less carbohydrate and a much more gel-like character than the mucus we have been comparing it with.

Reid: You were working with fresh bovine cervical mucus and Litt with reconstituted. Does reconstitution affect the viscoelastic properties of mucus?

Silberberg: Litt freezes and lyophilizes mucus, i.e. removes the water by sublimation, a mild technique which tends to leave structure fairly intact. Hence when water is restored the original structure may well be recovered.

Reid: To go back to the models, is there any evidence to favour one or the other?

Silberberg: No, but you must have an entanglement model consistent with the long time-scale. You recall that the DNA double helix can unravel very rapidly within the cell nucleus; a tremendous entanglement problem is here resolved in a fraction of a second and in a very confined space. In mucus, on the contrary, we have a lot of space—this is a very dilute system. As far as we can see, no hydrogen or hydrophobic bonds are involved which could delay matters, and the macromolecular entities are probably smaller; yet it takes a long time. Hence we have suggested the kind of interactions of Figs. 1 and 2. The interactions must, indirectly, involve the disulphide bridges, because they can be rapidly resolved if these bridges are broken. Trypsin, which detaches the bare peptide region from the glycosylated one, must have the same effect. Those are the starting elements with which one has to work. As already stressed, neither model is meant as a serious suggestion, but only as the kind of thing we should be looking for in a possible explanation.

Allison: Do chelators of divalent ions affect the rate of this process? Are calcium and magnesium ions involved, as they might be?

Silberberg: We haven't looked at that aspect as yet.

Guz: Can we deduce from your viscoelastic data what the optimum frequency of the ciliary beat might be? Presumably the ciliary beat is giving a regular rhythmic motion to the process.

Silberberg: Cilia beat about 1000 times a minute, corresponding to a frequency of about 17 cycles/s. Hence we have chosen this range of frequencies to see how mucus responds mechanically. In fact the elastic response of mucus increases rather rapidly in the region of 1 cycle/s so that at a frequency some ten times larger most of the mechanical relaxation mechanisms are too long-lived. Mucus, in other words, is responding elastically to the ciliary beat. We have, therefore, got about as much elasticity out of the system as it is capable of giving.

Guz: Do you accept the analogy that the beat may be imparting this cyclic force?

Silberberg: Very likely. The frequency of the beat is the characteristic frequency of the system. It is, of course, not a pure sinusoidal motion, so the beat will have other frequencies built into it. The fundamental beat frequency is clearly, however, the dominant frequency involved.

Allison: Could the nature of the mucus impose a restriction on the beat frequency of the cilia? Is there any indication of feed-back control of that sort?

Silberberg: We have looked at ciliary beat frequency as a function of depletion. Frequency goes down as depletion begins and in the frog it drops to about 50% of the initial frequency and then stays at that value, down to the point where one gets zero transport velocity (Gilboa & Silberberg 1975). So it doesn't really change all that much.

Moreover, cilia do not beat in mucus, but in a glycoprotein-free interciliary fluid. Nothing is really known about the rheological characteristics of this fluid. What we have done in this connection, however, is to change the viscosity of the environment in which cilia beat in tissue cultures of excised epithelia. Here we have an outgrowth of a monolayer of cells in a medium under our control, and can see the cilia very well under the microscope and measure the frequency of their beat. It is easy to change the environmental fluid and change its viscosity by adding macromolecules. We have used dextrans of various molecular weights. The molecular weight of the additive had no effect and only change in viscosity affected the ciliary beat. We had, however, to go up to very high viscosities—close to 0.1 N s m^{-2} (100 centipoises)—before ciliary beat frequency was reduced by a factor of 2. A dextran solution is potentially viscoelastic but at the frequencies of interest here it is predominantly viscous.

Davis: You find that ciliary beat doesn't change with changing viscosity and you have also shown with your synthetic molecule that changing the amount of water present with the molecule seems to change the physical properties. Do you think there is some property of the interaction of water with the mucin molecule or with your synthetic molecule that could regulate the transport properties of the system?

Silberberg: No, or not at any rate in a very direct way. A molecular structural feature will obviously be involved when we arrive at the final explanation of why the presence of mucus, or a substitute, which has a set of specified rheological properties (King *et al.* 1974), can translate ciliary beat (the metachronal wave) into the conveyance of loads. Before we can hope to find that explanation, however, we must be much clearer in our minds about the solution of the fluid mechanical problem and the features of the constitutive relationship of mucus which are essential. It is generally agreed that cilia are not actually moving within the mucus. We have shown, moreover, that mucus or its substitute must possess certain limited, gel-like characteristics. It is reasonable to assume, therefore, that mucus must react in an elastic, solid-like fashion with the ciliary wave. For this to occur there will have to arise certain interactions between the mucin molecules which will depend upon concentration and the presence, therefore, of an adequate amount of water. An aqueous environment may, in addition, be essential in order to produce the kind of interactions between mucin molecules in which we are interested. Moreover, when the amount and/or quality of the mucus declines the rate at which the load is carried along with the flow in the interciliary space is changed. However, since the nature of this mechanical effect is not understood, the manner in which mucus fails cannot properly be specified. It may well be that the effectiveness of the ciliary beat is impaired and that the effect of depletion is an indirect one.

Iravani: An increase in the viscosity of the interciliary fluid causes initially a decrease in the amplitude of the ciliary beat; the ciliary frequency remains fairly constant.

Sadoul: What is the influence of elasticity on transport by the cilia? You told us that viscosity may rise as high as 0.1 N s m^{-2} but do you keep the elasticity constant?

Silberberg: I would like to remind you that the fluid whose viscosity we were varying was the interciliary medium. Moreover, we were studying an artificial situation where there was no mucus blanket because our test systems were monolayers of cells and we were merely changing the viscosity of the culture medium and looking at the beat as cilia were moving in those media. In those circumstances we could increase the viscosity and in this way affect the beat frequency but, as Professor Iravani has pointed out, the amplitude could be changed by a much bigger margin than the frequency. We did not study amplitude. As I have already mentioned, the dextran solutions which we have used are probably not very 'elastic' at the frequencies of the ciliary beat.

References

BUSHANA RAO, K. S. P. & MASSON, P. L. (1977) A tentative model for the structure of bovine oestrus cervical mucin, in *Mucus in Health and Disease* (Elstein, M. & Parke, D. V., eds.), Plenum Press, London

GILBOA, A. & SILBERBERG, A. (1975) Characterization of epithelial mucus and its function in clearance by ciliary propulsion, in *Air Pollution and the Lung* (Aharonson, E. F. *et al.*, eds.), John Wiley, New York

GILBOA, A. & SILBERBERG, A. (1976) *In situ* rheological characterization of epithelial mucus. *Biorheology 13*, 59–65

KING, M., GILBOA, A., MEYER, F. A. & SILBERBERG, A. (1974) On the transport of mucus and its rheologic simulants in ciliated systems. *Am. Rev. Respir. Dis. 110*, 740–745

LITT, M. (1977) in *Mucus in Health and Disease* (Elstein, M. & Parke, D. V., eds.), Plenum Press, London

MEYER, F. A. (1977) Comparison of structural glycoproteins from mucus of different sources. *Biochim. Biophys. Acta, 493*, 272

SCAWEN, M. & ALLEN, A. (1975) The digestion of the glycoprotein from pig gastric mucin with pepsin and other proteolytic enzymes. *Biochem. Soc. Trans. 3*, 1107–1109

SILBERBERG, A., MEYER, F. A., GILBOA, A. & GELMAN, R. A. (1977) Function and properties of epithelial mucus, in *Mucus in Health and Disease* (Elstein, M. & Parke, D. V., eds.), Plenum Press, London

Nasal mucociliary clearance in man

DONALD F. PROCTOR*, G. KENNETH ADAMS*, IB ANDERSEN† and S. F. PAUL MAN†

** Department of Environmental Health Sciences, The Johns Hopkins School of Hygiene and Public Health, Baltimore, Maryland and † Institute of Hygiene, University of Aarhus, Aarhus, Denmark*

Abstract Nasal mucociliary clearance was measured in healthy young human subjects and tracheal clearance in the experimental animal under a wide variety of conditions. There is a broad range of clearance rates whether at standard ambient conditions (23° C, 50% relative humidity) or in the face of a number of environmental variables. The degree to which those differences are attributable to the effectiveness of ciliary beating or the character of airway secretions is not known. Studies of tracheobronchial secretions simultaneous with clearance measurement in the anaesthetized dog have not yet provided a definite answer. Variations in upper respiratory defence mechanisms may bear some relationship to the aetiology of small airway disease in the lungs.

The airways from nose or mouth to alveoli serve one main purpose, the exchange of oxygen and carbon dioxide between the ambient air and the blood. But that main purpose could not be effectively realized or long maintained were it not for the capacity of the airways to modify the physical condition of inspired air, cleanse it of impurities, protect their delicate alveolar terminations from airborne noxious materials, and continually clear their surfaces. In other words, under ideal circumstances, the respiratory tract makes it possible for us to enjoy the benefits of gaseous exchange while it prevents injury from toxic atmospheric influences. Unfortunately, the prevalence of airborne disease provides ample evidence that this physiological system of defences is not invulnerable.

Our investigations of respiratory defence mechanisms have been largely directed at the upper airways because, with nasal breathing, this is the region first exposed to the passage of ambient air. The fact that important defences

† *Present address:* Department of Medicine, University of Alberta, Edmonton, Alberta, Canada

of the lung lie in the nasal passages has been recognized for a long time, but the possible effects of impairment of those defences has received scant attention. The respiratory tract beyond the nasopharynx is a continuum from the point of view of inspired air and it is lined with a ciliated secretory epithelium comparable to that in the nose. Thus, it may not be unreasonable to draw some deductions regarding the lower airways from examination of the upper airway. The purpose of this paper is to summarize our findings and then to suggest that certain adverse changes in the small airways of the lung may be at least in part influenced by relative failure in upper airway defence mechanisms.

METHODS AND FINDINGS

During the past 15 years we have developed methods for studying nasal physiology, applied them to the establishment of normal values, and searched for factors adversely affecting normal function. We have used experimental animals (principally the dog), but have directed a large part of our effort towards the study of normal human volunteers in a climate chamber in Aarhus, Denmark. In those studies we have been able to keep most environmental parameters constant while measuring the effect of a single variable on function. Although we have investigated a number of factors, including nasal airflow resistance and inspired air modification, we have concentrated mainly on the exact measurement of nasal mucociliary clearance on the assumption that it may be an indicator of the efficacy of nasal physiology.

We have used a tagged particle technique to measure mucociliary clearance (Quinlan *et al.* 1969; Andersen *et al.* 1971). It yields highly accurate measures of clearance rate. During the past four years we have supplemented this with the saccharine method (Andersen *et al.* 1974*a*) which probably reflects some clearance in the superficial layer of periciliary fluid as well as mucus clearance. To what degree either method is comparable to the conventional aerosol method of measuring tracheobronchial clearance is not known.

The discovery of a wide range of nasal clearance rates led us to studies of tracheobronchial secretions and tracheal clearance (Proctor *et al.* 1973). These experiments were designed to yield data on the nature of normal airway secretions and to relate the nature of these secretions to efficiency of clearance. The technique has been fully described elsewhere (Adams *et al.* 1976). It involves collecting secretions in the upper trachea of dogs anaesthetized with intravenous pentobarbital (pentobarbitone) and breathing through the nose. It yields a measure of the quantity of fluid reaching that region per unit time from all parts of the lungs, and specimens for biochemical and rheological analysis. Particles are repeatedly placed in the lower trachea and their passage upwards is continuously tracked.

Not only is the nose the most accessible region of the airways, but it is also the region most immediately exposed to the vicissitudes of the ambient air and airborne disease. We therefore presume that the effects of environmental air are reflected there more than in the lower airways of the lung. In one of our early studies in man we defined normal function in the nasal passages in a controlled climate (Andersen *et al.* 1971). The average rate of nasal clearance is about 6 mm/min. In subsequent similar studies we measured changes in function associated with common variations in environmental air.

Our findings to date in healthy young adults are as follows:

1. Ambient humidity (9 to 70% relative humidity) in clean air at 23 °C has no effect on nasal mucociliary clearance (Andersen *et al.* 1974*b*).
2. Ambient temperature change either up or down from 23 °C (7 to 39 °C) is followed by a small reduction in nasal mucociliary clearance (Proctor *et al.* 1977).
3. Exposure to SO_2 as a gas in clean air for 3 h reduces nasal clearance at 1 part/10^6 and markedly impairs it at 5 parts/10^6 (Andersen *et al.* 1974*c*).
4. Our studies of exposure to inert particles and to SO_2 combined with particles (with and without vanadium added) have not yet been fully analysed. Preliminary analysis of the data indicates that particle exposure has no effect, and particles plus SO_2 (with or without vanadium) seem to have an effect similar to exposure to SO_2 alone.

In monozygotic twins (Andersen *et al.* 1974*d*) we have not found the similarity between twins in nasal clearance demonstrated by Camner for bronchial clearance (Camner *et al.* 1972). We found no correlation between nasal and bronchial clearance rates in the same individual (Andersen *et al.* 1974*c*); but, since the methods used in the nose differ from those used in measuring bronchial clearance, that observation may not be wholly justified. Laryngectomized patients, whose nasal passages have only a very limited exposure to ambient air, have average clearance rates higher than those found among healthy young adults (Quinlan *et al.* 1969; and unpublished data). Those findings are compatible with the hypothesis that, even among healthy young adults, some exhibit impaired nasal clearance which may be related to their years of exposure to the ubiquitous upper respiratory infection and the varied conditions of the ambient air. This degree of impairment in the young adult is apparently not sufficient to result in any obvious respiratory problems.

Perhaps our most interesting finding to date has been that, whereas among laryngectomized patients there is only a small variance in nasal clearance

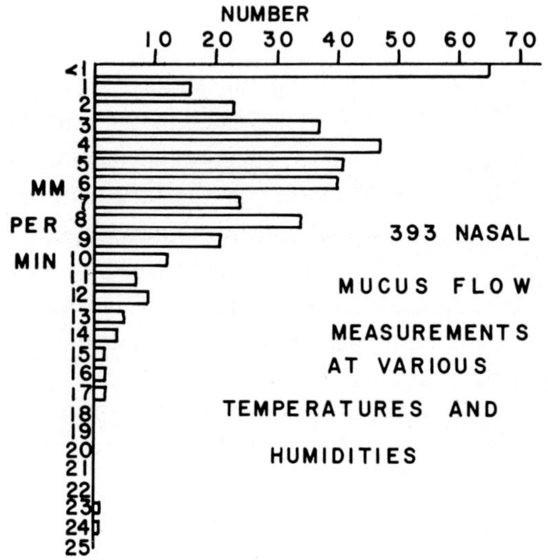

FIG. 1. Nasal mucociliary clearance rates found in our studies of 393 human subjects under various environmental conditions. (From Proctor 1977.)

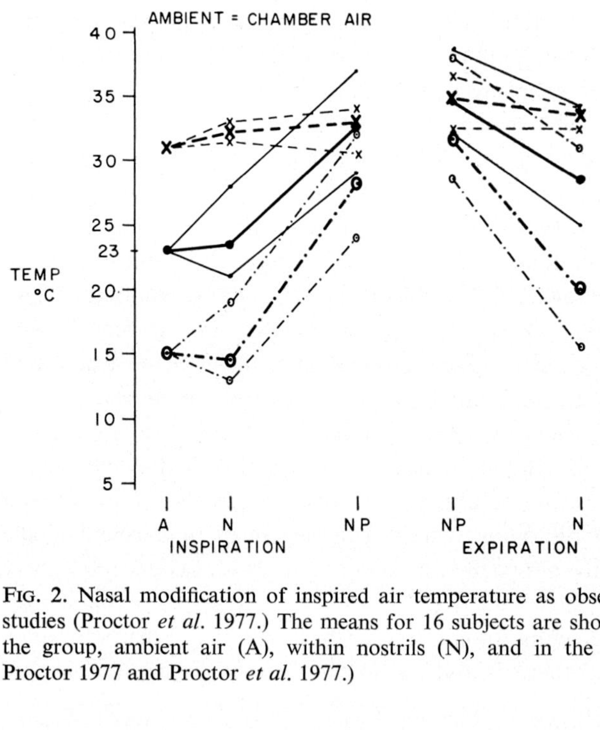

FIG. 2. Nasal modification of inspired air temperature as observed in one of the Aarhus studies (Proctor *et al.* 1977.) The means for 16 subjects are shown as well as the range for the group, ambient air (A), within nostrils (N), and in the nasopharynx (NP). (From Proctor 1977 and Proctor *et al.* 1977.)

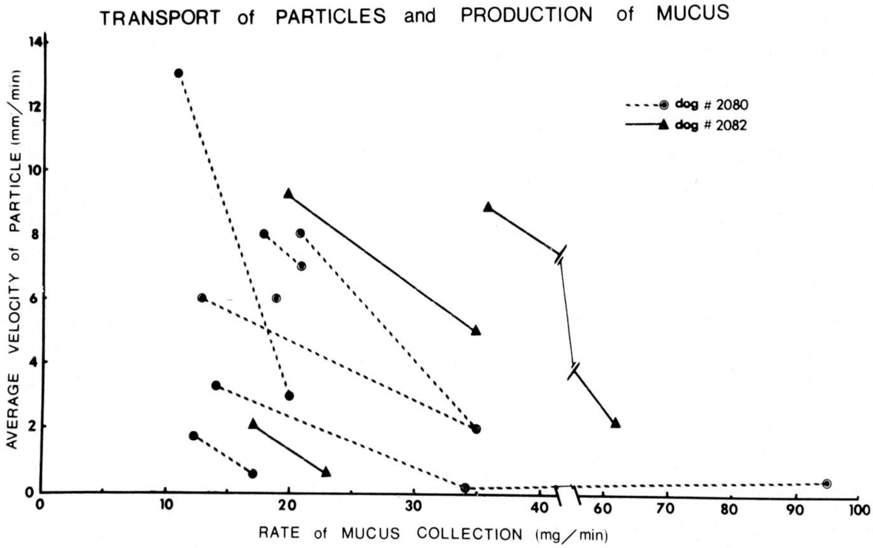

FIG. 3. Mucociliary clearance rate (vertical axis) in relation to secretion collection rate (horizontal axis) in the dog trachea. Repeated studies in two dogs are included. (From unpublished data from E. F. Aharonson and G. K. Adams.)

rates between individuals, in our healthy young adults (over 200 studied to date) nasal clearance varies between less than 1 mm/min and over 20 mm/min (Proctor 1977). Each individual has a fairly consistent rate characteristic of himself. The distribution of clearance rates is distinctly skewed, with about 20% of all healthy young subjects showing rates below 2 mm/min (Fig. 1). We have no data as yet on children, but are beginning work on them this year. That study should give us some indication of the relative importance of genetic and environmental influences in causing such variability in clearance rates.

It is of interest that the capacity of the nose to warm inspired air (Fig. 2) also varies among healthy young subjects (Proctor *et al.* 1977). It is probable that the efficiency of the nose in removing inhaled particles also significantly differs among healthy subjects.

When we investigated airway secretions in the dog, our first observation was that, in each dog, when the collection rate rose clearance rate fell. When methacholine was administered a marked increase in collection rate was accompanied by almost total stasis of surface particles (Fig. 3) (Adams *et al.* 1976). We have attributed these apparently paradoxical findings to increasing depth in the periciliary fluid and relative stasis in the mucus layer—now relatively remote from the cilia tips. In numerous instances we opened the trachea for direct observation. While surface particles were indeed seen to be motionless, a soluble dye placed lower down in the trachea could be seen to sweep upwards in the periciliary stream beneath the particles.

More recent studies of tracheobronchial secretions in the dog have involved measuring electrolyte concentrations and osmolarity. In the animals studied so far, the least variable characteristics have been the concentration of Na^+ and Cl^- ions and the osmolarity. The figures for all three have been higher than those for dog serum; and, in the face of a variety of changes in other constituents, they have remained remarkably constant from time to time and from dog to dog. When methacholine was administered the quantity of tracheobronchial fluid collected per unit time rose sharply and the protein concentration fell, but no significant alteration in Na^+ or Cl^- ions or in osmolarity occurred (G. K. Adams & S. F. P. Man, unpublished data).

We suspected that the high osmolarity was attributable to the contribution of surface water to inspired air humidification and we tested this hypothesis by allowing the dog to breathe through an oral airway instead of the nose. This resulted in an increase in osmolarity, suggesting that the tracheal epithelium may not be readily permeable to interstitial water.

From these data we tentatively conclude that water transport in the dog trachea *in vivo* is coupled with chloride and sodium transport but not with protein secretion. If isotonic transport of water is the mechanism by which water is moved from the interstitium to the airway surface, the site of that transport seems likely to be remote from the airway surface, perhaps in the mucous glands.

If current theories on mucociliary transport are correct it would appear that control of the exact depth of periciliary fluid, so that it reaches a level just below the tips of fully extended cilia, is one of the important factors in clearance of mucus and surface particles. We suggest that a chloride and/or sodium pump, perhaps located in the serous cells or in cells in the ducts of mucous glands, and combined with a tracheal surface epithelium relatively impermeable to water, may be important factors in the control of the depth of periciliary fluid. The high osmolarity of tracheal secretions may be attributable to the contribution of this region to humidification of inspired air. But these suggestions must remain hypothetical until further data are accumulated.

SPECULATIONS FOR FUTURE INVESTIGATION

To guide future investigations it may be fruitful to indulge in some purely speculative comments stemming from certain widely accepted facts. The fluids lining the respiratory tract in different parts of the airways differ in composition and serve multiple purposes—of which surface clearance is only one, and perhaps not the most important. The fluids reduce surface tension in alveoli and small airways. They also serve to humidify inspired air and maintain a fluid bath about the cilia. They act as a carrier of immunoglobulins, phagocytic cells and mast cells. They contain albumin which is capable of binding many solutes, and lysozyme which may play an antimicrobial role. Their glycoproteins serve to sweep the surface clear of particles, but these fibre systems probably also serve as important physical barriers protecting the underlying epithelium from surface agents.

On the one hand these facts should remind us that, in our studies of airway secretions, their role in clearance should by no means be our sole interest. On the other hand, numerous techniques for measuring clearance are now available and the adequacy of clearance rates may be an indirect measure of the normal nature of respiratory tract fluids and their function in other respects. Thus, if clearance is excessively slow, other factors may no longer suffice to impede penetration of surface materials to the epithelium, and the rate of replacement of surface water may not be sufficient to maintain inspired air modification.

We speak of adequate, effective, slow or fast clearance rates, but what is the optimum clearance rate at various levels in the respiratory tract? Is it the faster the better? And if so, how much better is 20 than 2 mm/min? How slow a clearance rate is compatible with the maintenance of respiratory defences? And is there any evidence that a specific biochemical or rheological character of airway fluids either enhances or diminishes clearance rate?

Thirty-four years ago Hilding (1943*a*) observed that '. . . a very heavy, tenacious mucin, so gummy that it could be picked up with thumb forceps, was moved up vertical surfaces by ciliary action with the greatest dispatch . . .'. Hilding (1943*b*) also showed that, *in vitro*, a chicken trachea could be plugged with a mass of thick mucus of this type and, when the trachea was connected with a manometer, the clearance of that plug by ciliary action was so effective as to develop negative pressures of 4 to 15 cmH_2O (0.4–1.47 kPa) (Fig. 4).

In the summary of their paper on rheological simulants of mucus, King *et al.* (1974) state that '. . . mucus from a number of sources can perform the same biological role'. They noted the '. . . biochemical similarities among mucus samples from various sources', and found that '. . . a number of materials chemically dissimilar to mucus were also capable of performing its transport function in the frog palate system'. Indeed there is now ample evidence from a variety of sources that ciliary activity in clearing mucus or its simulants—with varying biochemical and rheological characteristics, and with or without

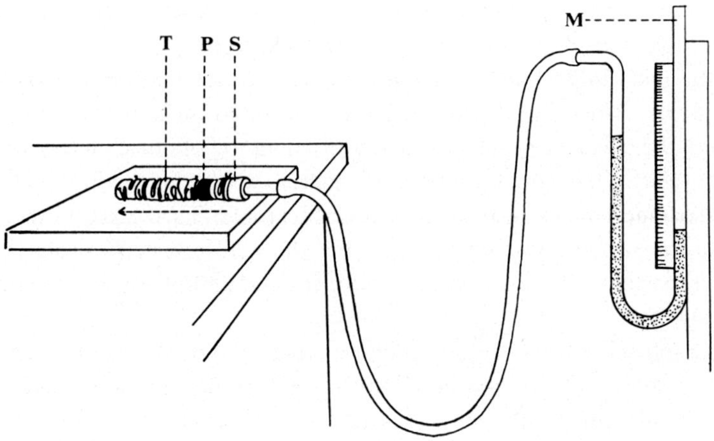

FIG. 4. Clearance of mucus plug through chicken trachea. After placement of the plug of mucus (P) filling the lower end of the trachea (T), the trachea was attached to a manometer (M). Movement of the mucus by ciliary activity produced negative pressures in the manometer. (From Hilding 1943*b*.)

the aid of gravity—is a remarkably hardy system. And there is little evidence that failure of ciliary activity is commonly involved in mucus stasis or slow clearance rates. There is our finding in the dog that a change in the character of tracheal secretions may be accompanied by slowing of surface clearance while cilia continue to clear periciliary fluid. Aspin and colleagues have recently found that, whereas in normal subjects tracheal clearance proceeds effectively against gravity, in cystic fibrosis there is often not only a slowing of clearance but also a falling backwards down the trachea of surface materials when the subject is upright (Wong *et al.* 1977). When this finding is taken in conjunction with Hilding's chicken trachea study (Hilding 1943*b*), it would appear that the failure of clearance against gravity in cystic fibrosis must indicate some change in the character of secretions other than simple 'thickening' (in the sense of altered viscoelastic properties). In conjunction with our findings in the dog, one might wonder whether that change might have been in the depth of periciliary fluid. Bang found that sufficient dehydration in birds resulted in mucus stasis although cilia continued to beat apparently normally in underlying periciliary fluid (Bang & Bang 1963).

Another instance of failure of clearance (and this one is repeatedly documented as a cause of human death) is the accumulation of obstructing plugs of mucus in the small airways of patients dying from chronic obstructive pulmonary disease, especially bronchial asthma—to which we shall now turn our attention.

Hilding (1932) reported experiments in which he surgically closed one nostril in the rabbit. After some time the animals were killed and the mucosal lining of the two nasal passages was examined. On the side left open no major changes had occurred; but, on the side shut off from airflow, 'the erstwhile ciliated columnar cells were all goblet cells and quite devoid of cilia'. In Hilding's words, 'These experiments indicate that the different forms of epithelium found in the upper part of the respiratory tract are not fixed types, but are more or less interchangeable, according to circumstances'. A dozen years after that interesting experiment on the rabbit, Hilding wrote a paper on death from asthma (Hilding 1943*c*) in which he said of the pathologist conducting a clinico-pathological conference on a patient dying of that disease, 'The pathologist then projected a section of bronchiole upon the screen, and there was the same picture that had occurred in the nasal epithelium of the rabbits behind the closed nostril. Every ciliated cell had become a goblet cell'. We shall return to that in a moment.

Thus, the nasal passage normally acts in defence of the lungs by removing a large part of all inspired particles and water-soluble gases and by adjusting the temperature and water vapour content of inspired air so that they are close to those of the body (Brain *et al.* 1977). The maintenance of a normal lining layer of liquid is an important part of the mechanism enabling the nose to carry out these functions.

Our findings in healthy young adults suggest, first, that in some subjects inspired air may pass beyond the nasal airway insufficiently modified, and, secondly, that this impaired function may be related to prior injury from relatively minor disease or from exposure to environmental air. To whatever degree inspired air reaches the pharynx carrying airborne pollutants, or with temperature and water vapour insufficiently modified, the remainder of the air modification must occur in the lower airways. Since the linear velocity of the air in the major tracheobronchial airways is relatively high, and the diameter of the air stream relatively large, it seems likely that little further modification will occur until the small airways are reached. There the very low linear velocity, the small diameter of the streams and the immense surface area provide an optimum opportunity for completion of the process left unfinished in the nose.

But the epithelial lining and surface fluids of these small airways differ in important respects from those of the nose and major tracheobronchial airways (Fig. 5). As we work outwards along the airways, cilia become increasingly sparse, mucus-secreting elements are reduced and then disappear, and the lining fluid may be largely the serous periciliary fluid.

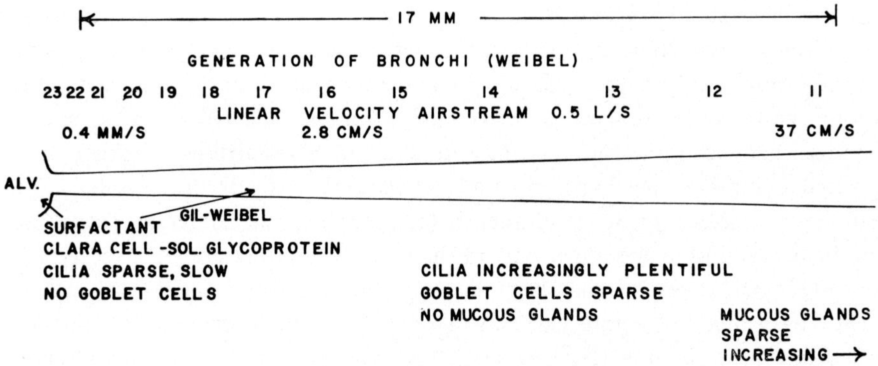

FIG. 5. Some of the presumed characteristics of the small pulmonary airway, shown here diagrammatically without the multiple branches. Alv.: alveolus. (From Proctor 1977.)

Is there any reason to believe that the epithelium in the lower respiratory tract may not be susceptible to change according to circumstances, as was the epithelium in the noses of Hilding's rabbits? If not, a number of possibilities arise. One of these is that, faced with an unaccustomed task of air modification, and in reaction to relatively dry, cool or polluted air, goblet cells may differentiate instead of being ciliated. A minor change in that direction could conceivably enhance the defence of these delicate airways. But, once a sufficient burden of mucus is being produced and the number of ciliated cells has sufficiently decreased, clearance will come to a halt and the airway will fill with accumulated mucus.

Another possible effect of insufficiently modified inspired air reaching these small airways could be that surface-active material becomes less effective in stabilizing their lumina. That could be followed by closure; and, when air passage was stopped through the rabbit's nose in Hilding's study, the ciliated cells metamorphosed into goblet cells. Might this occur in small airways which close intermittently?

CONCLUSION

It seems clear that some apparently healthy young adults have nasal defence mechanisms which are at least on the borderline of normal. It is also now recognized that the earliest change in many chronic lung diseases is failure of function in small pulmonary airways. Is it possible that there is a link between the two? Methods for experimental investigation of the small airways of the lung, a region of such difficult access, are badly needed. With appropriate techniques we could then determine whether impairment of upper airway defences can result in pathological changes in the small airway. Meanwhile, we suggest that indirect evidence can be obtained through the measurement of upper airway function in patients in the earliest stages of small airway disease.

ACKNOWLEDGEMENTS

We should like to thank the many investigators who have played key roles in our studies over the past fifteen years. Among them are E. F. Aharonson, K. Bucklen, P. L. Jensen, G. Lundqvist, M. Quinlan, M. J. Reasor, Y. Sakakura, S. Salman, D. L. Swift, Y. Takagi and H. N. Wagner, Jr. This work was supported by US Public Health Service grants ES00454 H1 14153 and HL 19157.

References

Adams, G. K., Aharonson, E. F., Reasor, M. J. & Proctor, D. F. (1976) Collection of normal canine tracheobronchial secretions. *J. Appl. Physiol. 40*, 247–249

Andersen, I., Lundqvist, G. & Proctor, D. F. (1971) Human nasal mucosal function in a controlled climate. *Arch. Environ. Health 23*, 408–420

Andersen, I., Camner, P., Jensen, P. L., Philipson, K. & Proctor, D. F. (1974*a*) Nasal clearance in monozygotic twins. *Am. Rev. Respir. Dis. 110*, 301–305

Andersen, I., Lundqvist, G., Jensen, P. L. & Proctor, D. F. (1974*b*) Human response to 78 hours exposure to dry air. *Arch. Environ. Health 29*, 319–324

Andersen, I., Lundqvist, G., Jensen, P. L. & Proctor, D. F. (1974*c*) Human response to controlled levels of sulfur dioxide. *Arch. Environ. Health 28*, 31–39

Andersen, I., Camner, P., Jensen, P. L., Philipson, K. & Proctor, D. F. (1974*d*) A comparison of nasal and tracheobronchial clearance. *Arch. Environ. Health 29*, 290–293

Bang, B. G. & Bang, F. B. (1963) Responses of upper respiratory mucosae to dehydration and infection. *Ann. N. Y. Acad. Sci. 106*, 625–630

Brain, J., Proctor, D. F. & Reid, L. (eds.) (1977) in *Respiratory Defense Mechanisms*, Dekker, New York

Camner, P. Philipson, K. & Friberg, L. (1972) Tracheobronchial clearance in twins. *Arch. Environ. Health 24*, 82–87

Hilding, A. C. (1932) Experimental surgery of the nose and sinuses. 1. *Arch. Otolaryngol. 16*, 9–18

Hilding, A. C. (1943*a*) Loss of cilia in the respiratory tract and its relation to death from respiratory disease. *Minn. Med. 26*, 272–275

Hilding, A. C. (1943*b*) The role of ciliary action in production of pulmonary atelectasis, vacuum in the paranasal sinuses, and in otitis media. *Ann. Otol. Rhinol. Laryngol. 52*, 816–834

Hilding, A. C. (1943*c*) The relation of ciliary insufficiency to death from asthma and other respiratory diseases. *Ann. Otol. Rhinol. Laryngol. 52*, 5–20

King, M., Gilboa, A., Meyer, F. A. & Silberberg, A. (1974) On the transport of mucus and its rheologic simulants. *Am. Rev. Respir. Dis. 110*, 740–745

Proctor, D. F. (1977) The upper airways 1. Nasal physiology and defense of the lungs. *Am. Rev. Respir. Dis. 115*, 97–129

Proctor, D. F., Aharonson, E. F., Reasor, M. J. & Bucklen, K. (1973) A method for collecting normal respiratory mucus. *Bull. Physio-Pathol. Respir. 9*, 351–358

PROCTOR, D. F., ANDERSEN, I. & LUNDQVIST, G. L. (1977) Human nasal mucosal function at controlled temperatures. *Respir. Physiol. 30*, 109–124

QUINLAN, M., SALMAN, S., SWIFT, D. L., WAGNER, Jr., H. N. & PROCTOR, D. F. (1969) Measurement of mucociliary function in man. *Am. Rev. Respir. Dis. 99*, 13–23

WONG, J. W., KEENS, T. G., WANNAMAKER, E. M., CROZIER, D. M., LEVISON, H. & ASPIN, N. (1977) The effect of gravity on tracheal mucous transport rates in normal subjects and in patients with cystic fibrosis. *Pediatrics 60*, 146

Discussion

Guz: I have studied a number of largyngectomized patients and I have never met one with normal airway function.

Proctor: But we don't know how many of them have abnormal airway function to begin with.

Guz: I have documented normal airway function on three occasions before surgery and twice I have taken biopsies from the IVth and Vth divisions with the fibre-optic bronchoscope at least one year after surgery; there now appears to be a gross excess of mucus-secreting cells.

Proctor: Griffith & Friedberg (1964) have studied the extensive change in the epithelium in laryngectomized patients. In my view, if air gets beyond the nose without being fully conditioned (or almost so), conditioning is unlikely to be done very well in the major conducting airways because of the diameter of the airstream, the linear velocity of the flow, the lack of turbulence, and so on; whereas in the small airways of the lung it will inevitably be completed because of the very low linear velocity and the small radius of the stream. But the small airways are peculiar and they may be particularly vulnerable to injury.

Thurlbeck: Yergin *et al.* (1977) use a system similar to yours but with the tracheobronchial tree. They found that in the trachea in normal non-bronchitic, healthy non-smoking subjects, a proportion will show no movement of particles, or the same subject from time to time will show no movement of the particles. When they express that group as a whole, they have normal tests of ciliary function, compared to smokers.

Proctor: We just need more information.

Iravani: Elimination of the upper airways leads to improper conditioning of the inspired air, and allows particles that are normally cleared by these airways to reach the more peripheral regions. The load is beyond the elimination capacity of the cilia in these small airways because of their lower transport velocity and sluggish clearance function (Iravani 1971).

Proctor: I am glad to hear you say that. It is my impression that some of the earliest manifestations of the transition from health to disease in chronic bronchitis, asthma and cystic fibrosis are changes in small airways. There may be some unitary factor here making a variety of people more susceptible to these changes.

Iravani: It is not necessary to have a feedback mechanism. On reaching a certain electrochemical gradient of chloride ions due to the pump action, a back-diffusion of these ions of equal magnitude might take place so that an equilibrium state results.

Proctor: In our dog preparations the most constant finding in our airway secretions is that sodium and chloride concentrations are higher than in dog plasma, as is osmolarity. Even when we grossly alter these secretions by giving the animal methacholine, which will stop particle movement entirely, those three remain constant. When methacholine is given and this gross change in the nature of secretion occurs, with the particles not moving, if the trachea is opened and a soluble dye is put in, the dye is swept up the trachea beneath the particles. So one is not stopping periciliary clearance; only the surface particles are being stopped. There is still the problem of how to control the thickness (depth) of mucus so that one gets the same chloride concentration and the depth of periciliary fluid remains the same.

Dr Sleigh (1977) feels that the depth of periciliary fluid should be just sufficient for the tips of the cilia to reach out at the top of the stroke and claw the mucus. If that is so, 2 μm difference in the thickness of that fluid could make a big difference.

J. G. Jones: Is the idea of these things scratching away at a layer of mucus over the top too simplistic a view? Could mucociliary transport be what the engineers call a two-phase problem, where there are two liquids adjacent to one another, one with slightly different physical properties from the other, and the motion of one is coupled to the other without these 'claws' actually scratching at the surface? The purpose of the cilia may simply be to move a layer of very low viscosity, and the movement of that layer is transformed into the movement of the mucus.

Silberberg: If the viscosity of that periciliary fluid is roughly that of water, we should not be able to put in enough energy to remove the mucus layer by flow induced in the fluid itself. Ciliary movement would have to be linked to the mucus blanket mechanically.

Richardson: Yoneda (1976) recently published some electron micrographs of airways of newly killed rats. He gave glutaraldehyde vapour into the lungs to fix the airway surface *in situ.* He found that there really seemed to be two layers of airway secretion—a periciliary layer which was electron-lucent, and above, just at the level of the tips of the cilia, the appearance of the fluid became more electron-dense.

Proctor: I am glad to hear that.

Cumming: There are some physiological data which may throw light on these questions. One might measure with a mass spectrometer the partial pressure of water vapour breathed out and take a vital capacity inspirate and vital capacity expirate in a normal subject. If 6.265 kPa (47 torr) is the alveolar concentration of water vapour and the ambient concentration is about 1.333 kPa (about 10 torr), one gets the sort of curve shown here in Fig. 1. The level changes continuously throughout the expirate and it always ends at 5.065 kPa (38 torr). In the alveolus it is 6.265 kPa so the vapour must cool as it comes out; the question is, where does this cooling happen? We took the known anatomy of the airways from a bronchial cast and tried to calculate from the asymmetry of the model how much of the lateral surface of the gel was available for transfer of heat and of fluid. In the cast, using chemical engineering techniques, we found that, during quiet breathing at about 500 ml tidal volume, the nasopharynx does about 30% of the work and the bronchial tree about 70%, which requires six orders of bronchi. If we put in a large

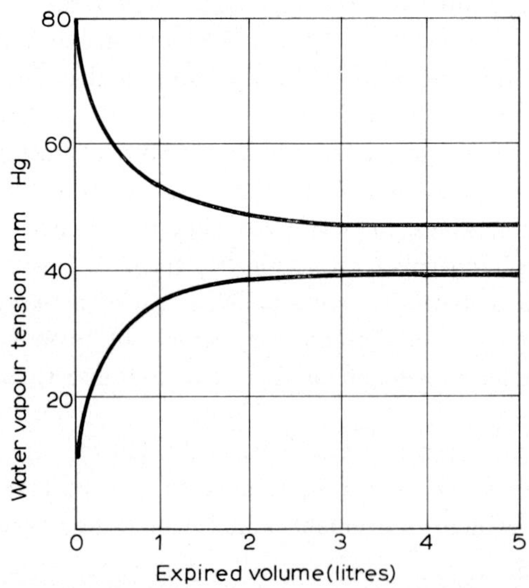

FIG. 1. (Cumming). Expired water vapour partial pressure during a vital capacity manoeuvre. The lower curve is inspiring ambient air, the upper curve air saturated at 100 °C, so that the inspired P_{H_2O} is 80 mmHg. The lower curve fails to reach alveolar partial pressure but the upper one achieves this value of 47 mmHg.

breath of hot air—4 litres at 100 °C, bone dry—it goes further down the bronchi, using 11 orders rather than 6. The answer seems to lie in the recruitment of further branches of the bronchial tree as the point of maximum saturation recedes and advances up and down the airways.

Proctor: I don't quite agree. Some excellent studies have demonstrated that in the average normal individual, both in the nasopharynx and in the subglottal region, inspired air is far closer to saturation than these figures would indicate. There is a gradient all along the airway, and to my mind the evidence is quite clear that in the average normal individual with nasal breathing most of the conditioning occurs along the nasal passage.

Cumming: Assuming that much of the conditioning goes on in the nose, and the air is fully conditioned by the time it gets to the trachea, then the trachea is receiving conditioned air, and if that air is breathed out through the mouth it will come out conditioned. So if inspiration is through the nose and expiration through the mouth, then the mouth gets only expired air and will only receive what comes up after conditioning. If it were true that the nose played an important part, the 4.932 kPa (37 torr) level should rise to about 6.265 kPa, but in 25 individuals we found no difference at all with a precision of measurement of about 0.066 kPa (0.5 torr).

Proctor: I don't accept that. The argument from expired air could have a number of possible explanations but when the measurement is made on inspired air it is hard to argue with what you find as long as the measurements are accurate. Several people have made such measurements and they have agreed pretty well. We really don't know what happens during expiration and what happens to the air in passing from the larynx through the mouth when a person is expiring through the mouth, so there may be other problems that we are not seeing in your findings. We need more studies of inspired air.

Silberberg: As regards the air that reaches down into the depths of the lung, wouldn't part of that air occupy a dead space?

Proctor: There would be dead space; there is no question about that.

Allison: That is presumably below the 11th order of bronchi.

Cumming: We can't talk about dead space in respect of water vapour. It is a meaningless abstraction.

Proctor: But in the dead space the temperature of the airway surfaces is not going to be the same as in the alveoli.

Cumming: You mean the dead space for the expirate gases or the dead space for water vapour?

Proctor: I mean the main tracheobronchial conducting airways; the surface temperature is going to be different there from the alveoli.

Cumming: Which is exactly what our calculations indicate.

Allison: Are there any biochemical data?

Kent: Points have been made about the use of SO_2 as an irritant and a great deal of work has obviously been done using that material. In fact we have found $^{35}SO_2$ to be more than an irritant; it is rapidly oxidized by the tracheal surface to a metabolite which is incorporated into the tracheal glycoproteins as ester sulphate.

Proctor: It is in the nasal glycoprotein because none of it gets past the nose, although some of it is excreted through the lung. We sampled pharyngeal air and could not detect any SO_2.

Kent: The same enzyme pattern will be present.

References

GRIFFITH, T. E. & FRIEDBERG, S. A. (1964) Histologic changes in the trachea following laryngectomy. *Ann. Otol. Rhinol. Laryngol. 73*, 882–892

IRAVANI, J. (1971) Physiologie und Pathophysiologie der Cilientätigkeit und des Schleimtransportes im Tracheobronchialbaum. *Pneumonologie 144*, 93–112

SLEIGH, M. A. (1977) The nature and action of respiratory tract cilia, in *Respiratory Defense Mechanisms* (Brain, J. *et al.*, eds.), ch. 8, Dekker, New York

YERGIN, B. M., GOODMAN, R. M., LANDA, J. F., GOLINVAUX, M. H. & SACKNER, M. A. (1977) Effects of cigarette smoking on tracheal mucous velocity in young smokers with and without small airway obstruction. *Am. Rev. Respir. Dis. 115*, 183

YONEDA, K. (1976) Mucous blanket of rat bronchus, an ultrastructural study. *Am. Rev. Respir. Dis. 114*, 837–842

Tracheobronchial clearance in health and disease: with special reference to interciliary fluid

JOSEF IRAVANI, G. NORRIS MELVILLE and GUNTER HORSTMANN

Department of Anatomy II, Ruhr University Bochum, West Germany

Abstract Rats were exposed to influenza B virus for 2 hours. Mucociliary function in the isolated airway preparation of these animals was studied from the first day after exposure and at regular intervals for up to 190 days. Transmission electron microscopy (TEM) studies were done at times corresponding to the mucociliary function studies.

TEM studies confirmed the results of the mucociliary function studies: pathological changes were first apparent three days after exposure and began in the distal bronchioles. The morphological studies further demonstrated that the infection progressed proximally to include the entire tracheobronchial tree by the 18th day. The alterations observed included an increase in the number of goblet cells, a decrease in the number of microvilli and a reduction in the amount of interciliary fluid. The last two changes were closely correlated with the severity of the infection. The abnormalities found in mucociliary function included hypersecretion of mucus, inactive and hypoactive zones, synchronization of cilia beating, and a sticking together of the cilia tips.

Lucas & Douglas (1934) suggested that the tracheobronchial secretion is composed of two layers: (a) a deep layer lying directly on the epithelium, now called interciliary or periciliary fluid (Iravani 1971; Horstmann *et al.* 1977), and (b) the mucus lying on the interciliary fluid layer.

The composition and physicochemical characteristics of the tracheobronchial fluid in healthy (Boat *et al.* 1973; Gallagher *et al.* 1975) and pathological conditions (Rasche *et al.* 1972; Lieberman & Gawad 1971; Lopez-Vidriero *et al.* 1973) are well known. Although the cells responsible for the production of mucus in the respiratory tract have been identified (Jeffery & Reid 1975) little is known about the mechanism of production, the place of production or the composition of the interciliary fluid. Recent studies have suggested that the microvilli-bearing cells could possibly be the site of origin of the fluid

(Horstmann *et al.* 1977; Iravani *et al.* 1977). The interciliary fluid appears to play a prominent role in the pathophysiology of airway clearance.

This paper presents results of experiments designed to clarify the role played by interciliary fluid and the microvilli in the development of lung disease.

MATERIALS AND METHODS

Seventy-four female Wistar rats, each weighing on average 160 g, were studied. Thirty-seven animals were exposed to influenza B virus (B/Mass/3/66, HA 1:1280, Behring); the other animals were exposed to physiological saline and served as controls. The virus and saline solutions were dispensed by means of a nebulizer (Dräger) driven by compressed air. Exposure lasted 2 h, during which about 9 ml of each solution was nebulized. The control and exposed animals were kept in separate cages and were killed on each of the following days after exposure: 1–14, 16–19, 21–27, 54, 61, 80, 110, 180, 188, 190. Two animals, one from each group, were killed on these days and mucociliary function was studied *in vitro* as previously described (Iravani 1967; Iravani & van As 1972; Melville & Iravani 1975). The airways of these animals were examined either by incident light microscopy or by cinematography. Films were made of representative areas for later analysis.

Two animals from each group were killed on the 3rd, 7th and 18th days after exposure and were prepared for transmission electron microscopy (TEM) as follows. The airway preparations were fixed in a mixture of 4% glutaraldehyde in 0.1M buffer (pH 7.4) for 12 h at 4 °C. The airways were then washed in buffered solution (0.22M-sucrose in 0.1M-phosphate, pH 7.4). Postfixation was done in 2.0% aqueous OsO_4 in buffer for 2 h and the tissue was dehydrated in increasing strengths of alcohol. Small areas of the trachea, bronchi and bronchioles were excised and embedded in Araldite. Ultrathin sections were obtained with a Reichert ultramicrotome (OmU_2) and stained with uranyl acetate and lead citrate on copper grids. The sections were examined in a Zeiss EM 9S.

RESULTS

Abnormalities of mucociliary function and micromorphological changes in the tracheobronchial mucosa were seen not only in the virus-exposed animals but also in the control group. The difference between the two groups was purely quantitative, that is, the abnormalities were more extensive and more frequent in the virus-exposed animals. The most severe changes, with peribronchitic reactions, were present only in the virus-exposed animals.

(a) Mucociliary function studies

The following changes in mucociliary function were observed.

(i) Disturbances in ciliary coordination, with whirlpool formation and reversal of the direction of mucus transport (see Iravani 1971).

(ii) Singly scattered or densely packed droplet-like microscopic homogeneous masses, that were either firmly or less firmly attached to the epithelial surface and were considered to be incompletely expelled cell contents. These protrusions, depending on their attachment, were moved to and fro by ciliary beat and were occasionally released to be transported with relatively high velocity.

(iii) Adhesive mucus: in spite of unimpaired ciliary activity the transport of certain mucus flakes was slow and jerky. This phenomenon was observed also in rats exposed to cigarette smoke and was considered to be due to the altered rheological characteristics of the mucus secretion (Iravani & Melville 1974).

(iv) Decreased ciliary activity, to the point of ciliostasis. The ciliary activity, especially the amplitude of ciliary beat, was markedly reduced in the areas with stagnant mucus. The amplitude was sometimes reduced so much that only under high microscopic resolution were vibrations visible. The epithelium of the adjacent areas showed normal ciliary activity. Whenever mucus was transported to one of these areas, it either remained bound in the upstream part of this area or was transported over it with decreased velocity. The most impressive observation in these areas was the synchronization of the cilia: that is, all the cilia appeared to be in the same beating phase, an observation not made in healthy epithelium (Iravani 1967, 1969). The synchronization phenomenon is probably the result of the cilia sticking together and of a change in the interciliary fluid layer. The epithelium could be freed of stagnant mucin by repeated washing with physiological saline (37 °C), and the cilia quite often recovered, showing increased amplitude. However the coordination of the cilia remained disturbed in that they appeared to beat independently of each other. Complete recovery was never observed.

(v) Inactive zones: ciliary activity was not present in these areas. A thick mucus film was almost always present and was considered to be a later stage of the abnormalities described in *(iv)* above. The major part of these inactive zones consisted of metaplastic epithelium.

All the above-mentioned abnormalities were observed in the entire tracheobronchial tree. As a rule it could be said that the more severe the peribronchitic reaction, the more severe the impairment of mucociliary function. The inactive zones were almost always confined to regions with severe peribronchitic reactions.

The nature, frequency, severity and extent of the abnormalities were identical in control animals and animals studied 24 and 48 h after virus exposure. In both groups the mucus production was sparse and only single mucus flakes were observed in the trachea and main bronchi. Small areas with protrusions and ciliary incoordination were present. Likewise, rats studied at 5, 7, 27, 54, 61, 80, 111 and 180 days after virus exposure did not differ from the control group. Increased mucus production was seen in both groups, in contrast to what is seen in specific-pathogen-free animals.

In rats killed 3 days after exposure to virus, several areas of stagnant mucus were observed in the trachea and larger airways. Many regions showed protrusions, ciliary incoordination and whirlpool formation in the entire tracheobronchial tree. At 4 days, rats showed ciliary incoordination and protrusions of similar proportions to the 3-day animals. In addition, marked hypersecretion and whirlpool formation were present in the medium-sized airways. At 6 days the trachea and main bronchi were completely filled with mucopurulent secretion which had to be removed before mucociliary activity could be studied. Many hypoactive areas with ciliary synchronization and single peribronchitic reactions at the branching sites of the bronchial tree were discernible. At 8 days the rat showed changes similar to the 6-day animal, but with reduced mucus secretion.

The 9–12-day animals showed, in contrast to the control animals, a slight hypersecretion, many densely packed protrusions and hypoactive regions in the entire tracheobronchial tree. In addition several peribronchitic areas were present in the larger and medium-sized airways. Changes were similar in the 13–19-day animals, except that the peribronchitic reactions were more extensive than in the 9–12-day animals.

The differences between the control and the reactive virus-exposed group were more pronounced from the 21st day onwards. Hypersecretion was present and abnormalities were confined to peribronchitic areas. These areas were more extensive as time after virus exposure increased, and they showed thickening of the walls of up to 1 mm or more. Rats examined at 188 and 190 days after exposure to virus showed many lung abscesses, marked pleural adhesions and bronchiectasis.

(b) Transmission electron microscopy

Changes were already evident in the bronchioles of rats at 3 days after virus exposure (Figs. 1*a*, 8*a–c*) and included protrusions of the serous Clara cells through the membrane and a thickening of the microvilli (Fig. 7*a*). These changes were not observed in animals treated with normal saline (Fig. 1*b*).

text continued p. 243

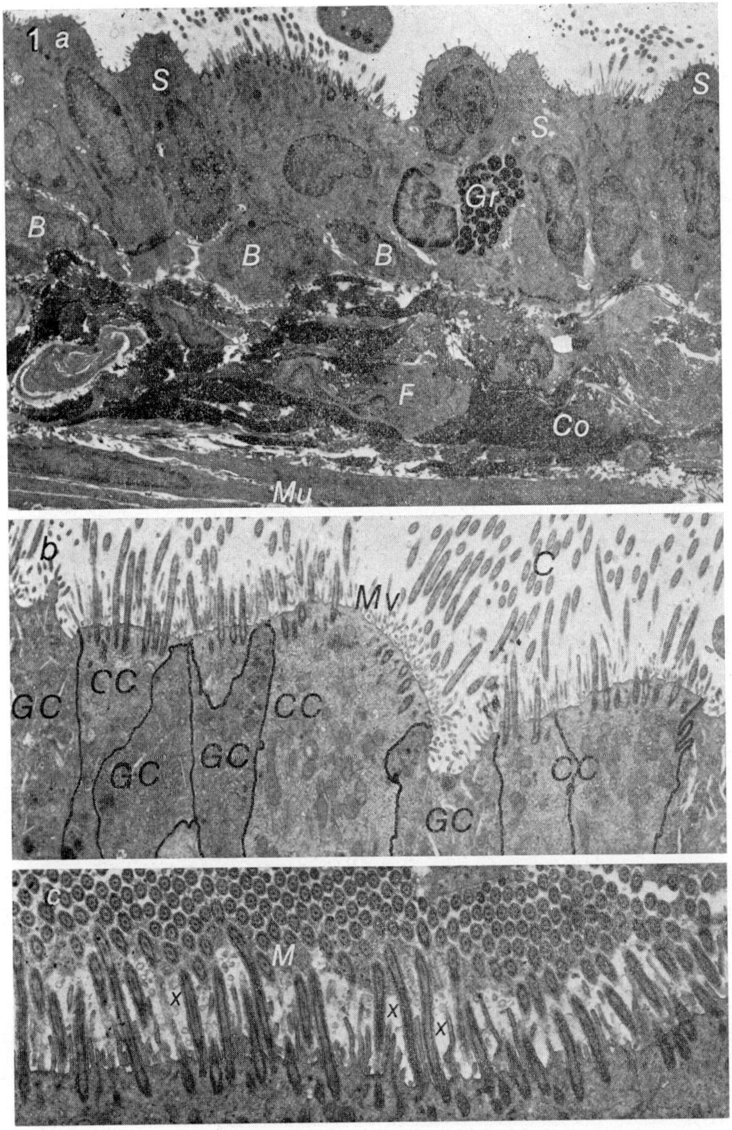

FIG. 1. *(a)* Transverse section of a proximal bronchiole of a rat 3 days after virus exposure to influenza B virus. The cytoplasmic droplet at the upper middle margin is probably transported by ciliary beat from the periphery. The first significant reaction of the tissue to the virus in this area is the wandering phagocyte (GR) between the epithelial cells. The Clara cells (S) are almost devoid of secretory granules. × 2900.
(b) Luminal border of the ciliated epithelium of normal rat bronchus. Note the lack of mature mucigen granules in the goblet cells (GC) and the abundant thin and long microvilli (Mv). × 5700.
(c) Luminal border of the tracheal ciliated epithelium of a rat 7 days after virus exposure. Many microvilli have already been altered by vesiculation. Cell debris is present at the upper middle margin. F = fibrocyte; Co = collagenous fibrils; Mu = smooth muscle cells; C = cilia; CC = ciliated cells. × 8000.

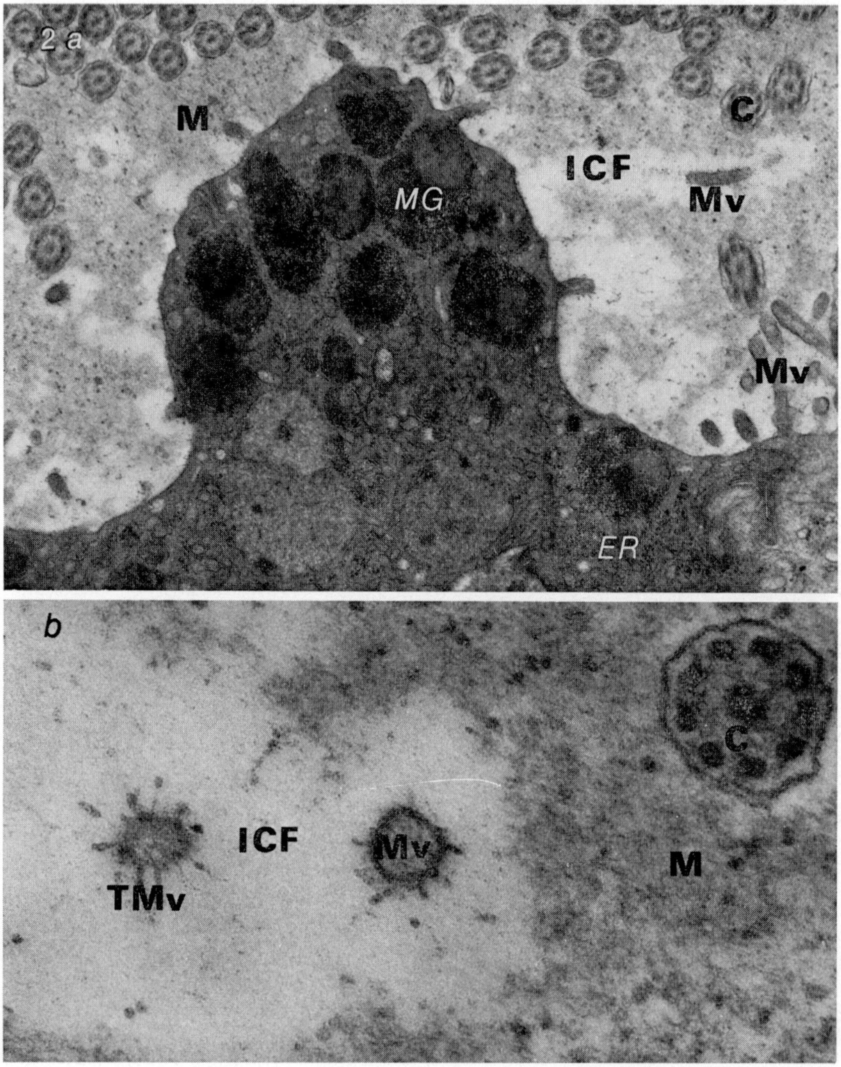

FIG. 2. *(a)* Apical part of a normal tracheal goblet cell (3 days after exposure to saline) with mature mucigen granules (MG), each with different electron opacity. The electron translucent areas around the microvilli (Mv) are probably the areas occupied by the interciliary fluid (ICF). The trachea was cooled (30 °C) for 90 min. × 24000.
(b) High power TEM of the same area as in Fig. 2*a*. The electron-dense mucus (M) reaches to the cilium (C) but not to the furry-coated microvillus (Mv). C = cilium in transverse section; ER = endoplasmic reticulum; ICF = interciliary fluid. × 80000.

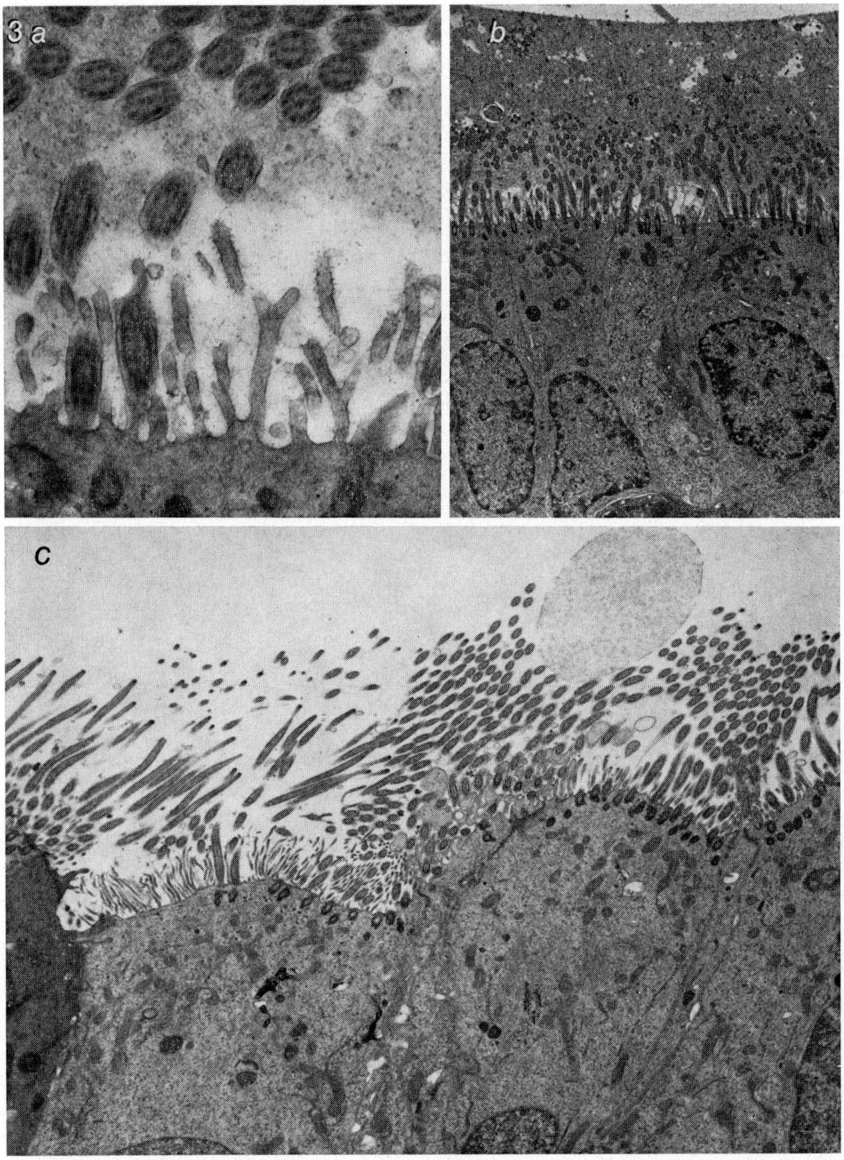

FIG. 3. *(a)* Luminal edge of a ciliated cell of a normal rat. Note the translucent space around the intact microvilli. × 24000.
(b) TEM showing the thickness of the mucus layer of rat 7 days after exposure to virus. The number of microvilli has decreased so that the mucus penetrates to the bases of the cilia. × 2900.
(c) Apical edge of a 7-day rat. The right half of the figure shows thicker microvilli and small cytoplasmic extrusions between the cilia. × 5700.

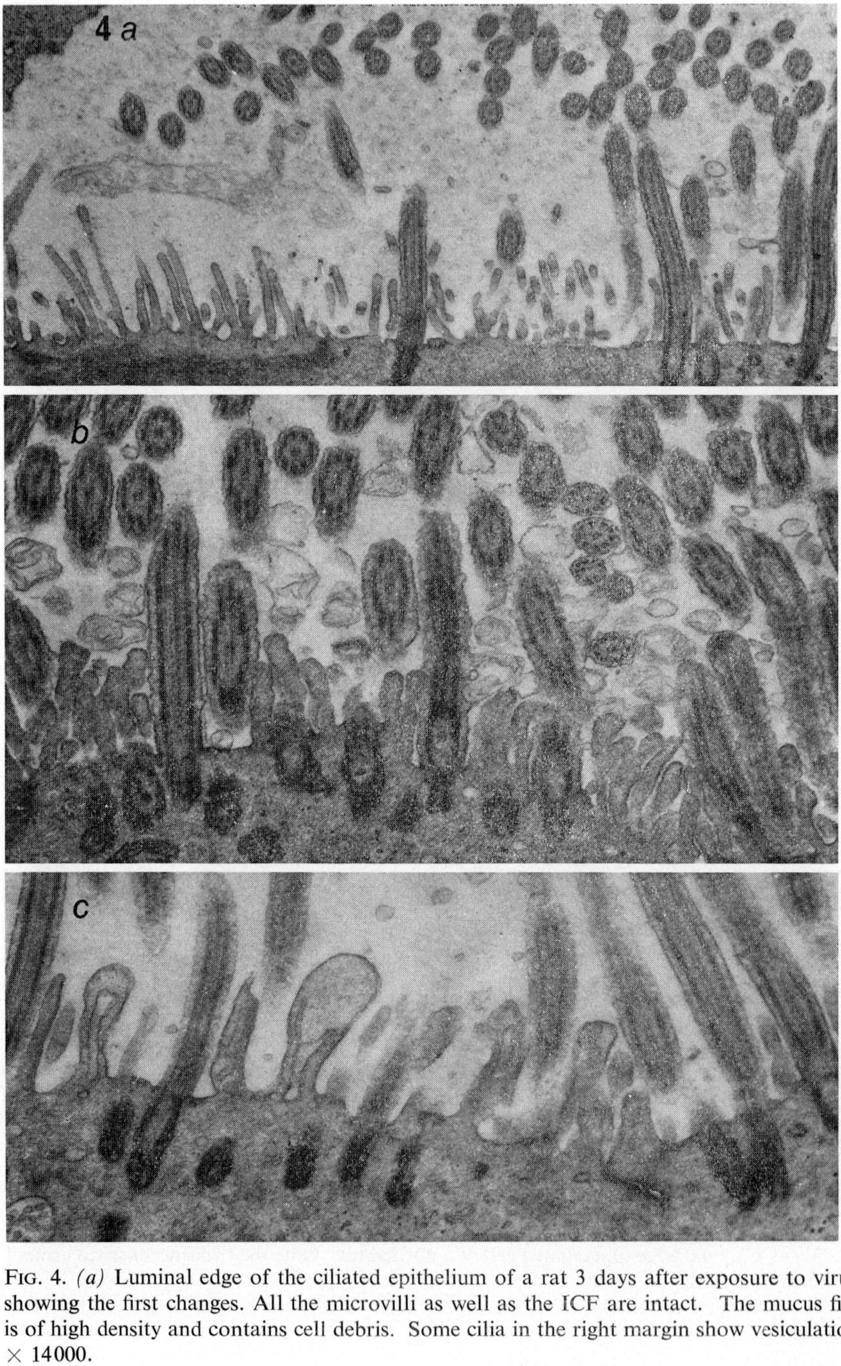

FIG. 4. *(a)* Luminal edge of the ciliated epithelium of a rat 3 days after exposure to virus, showing the first changes. All the microvilli as well as the ICF are intact. The mucus film is of high density and contains cell debris. Some cilia in the right margin show vesiculation. × 14000.

(b) Proximal branches of an 18-day animal. The microvilli are shorter, thicker and appear rough. Some are clustered together. Numerous vesicles occupy the spaces between the cilia. × 24000.

(c) Same animal as in *(b)* but a neighbouring area. Many microvilli have been destroyed. × 24000.

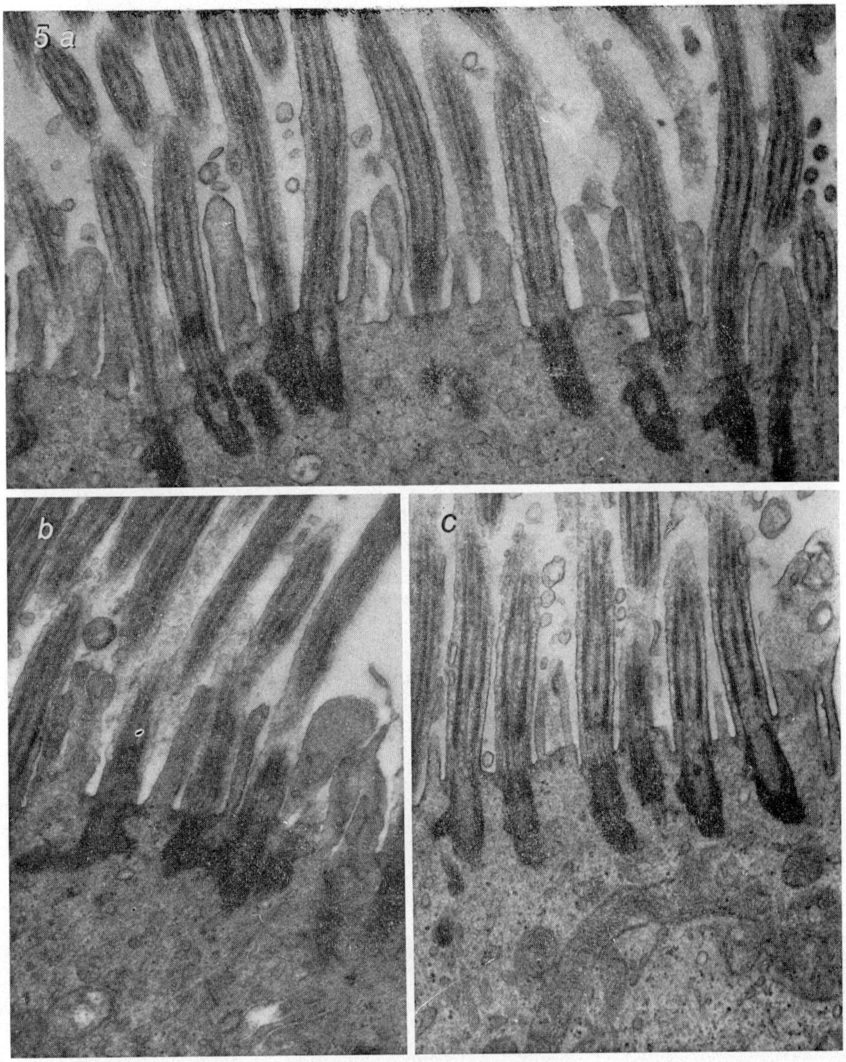

FIG. 5. *(a)–(c)* TEM of an 18-day rat showing different stages in the destruction of the microvilli. × 24000.

At 7 days, the microvilli showed vesiculation (Fig. 1*c*); a thick mucus film was present and the number of microvilli was decreased (Fig. 3*b*). The mucus was capable of penetrating to the base of the cilia which does not occur in normal animals. The areas around the microvilli are translucent and probably represent the interciliary fluid (Fig. 2*a*).

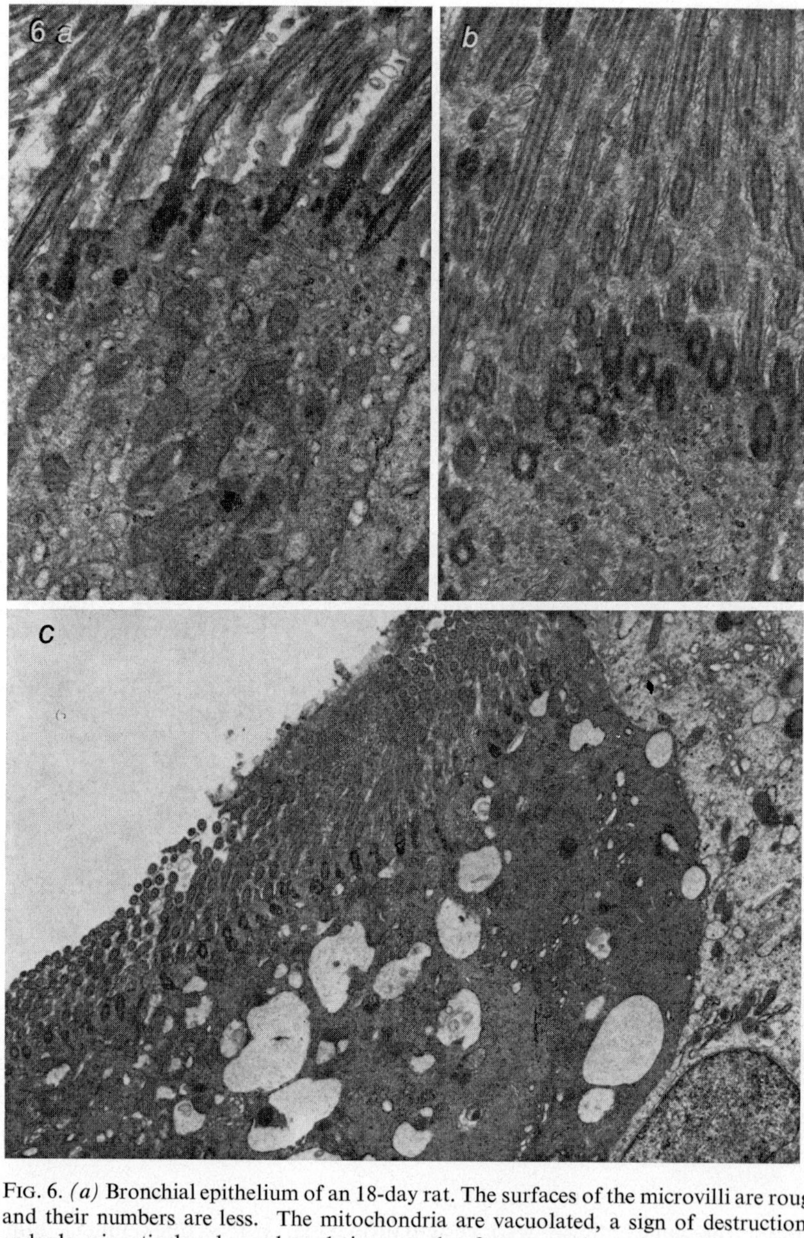

FIG. 6. *(a)* Bronchial epithelium of an 18-day rat. The surfaces of the microvilli are roughened and their numbers are less. The mitochondria are vacuolated, a sign of destruction. The endoplasmic reticulum has enlarged cisternae that form vacuoles. × 16000.
(b) Another area of the same animal. The infection is more marked, as evidenced by the absence of the interciliary fluid space and microvilli. The ICF space is filled with mucus vesicles. × 16000.
(c) Another area in the same animal, showing progression of the disease. The vacuoles are more translucent, probably due to water absorption. × 5700.

By 18 days the infection had progressed to include the main bronchi and trachea (Figs. 3*c*, 4*a–c*, 5*a–c*). Normal areas could be found between the bronchitic areas. Up to 7 days no increase in the number of goblet cells was observed (Fig. 3*b*). In some areas the first sign of infection was heralded by decimation or destruction of the microvilli-bearing cells (Fig. 6*b*). By the 18th day the number of goblet cells increased, the cisternae in the endoplasmic reticulum were enlarged and the surface of the microvilli appeared rough (Fig. 6*a*). Intercellular spaces were seen between the epithelial cells before they finally disintegrated.

The airways at this stage were blocked by mucus and cell debris. Many protrusions were also present.

In summary, as the infection progressed the number of goblet cells increased, the number of microvilli decreased and the interciliary fluid layer disappeared.

DISCUSSION

The mucociliary abnormalities observed in animals exposed to influenza B virus are almost identical to those reported in animals with spontaneous bronchitis and after exposure to cigarette smoke (Iravani 1971; Iravani & van As 1972; Iravani & Melville 1974). In those earlier studies we concluded that the protrusions represented a disturbance of the secretion process. Electron microscopic studies have now shown that protrusion formations are probably due to cellular damage. Whether the protrusions are the same as the globular bodies described by Scudi *et al.* (1951) remains open to question. The protrusions are certainly not *in vitro* artifacts of fixation, since they are found in similar numbers in airways fixed by perfusion (unpublished results). No definite changes were observed during the first 48 h after exposure. From this period up to two weeks after virus exposure the pathological changes consisted of hypersecretion of mucus, ciliary incoordination, protrusion formation, and single hypoactive and inactive zones in the entire tracheobronchial tree.

Electron microscope studies showed that the observed abnormalities began in the very distal areas of the bronchial tree and progressed proximally with time, so that by the 18th day after virus exposure the entire tracheobronchial tree was involved.

From the 3rd to 4th week after virus exposure, and onwards, the abnormalities in mucociliary function were mainly confined to the peribronchitic areas. The extent of the peribronchitic reaction was closely correlated with the time after exposure. The areas adjacent to the peribronchitic patches had generally normal mucociliary function, which supports earlier findings in animals with chronic bronchitis (Iravani 1971). No difference from control

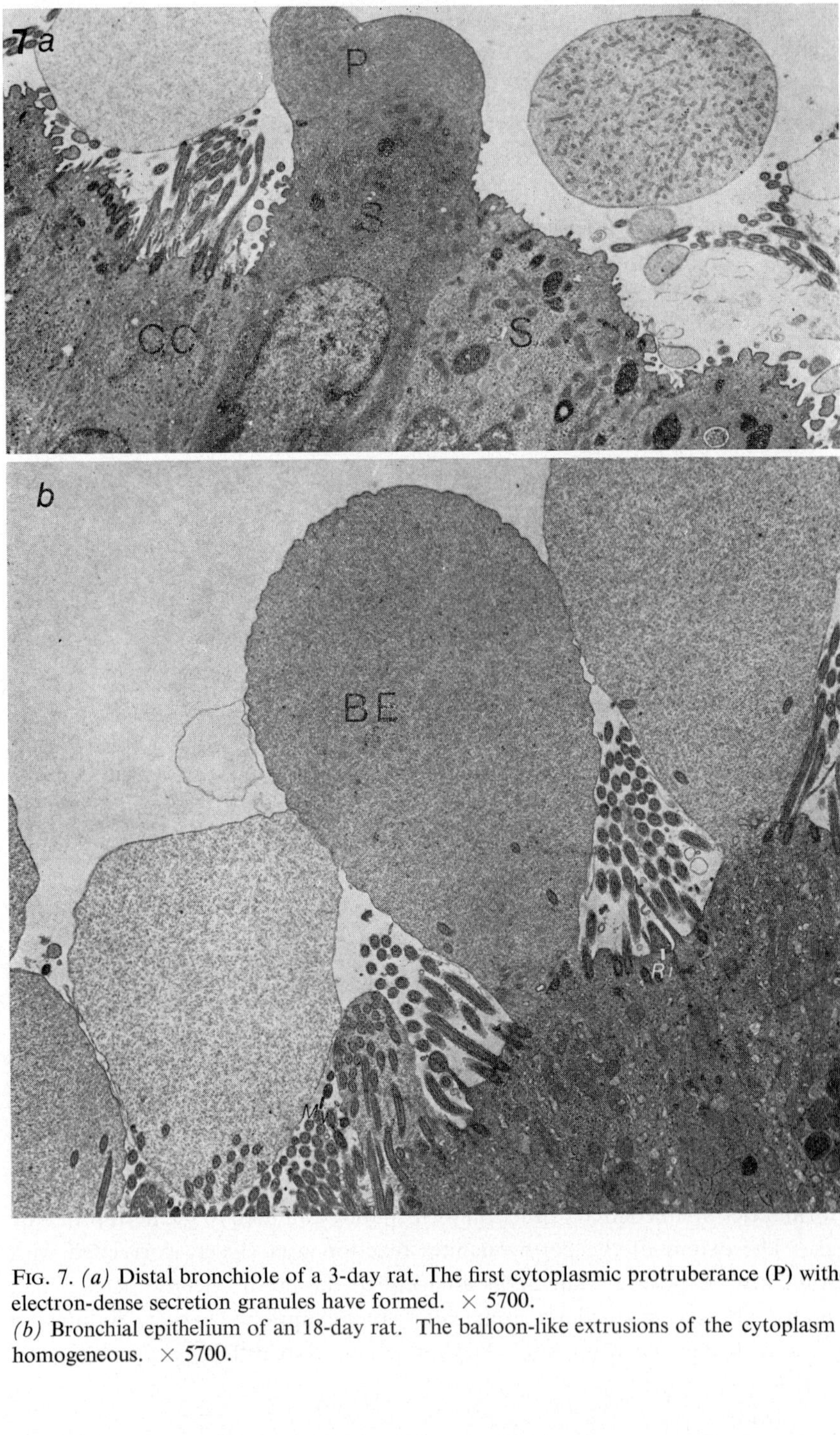

FIG. 7. *(a)* Distal bronchiole of a 3-day rat. The first cytoplasmic protruberance (P) without electron-dense secretion granules have formed. × 5700.
(b) Bronchial epithelium of an 18-day rat. The balloon-like extrusions of the cytoplasm are homogeneous. × 5700.

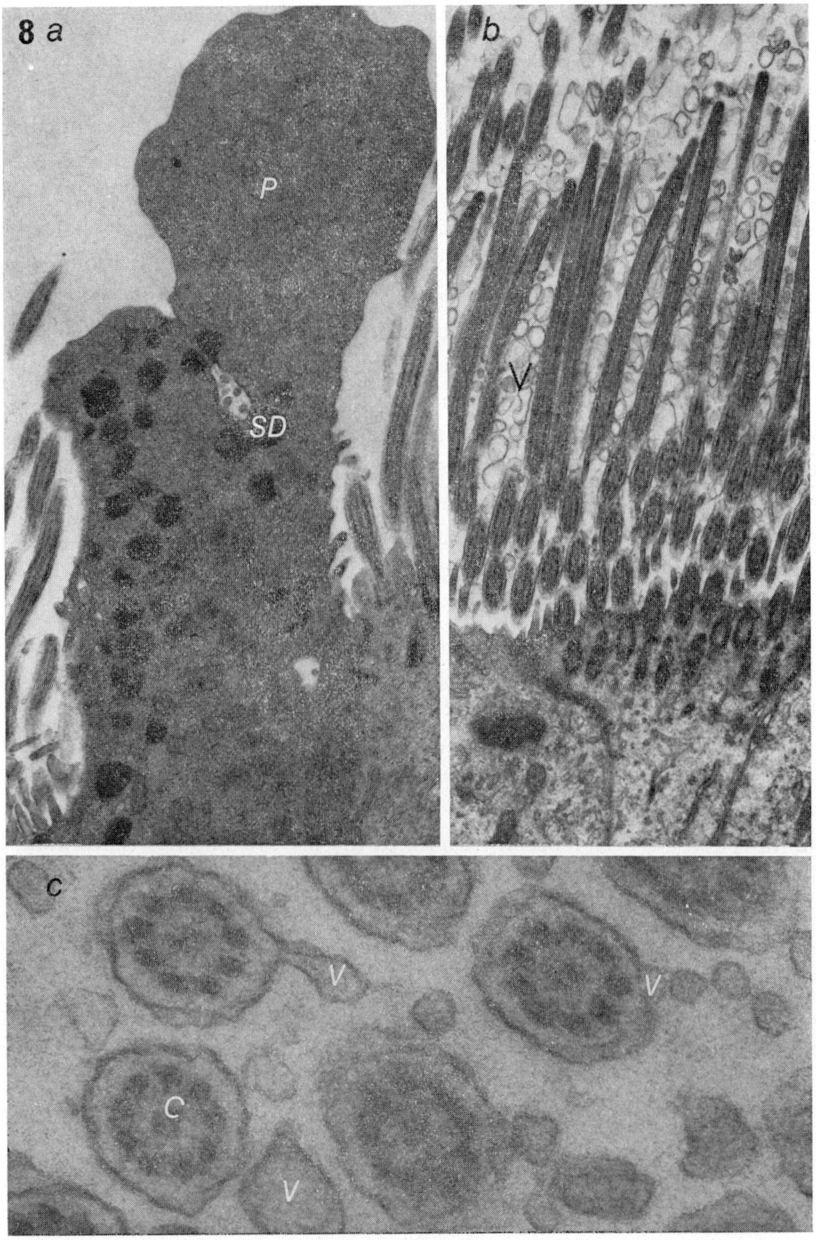

FIG. 8. *(a)* Three-day rat. Note the cytoplasmic protrusions (P) that are almost devoid of electron-dense secretion droplets (SD). × 14000.
(b) Eighteen-day animal. Numerous vesicles (V) fill the ICF space. They originate from the membranes of the microvilli and the cilia. × 14000.
(c) The same area as in *(b)* at higher magnification. C = cilia in transverse section with vesiculation (V). × 80000.

was observed in 10 virus-exposed rats; this could either be because the animals were not susceptible to the influenza virus or because they had completely recovered from bronchitis.

The morphological substrate of the abnormalities of mucociliary function consists initially of microvilli swelling and the formation of protrusions with cell contents. At later stages the number of microvilli progressively decreases and numerous protrusions are found on the bronchial epithelium. The cells, especially the ciliated cells, show vacuolization and signs of degeneration. This could be interpreted as the earliest stage of chronic bronchitis (Horstmann *et al.* 1977). Increased vacuolization of the epithelial cells, abnormal ciliated cells with membranous protrusions, sticking together of the cilia, metaplasia, membranous formations with the degenerated cell contents, and areas without microvilli-bearing cells could be seen at this stage. The reason for the ciliary incoordination in the initial stages is unknown, although the protrusions, the decrease in the number of microvilli and the reduction in the interciliary fluid layer (Iravani *et al.* 1977) might be partly responsible. The hypoactive zones with synchronization of the cilia could have their origins in the decreased interciliary fluid layer.

The decrease in the interciliary fluid layer and its replacement by more viscous cell contents from the protrusions, or probably by transudation between the surface cells, could lead to an alteration in the fluid surrounding the cilia, with clumping together of the cilia and alteration in their membranes leading to synchronization. At a later stage the cilia are stuck together along their entire length (Fig. 6).

The morphological evidence corroborates the *in vitro* findings that animals exposed to influenza B virus do not differ from control animals for up to 48 h and that after 72 h pathological changes are found in the most distal airways of the virus-exposed animals. The disease progresses over the next three weeks to include the entire tracheobronchial tree. In addition, the progression of the disease is marked by an increase in the number of goblet cells, a decrease in the number of microvilli-bearing cells and a diminution in the interciliary fluid layer.

References

BOAT, T. F., MATHEW, L. & LEROY, W. (1973) Chemical composition of human tracheobronchial secretions, in *Sputum: Fundamentals and Clinical Pathology* (Dulfano, M. J., ed.), pp. 243–274, Thomas, Springfield, Ill.

GALLAGHER, J. T., KENT, P. W., PASSATORE, M., PHIPPS, R. J. & RICHARDSON, R. J. (1975) The composition of tracheal mucus and the nervous control of its secretion in the cat. *Proc. R. Soc. Lond. B Biol. Sci. 192*, 49–76

HORSTMANN, G., IRAVANI, J., MELVILLE, G. N. & RICHTER, H.-G. (1977) Influence of temperature and decreased water content of inspired air on the ciliated bronchial epithelium. *Acta Oto-Laryngol. 84*, 124–131

IRAVANI, J. (1967) Flimmerbewegung in den intrapulmonalen Luftwegen der Ratte. *Pflügers Arch. Gesamte Physiol. Menschen Tiere 297*, 221–237

IRAVANI, J. (1969) Coordination of ciliary movement in the bronchial epithelium of the rat. *Pflügers Arch. Eur. J. Physiol. 305*, 199–209

IRAVANI, J. (1971) Physiologie und Pathophysiologie der Cilientätigkeit und des Schleimtransportes im Tracheobronchialbaum. *Pneumonologie 144*, 93–112

IRAVANI, J. & VAN AS, A. (1972) Mucus transport in the tracheobronchial tree of normal and bronchitic rats. *Pathology 116*, 81

IRAVANI, J. & MELVILLE, G. N. (1974) Long-term effect of cigarette smoke on mucociliary function in animals. *Respiration 31*, 358–366

IRAVANI, J., MELVILLE, G. N. & HORSTMANN, G. (1977) Interciliary fluid and its possible role in bronchitis. *Lung (Pneumonologie)*, in press

JEFFERY, P. K. & REID, L. (1975) New observations of rat airway epithelium: a quantitative and electron microscopic study. *J. Anat. 120*, 295–320

LIEBERMAN, J. & GAWAD, M. A. (1971) Inhibitors and activators of leukocytic proteases in purulent sputum. *J. Lab. Clin. Med. 77*, 713–727

LOPEZ-VIDRIERO, M., CHARMAN, J., KEAT, E., DE SILVA, D. J. & REID, L. (1973) Sputum viscosity: correlation with chemical and clinical features in chronic bronchitis. *Thorax 28*, 401–408

LUCAS, M. A. & DOUGLAS, L. C. (1934) Principles underlying ciliary activity in the respiratory tract. II. A comparison of nasal clearance in man, monkey and other mammals. *Arch. Otolaryngol. 20*, 518–541

MELVILLE, G. N. & IRAVANI, J. (1975) Factors affecting ciliary beat frequency in the intrapulmonary airways of rats. *Can. J. Physiol. Pharmacol. 53*, 1122–1128

RASCHE, B., MARCIC, I. & ULMER, W. T. (1972) Zusammensetzung des Bronchialschleims bei langzeitig vorbehandelter chronisch obstruktiver Bronchitis und bei unvorbehandelter Bronchitis in Abhängigkeit von der Therapie. *Pneumonologie 146*, 321

SCUDI, J. V., KIMURA, E. T. & REINHARD, J. F. (1951) Study of drug action on mammalian ciliated epithelium. *J. Pharmacol. Exp. Ther. 102*, 132–137

Discussion

J. G. Jones: I am puzzled about the arrangement of these layers in the normal situation. You show a clear layer between the villi but in one of your electron micrographs there was a fairly granular appearance between the cilia—the clear layer didn't go to the top of the cilia.

Iravani: The granular appearance is due to vesiculations between the cilia whose exact origin cannot at present be explained.

Allison: But the vesiculations are abnormal whereas you had electron-dense material between the tips of the cilia in mucus in the normal.

Iravani: The depth of penetration of mucus between the cilia might not correspond exactly to normal conditions because the airway preparations were cooled to 30 °C. This artificial method allowed us to look at the interciliary fluid.

Jeffery: But how artificial is it? Are you just maintaining mucus or are you causing a build-up of mucus which is not normally present at this site and which causes the mucous layer to sink between the cilia? And again, underneath this mucus are we actually seeing the 'periciliary layer', by your method?

Iravani: Cooling causes a decrease in ciliary activity (Iravani 1967) and leads to accumulation of mucus. This explains the presence of a continuous mucus layer in the airway preparations I discussed, in contrast to airways studied at body temperature (Iravani & van As 1972). I do not think that the depth of penetration of the mucus between the cilia is significantly affected by this method. The interciliary fluid located underneath the mucus is electron-translucent.

Jeffery: Yes. It doesn't seem to be visible in your pictures.

Iravani: In electron micrographs the areas around the microvilli are electron-translucent. Obviously these areas could not contain air; hence the most likely constituent must be a water-like fluid.

Silberberg: Aren't cilia usually very closely spaced, only about 50 nm from wall to wall? In those circumstances it would be impossible for the size of macromolecules that we think are present in mucus to infiltrate between the cilia. In the pictures you showed the cilia were far apart. Perhaps these were abnormal regions as far as ciliation is concerned.

Reid: We seem to have several ideas which we could put together as a hypothesis. First there is the layer closest to the cell, then the perivillous layer, which stains in the light microscopic sections but which is now showing up as space; then there is the periciliary layer. More superficially we come to the 'structure' that Jennifer Sturgess (1977) has worked on in rabbit. She has shown that there seems to be a layer on the surface which can really be identified—call it the 'blanket' or the 'sheet' or something like that. From the small airways right to the trachea you can see this extra layer which is discrete and separate from the tips of the cilia. It is obviously superficial to them and it changes in character from the depths of the lung to the trachea. In the small airways it looks fairly smooth and is fairly thin; in the rabbit it is probably protein and it doesn't stain for acid glycoprotein. As you reach the larger airways it becomes filamentous and mesh-like. Under the conditions of preparation by drying you see some holes in it. Finally, somewhere on top of this layer we have 'rafts' and discrete collections of really 'gluggy' stuff. So there are about five layers to be considered.

Godfrey: Surprisingly large particles of dirt, hundreds of microns in diameter, are successfully transported by the surface rafts of mucus in large airways.

J. G. Jones: Professor Iravani, to what extent is this layer due to the ciliary activity itself? You suggested that somewhere the interciliary fluid layer may be reduced so that the cilia stick together. I think the opposite happens and the whole thing is in fact a function of ciliary activity. When ciliary activity is reduced, the mucus tide comes in, so to speak, the mucus blanket drops, and the whole of the clear layer vanishes. If you dropped a ciliated organism into some mucus, would you see a clear layer around it where the cilia beat in the mucus?

Iravani: In my talk I mentioned that removal of the secretion by washing the epithelial surface with normal saline led to a recovery of the ciliary activity to normal values; this finding caused me to conclude that the decrease in ciliary activity is the consequence and not the cause. The second part of your question is under investigation.

Allison: I believe that we are talking about two different things. Dr Jones is asking about the normal situation and Professor Iravani is talking about what happens in animals exposed to influenza virus where marked changes occur in the microvilli.

Iravani: We also found a reduction of the interciliary fluid in rats with chronic bronchitis.

J. G. Jones: So you can put the two together and say that virus infections primarily alter ciliary activity and consequentially you get changes in these layers and also loss of villi.

Iravani: That is not so; the reduction in ciliary activity can be reversed by removing the secretion.

J. G. Jones: The frequency may not alter but you said that the amplitude was greatly diminished. Is the amplitude diminished primarily or is it because the tide has gone out and left nothing for the cilia to beat in?

Iravani: I think the amplitude is diminished because of the viscous fluid between the cilia.

Allison: So it is cause rather than effect.

Guz: What is known about the coordination of the ciliary beat?

Iravani: There are two possible modes of coordination of the cilia: neural and mechanical (Kinosita & Murakami 1967). In the bronchial epithelium there is evidence that the coordination is mechanically induced (Iravani 1969).

Jeffery: I think Sleigh (1974) has postulated that if a cilium starts to move, by whatever mechanism, then that cilium has a direct effect through the surrounding fluid medium on its immediate neighbour (i.e. a hydrodynamic effect), causing metachronal coordination in that way.

Guz: Then a disordered pattern may be due to the fact that there are patchy areas of damage.

Iravani: The incoordination found in bronchitis might be caused by the cellular protrusions. These protrusions are much larger and more inert than the cilia, and due to these mechanical differences they disturb the metachronal coordination of the ciliary movement.

Silberberg: I have heard it said that the coordination is discharge-dependent, very much like nerve action is discharge-dependent. The bending of the cilium is definitely an ATP-controlled process which has to be initiated at the root and then proceeds upwards.

Allison: This has been extensively studied in protozoa where there are mutants that are defective, in particular in calcium transport mechanisms which affect ciliary function (Eckert 1972). Control could be transferred from one cell to another by way of gap-junctional systems. If there is a dead cell in the middle, or a cell which is highly damaged, this type of coordination will cease. Although we have a lot of information on protozoa, we have no comparable information on mammalian systems and are really guessing about what is going on.

References

ECKERT, R. (1972) Bioelectric control of ciliary activity. *Science (Wash. D.C.) 176*, 473–481

IRAVANI, J. (1967) Flimmerbewegung in den intrapulmonalen Luftwegen der Ratte. *Pflügers Arch. Gesamte Physiol. Menschen Tiere 297*, 221–237

IRAVANI, J. (1969) Coordination of the ciliary movement in bronchial epithelium of the rat. *Pflügers Arch. Eur. J. Physiol. 305*, 199–209

IRAVANI, J. & VAN AS, A. (1972) Mucus transport in tracheobronchial tree of normal and bronchitic rats. *J. Pathol. 106*, 81–93

KINOSITA, H. & MURAKAMI, A. (1967) Control of ciliary motion. *Physiol. Rev. 47*, 53–82

SLEIGH, M. A. (1974) Metachronism of cilia of metazoa, in *Cilia and Flagella*, Pergamon Press, Oxford

STURGESS, J. M. (1977) The mucous lining of major bronchi in the rabbit lung. *Am. Rev. Respir. Dis. 115*, 819–827

The isolation and partial characterization of the major bronchial glycoproteins

J. SCHRAGER and G. CUMMING

Midhurst Medical Research Institute, Midhurst, Sussex

Abstract Partial characterization of glycoprotein obtained from mucous secretion of the bronchi and stomach has been attempted. The isolated glycoproteins and the glycoproteins from gastric aspirates showed similar carbohydrate and amino-acid composition. They consist of a protein core to which are attached carbohydrate side chains of galactose, *N*-acetylglucosamine and *N*-acetylgalactosamine in the ratio of 4 : 3 : 1. Superimposed on this structure were additional sugar residues, the blood group determinants. The carbohydrate side chains are linked by an alkali-labile *O*-glycosidic linkage to the threonine and serine residues of the protein core, with *N*-acetylgalactosamine forming the link.

The human bronchial tree is lined by a thin film of mucus secreted by the epithelial goblet cells and the submucosal tracheobronchial glands. The mucus layer is propelled upwards and outwards by cilia lining the trachea and bronchi and passes over the larynx into the oesophagus and stomach. Dust particles, bacteria and other debris trapped by the mucus layer are thus removed and the airways kept clear.

The biologically protective action of mucociliary clearance may be disturbed by a variety of pathological conditions in which the mucus secretions become detrimental to ventilatory function.

Despite the importance of the bronchial mucus to the physiology and pathology of the respiratory system, very little is known about the composition and structure of its components. No quantitative studies on individual bronchial secretions obtained directly from the bronchi are, as far as we know, available. Previous work (Brogan 1959; Atassi *et al.* 1959*a*, *b*; Roussel *et al.* 1972; Lamblin *et al.* 1972) was carried out on pooled sputum from patients with chronic bronchitis.

A recent paper from this laboratory (Schrager & Oates 1974*a*) described the isolation and partial characterization of glycoproteins from gastric aspirates and from extracts of gastric mucosae. This paper describes the isolation and composition of glycoproteins from individual bronchial aspirates using similar methods.

MATERIALS AND METHODS

Individual aspirates from bronchial mucus were investigated. Thirty specimens were aspirated into an ice-cooled trap during bronchoscopy, neomycin was added (final concentration 0.05%), and the aspirates were stored at —20 °C until used. A further ten specimens were obtained at autopsy within a few hours after death and treated in a similar manner.

To each bronchial aspirate was added solid guanidine chloride adjusted to an approximate concentration of 2 M. The resulting mixture was gently agitated at room temperature until the gel had dispersed to give a uniform solution. The dissolved mucus was centrifuged at 2500 **g** for 30 min at room temperature. The deposit, consisting of cell debris, as shown by stained smears, was discarded. The supernatant was eluted with 2 M-guanidine chloride on Sepharose 2B-CL, and was resolved into fractions A and B. Fraction A contained the bulk of the carbohydrate content and this was dialysed against water for two days at 4 °C, concentrated and re-chromatographed on Bio-gel A15M. It was eluted with 0.05M-sodium chloride just within the retarded area as one peak.

Gel filtration and preparation of the column

The preparation of the Bio-gel column, the carbohydrate and amino acid analysis, sulphate and sialic acid determinations, technical details of gas–liquid chromatography, periodate oxidation, Smith degradation and alkaline borohydride treatment have been described by Schrager & Oates (1974*a*, *b*).

Release of sialic acid by neuraminidase (EC 3.2.1.18)

Each solution of glycoprotein (5 ml) isolated from a bronchial aspirate was made 0.1 M with respect to NaAc, pH 5.5; NaCl and $CaCl_2$ were then added to make final concentrations of 0.9% and 0.1% respectively. Neuraminidase (0.25 ml B.D.H. material from *Vibrio cholerae*, 125 units) was added to the resulting solutions which were then incubated at 37 °C. Samples were removed at intervals for estimation of free sialic acid.

RESULTS

Chromatography on Sepharose 2B-Cl resolved the bronchial aspirates into non-retarded and retarded fractions. The non-retarded fraction containing the bulk of the carbohydrate content was re-chromatographed on Bio-gel A15M, and eluted just within the retarding area as one peak; its components were designated 'bronchial glycoproteins'.

The carbohydrate composition of the 'bronchial glycoproteins'

Table 1 summarizes the yields and molar composition of the carbohydrate content of the 'bronchial glycoproteins'. Each glycoprotein yielded, on acid hydrolysis, galactose, fucose, *N*-acetylglucosamine and *N*-acetylgalactosamine. In addition the glycoproteins contain quantities of *N*-acetylneuraminic acid and sulphate end-groups in variable amounts. The ratio of galactose to *N*-acetylglucosamine to *N*-acetylgalactosamine was found to be 4:3:1. Superimposed on this basic composition of the glycoproteins were additional sugar residues—the blood group determinants. Fucose was associated with blood group specificity Le^a (non-secretor), an additional fucose residue with H, a further *N*-acetylgalactosamine with A and a further galactose with blood group specificity B.

Periodate oxidation

Periodate oxidation (Table 1) destroyed all the fucose and sialic acid residues, about half of the galactose of glycoproteins with blood group specificity H or Le^a (non-secretor), and only one-third to one-fourth of the galactose residues of glycoproteins with blood group specificity A. Oxidation did not significantly alter the *N*-acetylglucosamine and *N*-acetylgalactosamine content of the glycoproteins with blood group specificity H or Le^a, but destroyed the terminal residues of *N*-acetylgalactosamine associated with blood group specificity A. Thus, after periodate oxidation blood group specificity A was lost, and the *N*-acetylglucosamine to *N*-acetylgalactosamine ratio was found to be 3:1, similar to the *N*-acetylglucosamine to *N*-acetylgalactosamine ratio of glycoproteins with blood group specificity H, B or Le^a. After periodate oxidation *N*-acetylgalactosamine was approximately equimolar with the sum of the threonine and serine residues in all the glycoproteins investigated.

TABLE 1

The carbohydrate composition of glycoproteins isolated from 13 bronchial aspirates (a) before and (b) after periodate oxidation. The quantities are in mmol/l. The data in brackets show the quantitative relationship between galactose, fucose, *N*-acetylglucosamine and *N*-acetylgalactosamine.

	Sulphate	*Sialic acid*	*Galactose*	*Fucose*	*N-acetylglucosamine*	*N-acetylgalactosamine*	*Blood group specificity*
1 a)	0.18	0.05	0.59 (4.0)	0.57 (3.8)	0.46 (3.00)	0.15 (1.00)	H sec
b)			0.32	—	0.43	0.13	
2 a)	0.13	0.004	0.38 (3.8)	0.27 (2.7)	0.30 (3.00)	0.11 (1.1)	H sec
b)			0.23	—	0.29	0.10	
3 a)	0.12	0.025	0.28 (4.00)	0.19 (2.71)	0.22 (3.00)	0.08 (1.14)	H sec
b)			0.16	—	0.20	0.06	
4 a)	0.36	0.12	2.12 (4.24)	1.80 (3.60)	1.50 (3.00)	0.94 (1.88)	A & H sec
b)			1.30	—	1.58	0.52	
5 a)	0.24	0.033	0 65 (4.06)	0.30 (1.87)	0.50 (3.00)	0.16 (1.00)	H sec
b)			0.36	—	0.52	0.16	
6 a)	0.17	0.092	1.52 (4.00)	0.72 (1.89)	1.16 (3.00)	0.40 (1.05)	H sec
b)			0.80	—	1.16	0.39	
7 a)	0.26	0.23	1.84 (3.91)	1.44 (3.06)	1.42 (3.00)	0.76 (1.61)	A & H sec
b)			1.17	—	1.36	0.46	
8 a)	0.04	0.20	1.20 (3.87)	0.75 (2.42)	0.95 (3.00)	0.52 (1.67)	A & H sec
b)			0.80	—	0.90	0.34	
9 a)	0.11	0.09	0.83 (4.00)	0.59 (2.81)	0.64 (3.00)	0.37 (1.76)	A & H sec
b)			0.57	—	0.58	0.25	
10 a)	0.10	0.14	0.49 (3.77)	0.27 (2.07)	0.38 (3.00)	0.14 (1.07)	H sec
b)			0.40	—	0.40	0.15	
11 a)	Nil	0.09	0.44 (4.00)	0.33 (3.00)	0.33 (3.00)	0.19 (1.72)	A & H sec
b)			0.30	—	0.32	0.14	
12 a)	0.22	0.85	1.95 (3.75)	0.85 (1.63)	1.57 (3.00)	0.66 (1.27)	Non-sec
b)			1.70	—	1.52	0.52	
13 a)	0.22	0.08	0.84 (4.66)	0.54 (3.00)	0.54 (3.00)	0.24 (1.33)	H sec
b)			0.39	—	0.60	0.22	

Amino acids of the protein core

The amino acid composition (Table 2) of bronchial glycoprotein was similar to that of salivary and gastric glycoprotein.

Threonine and serine constituted between 45 and 50%, and these together with proline, alanine and glycine accounted for 75–80% of the total amino

TABLE 2

Amino acid compositions of three representative specimens of bronchial glycoproteins. Values are in molar proportions (threonine = 10.0)

	(1)	*(2)*	*(3)*
Aspartic acid	1.5	0.8	1.60
Threonine	10.0	10.0	10.0
Serine	5.0	5.6	5.30
Glutamic acid	2.4	1.9	2.00
Proline	—	4.6	5.80
Glycine	1.8	2.8	3.60
Alanine	4.2	4.6	4.80
Valine	1.2	—	—
Isoleucine	—	0.5	0.60
Leucine	1.2	1.2	1.20
Tyrosine	0.9	—	—
β-Phenylalanine	0.3	—	—
Lysine	0.6	0.9	—
Histidine	—	1.2	1.10
Arginine	—	—	0.80

acid content. The ratio of threonine to serine was approximately 2:1. The sum of threonine and serine was approximately equimolar with *N*-acetylgalactosamine in glycoproteins with blood group specificity Le^a and H.

Treatment with alkaline borohydride

Treatment with alkaline borohydride (Table 3) gave results similar to those obtained with gastric aspirates in extracts of gastric mucosae (Schrager & Oates 1974*b*): we found that 85–90% of threonine, 75–90% of serine and 90–95% of *N*-acetylgalactosamine were selectively destroyed, and the loss of threonine and serine was roughly equimolar with a loss of *N*-acetylgalactosamine residues (except in glycoproteins with blood group specificity A). The loss of *N*-acetylgalactosamine was accompanied by an equivalent formation of *N*-acetylgalactosaminitol.

Sialated bronchial glycoproteins

Fourteen bronchial glycoproteins were incubated with neuraminidase. Each glycoprotein was treated with periodate before and after removal of sialic acid by neuraminidase or mild acid hydrolysis. Ten glycoproteins were

TABLE 3

Amino acid composition of two specimens of bronchial glycoproteins before (a) and after (b) treatment with alkaline borohydride. The quantities are in mmol/l.

	1		*2*	
	(a)	*(b)*	*(a)*	*(b)*
Aspartic acid	0.08	0.08	0.07	0.06
Threonine	0.29	0.03	0.35	0.05
Serine	0.17	0.04	0.19	0.05
Glutamic acid	0.09	0.09	0.09	0.08
Proline	0.19	N.D.	0.20	N.D.
Glycine	0.11	0.12	0.08	0.09
Alanine	0.17	0.28	0.12	0.22
Valine	0.06	0.06	Trace	0.44
Cystine	0.06	—	—	—
AB	—	0.16	—	0.15
Isoleucine	0.02	0.02	0.02	0.02
Leucine	0.06	0.07	0.07	0.06
Tyrosine	0.01	0.02	0.02	0.01
β-Phenylalanine	0.02	0.02	0.04	0.03
Lysine	0.05	0.03	0.03	0.02
Histidine	0.02	0.02	0.03	0.02
Arginine	0.04	0.02	0.04	0.03
N-acetylgalactosamine	0.42	0.05	0.44	Trace
N-acetylgalactosaminitol	—	0.30	—	0.43
N-acetylglucosamine	0.68	0.62	1.23	1.10
Fucose	0.58	0.61	0.70	0.30
Galactose	0.95	0.93	1.60	1.47
Galactitol	—	0.02	—	Trace

N.D. = Not determined

neuraminidase-sensitive, and three were partially resistant but cleaved with mild acid hydrolysis (Table 4). The removal of sialic acid followed by periodate oxidation increased the destruction of galactose. The resistance of the galactose residues to periodate oxidation indicate that sialic acid was linked to C-3; with the removal of sialic acid by neuraminidase or mild acid hydrolysis galactose became exposed to the action of the reagent. In nine samples, the increased loss of galactose was approximately equimolar with the free sialic acid residues, while in the remaining specimens the free sialic acid residues were in excess of the destroyed galactose. The observation that neither *N*-acetylglucosamine nor *N*-acetylgalactosamine were subjected to attack by

TABLE 4

The carbohydrate composition and sialic acid content of 14 bronchial aspirates before and after incubation with neuraminidase (a) before and (b) after periodate oxidation. The quantities are in mmol/l.

	Sul-phate	*Sialic acid*		*Galac-tose*	*Fucose*	*N-acetyl-glucos-amine*	*N-acetyl-galac-tos-amine*	*Blood group specificity of extract*
		Free	*Bound*					
1(a)	0.23		0.22	0.70	0.50	0.58	0.32	A & H sec
(b)				0.54	—	0.54	0.20	
After incubation with neuraminidase:								
(a)		0.11		0.70	0.50	0.58	0.32	
(b)				0.42	—	0.45	0.15	
2(a)	0.15		0.17	0.81	0.54	0.52	0.30	H sec
(b)				0.52	—	0.50	0.23	
After incubation with neuraminidase:								
(a)		0.14		0.81	0.54	0.52	0.30	
(b)				0.40	—	0.56	0.27	
3(a)	0.30		0.47	1.16	0.91	0.87	0.52	A & H sec
(b)				0.78	—	0.84	0.30	
After incubation with neuraminidase:								
(a)		0.45		1.16	0.91	0.87	0.52	
(b)				0.80	—	0.85	0.34	
4(a)	0.10		0.20	0.56	0.32	0.40	0.16	H sec
(b)				0.40	—	0.43	0.16	
After incubation with neuraminidase:								
(a)		0.20		0.56	0.32	0.40	0.16	
(b)				0.27	—	0.42	0.15	
5(a)	0.06		0.33	0.53	0.24	0.42	0.19	Non-sec
(b)				0.44	—	0.41	0.15	
After incubation with neuraminidase:								
(a)		0.25		0.53	0.24	0.42	0.19	
(b)				0.37	—	0.39	0.13	
6(a)	0.02		0.22	0.40	0.20	0.27	0.13	Non-sec
(b)				0.34	—	0.25	0.12	
After incubation with neuraminidase:								
(a)		0.13		0.40	0.20	0.27	0.13	
(b)				0.19	—	0.26	0.12	
After HCl 80 °C, 90 min		0.19		0.19	—	0.26	0.12	
7(a)	Nil		0.27	0.88	0.55	0.66	0.31	H sec
(b)				0.55	—	0.63	0.30	
After incubation with neuraminidase:								
(a)		0.30		0.88	0.55	0.66	0.31	
(b)				0.31	—	0.60	0.27	

TABLE 4 (continued)

	Sulphate	*Sialic acid*		*Galactose*	*Fucose*	*N-acetylglucosamine*	*N-acetylgalactosamine*	*Blood group specificity of extract*
		Free	*Bound*					
8(a)	0.06		0.31	1.16	0.84	0.86	0.33	H sec
(b)				0.71	—	0.87	0.26	
After incubation with neuraminidase:								
(a)		0.29		1.16	0.84	0.86	0.33	
(b)				0.56	—	0.91	0.28	
9(a)	0.02		0.11	0.36	0.25	0.26	0.17	H sec
(b)				0.24	—	0.28	0.14	
After incubation with neuraminidase:								
(a)		0.11		0.36	0.25	0.26	0.17	
(b)				0.19	—	0.25	0.14	
10(a)	0.13		0.18	0.95	0.70	0.74	0.31	Non-sec
(b)				0.50	—	0.77	0.24	
After incubation with neuraminidase:								
(a)		0.13		0.95	0.70	0.74	0.31	
(b)				0.38	—	0.70	0.23	
11(a)	0.20		0.30	1.19	0.76	0.85	0.33	Non-sec
(b)				0.62	—	0.85	0.30	
After incubation with neuraminidase:								
(a)		0.25		1.19	0.76	0.85	0.33	
(b)				0.52	—	0.86	0.31	
12(a)	0.12		0.21	0.91	0.74	0.67	0.27	H sec
(b)				0.48	—	0.64	0.22	
After incubation with neuraminidase:								
(a)		0.09		0.91	0.71	0.67	0.27	
(b)				0.40	—	0.67	0.24	
After HCl 80 °C, 90 min		0.21		0.40	—	0.67	0.24	
13(a)	0.04		0.12	0.39	0.28	0.28	0.12	H sec
(b)				0.19	—	0.26	0.09	
After incubation with neuraminidase:								
(a)		0.10		0.39	0.28	0.28	0.12	
(b)				0.14	—	0.25	0.09	
14(a)	N.D.		0.16	0.69	0.55	0.53	0.28	A & H sec
(b)				0.57	—	0.53	0.17	
After incubation with neuraminidase:								
(a)		0.17		0.69	0.55	0.53	0.28	
(b)				0.42	—	0.54	0.17	

periodate strongly suggests that these hexoses were protected from this reagent by suitable linkage.

Smith degradation

Only one cycle of Smith sequential periodate degradation (Schrager & Oates 1974*a*) was possible with the small amount of material available. Sugar and amino sugar values remained the same as after initial oxidation. The only polyol formed in appreciable amounts in the glycoproteins after removal of sialic acid with neuraminidase was glycerol.

DISCUSSION

The results of this study demonstrate fundamental similarities between bronchial glycoproteins and the gastric and salivary glycoproteins studied previously (Schrager & Oates 1974*a*, *b*), but also revealed significant differences between the three types of glycoproteins.

The data obtained show that bronchial mucus is made up of neutral, sialated and sulphated glycoproteins. Previous studies of gastric mucus and saliva suggest that the former contains only neutral, and the latter neutral and sulphated glycoproteins (Schrager & Oates 1974*a*, *b*).

Sialic acid is an important component of bronchial glycoproteins. Because the p*K* value of the average residue is about 2.6 an acidic character is imparted to the macromolecule. Electrostatic repulsion of ionized carboxyl groups near neutral pH results in distension of the average conformation of the macromolecule. Thus, these glycoproteins may be classed as polyanionic polyelectrolytes. Sulphate groups enhance the polyanionic character of the macromolecule.

The total release of the sialic acid by neuraminidase or by mild acid hydrolysis insufficient to affect any other component strongly suggests its terminal location. Neuraminidase is known to cleave the (2–3) linkage of *N*-acetylneuraminic acid to galactose, and the (2–6) linkage of *N*-acetylneuraminic acid to *N*-acetylgalactosamine (Gottschalk 1960).

The results of periodate oxidation after the removal of sialic acid by neuraminidase divided the sialated glycoproteins into two groups: (a) Glycoproteins in which all the sialic acid is linked to the subterminal galactose residues by $(2 \rightarrow 3)$, the sialic acid shielding the latter from oxidation. This protection would be lost after neuraminidase incubation or mild acid hydrolysis and the released sialic acid would be approximately equimolar with the destroyed galactose residues. (b) Glycoproteins in which some of the sialic acid is linked via (2→ 3) to galactose and some via (2→ 6) to galactosamine. Thus, only a part of the sialic acid content was shielding the subterminal galactose residues which became exposed to the action of this reagent after neuraminidase oxidation; as neuraminidase releases the sialic acid linked to both galactose and *N*-acetylgalactosamine, this would result in an excess of freed sialic acid over destroyed galactose.

Some of the galactose residues may have been protected by sulphate groups linked to C–3. This linkage has been suggested previously in salivary glycoproteins (Schrager & Oates 1974*a*, *b*). Glycoproteins with blood group specificity A and H would have an *N*-acetylgalactosamine at the non-reducing end of the carbohydrate side chains shielding the sub-terminal galactose after the removal of sialic acid (Table 2, sample 3).

The observation that neither *N*-acetylglucosamine nor *N*-acetylgalactosamine were subject to attack by periodate strongly suggests that these hexoses were protected from this reagent by suitable linkage. This could only be achieved if galactose is linked to C–3 or C–4 of *N*-acetylgalactosamine and *N*-acetylglucosamine.

The values of *N*-acetylgalactosamine are of particular interest. This component attaches the carbohydrate side chains to threonine and serine of the protein core. The results of alkaline borohydride treatment show that there is only one *N*-acetylgalactosamine residue for each carbohydrate side chain, as almost all *N*-acetylgalactosamine residues are destroyed by this treatment.

These results and the data on the molar ratios of the three major sugars, galactose/*N*-acetylglucosamine/*N*-acetylgalactosamine (4:3:1), facilitate calculation of the average size of the side chains. The calculated size would be a statistical average and compatible with variations in the size of these chains but, on the basis of the results which show constant ratios, one would expect these variations to form a regular pattern of long chains (peaks) and short chains (troughs), which would constitute the intrinsic structure of the bronchial glycoproteins.

References

Atassi, M. Z., Barker, S. A., Houghton, L. E. & Stacey, M. (1959*a*) Neuraminic acid and its relation to chronic bronchitis II. *Clin. Chim. Acta 4*, 741–747

Atassi, M. Z., Barker, S. A. & Stacey, M. (1959*b*) Neuraminic acid and its relation to chronic bronchitis. III. Carbohydrate constituents of sputum. *Clin. Chim. Acta 4*, 823–827

Brogan, R. D. (1959) The carbohydrate complexes of bronchial secretion. *Biochem. J. 71*, 125–131

GOTTSCHALK, A. (1960) *The Chemistry and Biology of Sialic Acids and Related Substances.* Cambridge University Press, London

LAMBLIN, G., DEGAND, P., ROUSSEL, P., HAVEZ, R., HARTEMANN, E. & FILLAT, M. (1972) Les glycopeptides du mucus bronchique fibrillaire dans la mucoviscidose. *Clin. Chim. Acta 36*, 329–340

ROUSSEL, P., LAMBLIN, G., DEGAND, P. & HAVEZ, R. (1972) Isolement des mucines bronchiques secrétées au cours de la mucoviscidose. *Clin. Chim. Acta 36*, 315–328

SCHRAGER, J. & OATES, M. D. (1974*a*) The isolation and partial characterization of a glycoprotein isolated from human gastric aspirates and from extracts of gastric mucosae. *Biochim. Biophys. Acta 372*, 183–195

SCHRAGER, J. & OATES, M. D. (1974*b*) The chemical composition and some structural features of the principal salivary glycoprotein isolated from human mixed saliva. *Arch. Oral Biol. 19*, 1215–1220

Discussion

Kent: Can you say any more about the part played by sialic acids in the original secretion that you described? Was there sialic acid in the blood group-reactive fractions?

Cumming: The values varied between 0.004 and 0.23 and are set out in Table 1 (p. 256).

Allison: I should point out that many bronchial carcinomas have carcino-embryonic antigens which are slightly different from those in the gastrointestinal tract. Blood-group precursors are also found and it is a complicated situation.

Davis: Did you find any differences between the mucus collected by aspiration through a rigid bronchoscope and the mucus from the airways at autopsy?

Cumming: No. All the 50 analyses gave similar results, which was surprising, and this may support the view that there is a glycoprotein which can be handled.

Silberberg: Have you studied the molecular weight of this material?

Cumming: Not yet, but clearly we shall have to.

Kent: To take up Dr Cumming's point about using antibodies to fractionate bronchial secretion, Dr Winterborne in our laboratory has been studying some fluorosugars which have been synthesized in a radioactive form, incorporated into the various secretions, and then the soluble secretions are fractionated. He found that, as a result of introducing these sugar analogues biosynthetically, certain glucosamine residues carry *N*-fluoroacetyl substituents producing a form of hyaluronic acid with increased resistance to hyaluronidase. On further analysis glycoproteins were present which contained not only *N*-acetylneuraminic acid but also *N*-fluoroacetylneuraminic acid and we think that this also is much more resistant to neuraminidase. So by biosynthetic manipulation one can probably produce secretions with very much altered mechanical properties and possibly antigenic properties as well.

Allison: Could you change the pool sizes of some intermediates?

Kent: Almost certainly. The pool sizes of the UDP-*N*-acetylglucosamine and CMP sialic acid are remarkably influenced by the presence of these false sugars. They are incorporated into the nucleotide pools, which are substantially diluted as a result.

Allison: So it might be possible to see how important they are in controlling synthesis.

Kent: The work has not yet been done but it is possible. We can see that by putting in the appropriate analogue, the extension of oligosaccharide can be blocked, since no further sugars can be added except in most extreme circumstances.

Cumming: How are those analogues incorporated into protein?

Kent: They are added to the growth media in cultured cell lines or organ cultures.

General discussion IV

Allison: Has the relationship of blood groups to respiratory disease been looked at?

Proctor: Yes, but we have not reached the point where we can draw broad conclusions. Camner *et al.* (1972) have found that there is a remarkable similarity in bronchial clearance in monozygotic twins but not between unrelated individuals or siblings who are not twins.

J. G. Jones: Pneumoconiosis has been looked at but I do not believe there is any association between susceptibility to pneumoconiosis and blood groups (Higgins 1963).

Godfrey: Edfors-Lubs (1971) studied asthma in monozygotic twins and found a concordance rate of only 19%.

Allison: There were claims that histocompatibility antigens are related to proneness to develop asbestosis in exposed persons, but these have not been confirmed. Blood group characteristics are associated with the presence of particular glycosyltransferase enzymes, and it would be interesting to have some clear indication of what these do; the resulting chemical differences may well affect functions of mucus and other systems.

Kent: Could you comment on the presence and role of immunoglobulins in the bronchial secretion?

Allison: They are there. There was a wide feeling a few years back that for defence against influenza virus, secretory IgA antibody was needed. The evidence is now against that; serum IgG antibodies reacting with variant-specific determinants of haemagglutinin appear to be more important in protection than secretory antibodies (Virelizier 1975). In IgA deficiencies there is sometimes, but not always, increased susceptibility to respiratory and gastrointestinal infections.

Reid: The cases I have seen with impaired ciliary clearance have been very like the old-fashioned surgical bronchiectasis, i.e. there was one incident of acute damage to the lung with resulting bronchial distortion. This is a very different pattern from that seen with the increased susceptibility to infection associated with immunoglobulin deficiencies, or even in cystic fibrosis. The immunoglobulin deficiencies mostly tend to be chronic pneumonitis and bronchiolitis. If one had to localize this, or cystic fibrosis, at a particular airway level it would be the small airways. Whatever the deficiency is in cystic fibrosis it is not primarily in the mucus because these children have normal glands. I believe that whatever is going wrong is caused by the susceptibility to infection and it is the infection that starts off the vicious circle of infection, mucus hypersecretion and gland hypertrophy. So there are differences in these three deficiency diseases. The ciliary clearance story doesn't seem to produce the sort of chronic recurrent infection that we think of as typical of impairment of the immune system.

Nadel: Is it possible that in IgA deficiency states, instead of there being an abnormal immunological response, the same cell that has the deficiency in the secretory piece may play a different role in infection? Do these cells secrete abnormally?

Allison: About two-thirds of people who have no demonstrable IgA in their secretions have no trouble with infection, but one-third do and they are often found to have associated abnormalities. Particularly in the gastrointestinal tract, the amount of lymphoid tissue may be markedly deficient, so the simple notion that IgA is necessary for protection of sero-mucous surfaces may have to be qualified.

Cumming: We treat a large number of children with cystic fibrosis. We determine the specific circulating antibodies when they have an infection and as far as we can see the immune system seems to be fairly competent.

Reid: I agree. Every test that has been done on them indicates that their immune system is mature but we still do not know why they are susceptible to infection.

Silberberg: How do you visualize this immune reaction taking place in the epithelium? How are the antibodies supposed to function there?

Allison: In the gastrointestinal tract it looks as though secretory antibodies are involved in the prevention of attachment of certain bacteria, for example cholera organisms, to the epithelium. There is no evidence for a role of secretory antibodies with leucocytes in killing bacteria. For example, there are no receptors for IgA on the surface of the macrophages so there is no reason to believe that IgA could collaborate with alveolar macrophages in killing, or indeed with infiltrating polymorphs, as happens with IgG antibodies. What Professor Reid was talking about is classical IgG deficiency where there is a tendency towards recurrent bacterial infections of the lung unless IgG is given; then there is collaboration between antibody, complement and leucocytes, with the antibody and complement providing opsonization for uptake.

Reid: One of the advantages of these substances in sputum—and in other secretions—is that they provide a marker of the serum component which is very important in studies of total secretion in diseases like asthma or viral infection.

Nadel: An abnormality in the IgA secretory piece could just be the marker of another abnormality in the epithelial cell.

Allison: That is possible. It ought to be looked at in the respiratory system.

Reid: Professor Silberberg, did you say that you were not getting any change in bovine cervical mucin by treating with urea?

Silberberg: We used 6M-guanidinium hydrochloride and purified mucin. This medium did not affect the final size of the breakdown product of the mucin aggregate nor the rate at which breakdown was occurring (Meyer 1976).

Reid: That is an important difference between bronchial and bovine cervical material. If you add urea to total bronchial secretion you will achieve the equivalent of having sheared at about 10 cycles/s, which means that you have begun to reduce viscosity and change elasticity.

Cumming: What about relating the constituents of normal mucus to the blood groups?

Allison: It would be more interesting to relate them to susceptibility to disease.

Reid: Dr Lamb (Lamb & Reid 1972) looked at various levels in the bronchial tree in a series of individuals and found a wide range between subjects of the sort of glycoproteins that Mrs Jones mentioned (pp. 175–188). But in a series of subjects, either normal or bronchitic, there is an extraordinarily similar distribution between different regions of the same bronchial tree. So perhaps it is not surprising that we seem to get such similar results from different individuals on different occasions, but I suspect that you will get differences between individuals.

Allison: We accept that different individuals vary in their susceptibility to respiratory infections; every clinician believes that. The situation is not static, because people can change; they may be susceptible for a number of years and then develop resistance, which implies that susceptibility isn't only genetically controlled; but we know next to nothing about its physiopathological basis. Are any of the tests or observations that we have discussed relevant to this problem and, if not, what should we be doing?

Proctor: Almost any of the studies of the functional defence mechanisms would be worth doing in individuals over a period of years. We are planning to start a study like this in cystic fibrosis patients and others. Certainly, in the practice of otolaryngology, we see patients with remarkable susceptibility to infections over a period of years who then go for another period of years without having any trouble. One would think that there must have been some change in their defence mechanisms.

Godfrey: Many studies on IgA and lymphocyte sensitization to antigens have proved disappointingly negative in people susceptible to recurrent chest infections.

Allison: Let us return to the question of the chemistry of mucin.

Carlstedt: One problem in the biology of mucus is how to remove the mucins from the mucus gel for further biochemical and physicochemical studies. A prerequisite to claiming that one has a representative sample of the mucins under study is that extraction must be carried out in a good yield. I think recovery and extraction yield are among the most neglected concepts in this field (see however Robson *et al.* 1975; Snary & Allen 1971, 1972). The reason is probably that mucins are difficult to quantitate. Mucins can be measured, for instance, as polymer-bound hexosamine (or as any sugar constituent known to be present in mucins) or by recovery of radioactive glycoprotein precursors in polymeric form. However, none of these methods measure mucins specifically.

Proteolytic digestion of the tissue was earlier the method of choice to extract mucins. We now know that a degradation product is obtained by this treatment, representing only the oligosaccharide domains of the nascent macromolecules. One advantage, however, is that proteases can accomplish total solubilization of the tissue, thus allowing us to isolate at least the glycopeptides derived from the mucins in full yield.

In a study of mucins from rat small intestinal mucosa, mucins were operationally defined as those macromolecules in the tissue giving rise to high molecular weight, polyanionic glycopeptides after papain digestion of the tissue. These 'marker' glycopeptides were prepared by ion-exchange chromatography (DEAE-cellulose) and gel chromatography (Sepharose 6B). Since papain accomplished total solubilization of the tissue the amount of 'marker' solubilized by this method was set to 100%.

I was able to show that guanidine-HCl, urea, neutral salts and various detergents over broad concentration ranges and at different pH values did not solubilize more than 20% of the mucins. Mucins were extracted by gentle stirring in the cold for 24 h. After centrifugation the amount of 'marker' glycopeptides was determined in the supernatant and compared to the amount of 'marker' solubilized from a corresponding amount of tissue by papain.

Apart from papain digestion, digestion with pronase, treatment with dithiothreitol (DTT) and the shear produced in a Waring Blender will give rise to 'good' solubilization. None of these methods appear attractive to me. Proteases will destroy the protein part of the mucins, DTT must involve some kind of modification and the Waring Blender probably breaks covalent bonds in the mucins from this mucosal tissue.

After the tissue had been extracted with deoxycholate, I noticed that only a very small residue was left despite the fact that only 20% of the mucins had been extracted. Consequently the tissue was subjected to repetitive extractions with deoxycholate. After each extraction cycle the *insoluble* part of the material was recovered by centrifugation. The residue was finally washed free from detergent and salt and was stored either lyophilized or deep-frozen. The residue (RI-DOC) is an almost pure insoluble complex of mucins representing about 80% of the total determined on the basis of 'marker' glycopeptides as described earlier. No (i.e. less than 1%) collagen, nucleic acids, phospholipids or residual deoxycholate could be detected.

Antibodies produced by rabbits against RI-DOC have been localized to the goblet cells and over the intestinal mucosal surface (I. Carlstedt & F. Sundler, unpublished work, 1976).

My attitude is to handle this insoluble glycoprotein complex just as an ordinary protein, trying to degrade it with various agents in the hope that overlapping fragments will provide sufficient information about its structure to tell what makes it really insoluble.

One obvious way to attack the structure of any protein or glycoprotein, insoluble or not, is to reduce disulphide bridges and see what fragments come out. DTT proved very effective and accomplished total solubilization of RI-DOC, as might be expected (extraction data). However, reproducible chromatograms of the split products were never obtained. Since the results might be interpreted as if a proteolytic enzyme had been working in concert with DTT, I started to look for such enzymes in RI-DOC using artificial substrates of low molecular weight. Activity was found against BAEE (benzyl-arginyl-ethyl-ester) and this activity could be suppressed by DFP (diisopropyl-fluorophosphate). Once this 'endogenous' protease was inhibited, I had no problem in obtaining well-defined fragments from RI-DOC in a reproducible manner with various techniques. How effective this 'endogenous' protease is can be illustrated by the fact that if RI-DOC is pretreated with DFP, no solubilization is obtained with DTT alone but full solubilization is obtained with DTT in 6M-guanidine-HCl. Guanidine-HCl alone does not solubilize RI-DOC as would also be expected (extraction data).

A major glycoprotein fragment has been isolated from RI-DOC after reduction of the DFP-pretreated complex with DTT in 6M-guanidine-HCl.

Purification was accomplished by isopycnic density gradient centrifugation in CsCl. The glycoprotein was banding at $\rho = 1.45$; it represents about three-quarters of the RI-DOC and contains all the carbohydrate.

I think this work illustrates two possible pitfalls. First, if extraction yield had not been determined in this case, probably only one-fifth of the mucins would have been studied further. This part of the macromolecules *might* represent material undergoing degradation and thus not constitute the physiologically relevant part of the total. Second, tissue proteinases could modify the structures we want to examine and we would end up with a structural and physicochemical picture that is not prevalent in the tissue.

Silberberg: We had a lot of difficulty when we started in this field, trying to solubilize bovine cervical mucus and get reproducible results. Until we established our methods we were getting all kinds of strange results, seemingly insoluble residues and so on. For example, when we concentrate bovine cervical mucus by a factor of two, this material is no longer solubilized by dithiothreitol, although it can still be solubilized by trypsin. All we have done is to take out half the water and we have changed the structure so that this reagent no longer attacks it. Consequently, when one takes material through a lyophilization stage one may be introducing blockages or structural changes that might affect its ability to respond to certain reagents. As I have stressed, a common basic structure seems to be characteristic of the mucins from epithelial mucous secretions. There seems to be a single amino acid sequence and they have certain characteristic structural features in common. These building blocks may, however, be used in different ways in different secretions. In bovine cervical mucus, there seems to be a supermolecular aggregate of about 15 million. In other materials, there may well be different structural combinations. While I believe that we are right in trying to emphasize the similarity at the lower level, we must first make sure of this, in any particular system, and then look at the higher level, as close to the native secreted material as possible to see what organization exists at that level and how it reflects itself in relation to the function of that particular secretion. Moreover, any manipulation is apt to produce artifacts. For example, while mild shearing of a dilute solution of macromolecules is not going to degrade them, mild shearing of a strongly aggregated system of macromolecules will most certainly affect structure. In this case long sequences of macromolecules are 'hand in hand' with each other and, therefore, the pull of the flow is over a very large surface. Much larger forces can, therefore, be built up than over a single macromolecule in isolation in a dilute solution.

Carlstedt: My extraction study does not include any lyophilization step. The tissue is just gently stirred with the extractant under study and the amount of mucin 'marker' is determined in the supernatant after unsolubilized material has been removed by centrifugation.

The kind of shear produced in a Waring Blender will solubilize RI-DOC. To judge from gel chromatographic data, degradation of the constituent macromolecules is obtained. Gentle homogenization in a Potter-Elvehjem or Dounce type of homogenizer does not even solubilize RI-DOC.

Silberberg: This is indeed one of the things that has always worried me. We found that when we sheared mucus we got solubilization. As I have just stressed, in very large molecules (and a gel is one enormous molecule), even mild shear can build up forces which can break covalent bonds. Therefore, do the structures that we get in that way really reflect the unaltered chemistry of this material? Apparently they do. We arrive, by shear, at essentially the same unit that we can also obtain by doing nothing more dramatic than leaving the material to stand.

Carlstedt: How do you distinguish between one preparation and the other? If you use S values or molecular weight you could cut off say 50% of the lateral portion of the protein moiety in these macromolecules and still not see the difference. You have to do detailed chemical analysis of the protein part of the molecules because the many oligosaccharide chains dominate the physical properties.

Silberberg: I think you are right. If we were missing a bit of the bare portion of the protein backbone we would not see it very easily by physicochemical means.

Carlstedt: I was talking about proteases earlier. Papain, which is a rather unspecific enzyme, produces well-defined fragments from immunoglobulins, for example. The fragments produced by the action of papain or pronase on RI-DOC look really homogeneous on gels. There might be steric reasons for this. The fact that a certain extraction procedure gives rise to well-defined glycoproteins cannot be taken as evidence that a protease has not been present and modified the structure.

Although a great deal of interesting and detailed work is coming along it is probably still premature to generalize. We still need to study a variety of glycoproteins and tissues.

Phelps: I agree; there are great dangers in over-simplification. I commend this scheme because we all know how difficult it is to get an entry into the system, and one attraction of Dr Carlstedt's procedure is that it gets rid of the nucleic acid.

Guz: I have a clinical question which the physical chemists may be able to help with. People whose cilia have packed up are able to move mucus up by coughing, and this prevents a lot of disasters. Now we do not know why mucus is sticky and we do not know what mucus is sticking to in the bronchial surface layer. What are the primary physical qualities that define stickiness and what ought we to do to mucus, to help a cough to displace it?

Silberberg: In what part of the lung does the coughing mechanism really operate, and how far does it go down into the lung? Is the effectiveness of clearance by coughing really the whole problem or are these people still dependent on getting the stuff out from deeper portions of the lung?

Proctor: A cough is most effective in the extrapulmonary airway.

Guz: I have put particles down the fibre-optic bronchoscope right into the divisions of the major bronchi deep in the lung and coughing is a major factor in moving them up; that however is not very far down.

Nadel: The cough receptors are mainly located in the larynx, the bifurcation of the trachea and the bifurcation of the major bronchi. The reflex secretory mechanisms associated with the cough involve the glands. Stimuli that produce cough may also stimulate reflex secretion. The major shearing effects of cough are normally in the trachea and the major bronchi. It seems rational to me to have reflux secretion tied to reflex cough, and located in large airways where cough is most effective.

Silberberg: Does the mucus have to be floated off?

Nadel: You have to shear it off.

Silberberg: The stream of air does that, but to make it glide easily over the epithelium one needs to float it off. You are operating against viscosity. Let us stick to our model that the mucus is involved with the tips of the cilia. This is good for moving it along with the ciliary beat but bad for trying to move it faster than ciliary motion because then there would be resistance. But if you imagine that the serous layer is temporarily increased by local excessive secretion of the thin flowing material, this would tend to float mucus off the cilia and then the airstream induced by coughing would be able to take it along and blow it upwards.

Guz: During fibre-optic bronchoscopy, especially in a chronic bronchitic, you can often see blobs of mucus and, if you mark a specimen with India ink, you can actually see that a lot of cough will suddenly cause the thing to jump up. It seems sticky but quite suddenly a sequence of coughs will cause the blob to move a few centimetres.

Thurlbeck: How far down the tracheobronchial tree?

Guz: Certainly two or three divisions.

J. G. Jones: S. W. Clarke and I have studied some effects of air flow rate on the clearance of sputum and simulated mucus from glass models of the tracheobronchial tree (Clarke *et al.* 1970). There are two points to be made. The first is the interaction between the velocity of air flow and the thickness of the lining layer, and the second is the role of the viscoelastic properties of the liquid in this interaction. With liquid layers greater than 0.5 mm in thickness small waves appear in the surface at a particular air flow rate, determined by the thickness and viscoelastic properties of the lining layer. Further small increases in flow lead to rapidly increasing gas–liquid interaction, a large rise in resistance to flow followed by a sudden expulsion of the liquid layer from the trachea. With increasing layer thickness the expulsive effect occurs at lower flow rates. This tracheal air flow rate may be quite modest, for example 2 litres per second, giving a linear velocity of 1000 cm/s, which contrasts with the almost sonic velocities (30 000 cm/s) which are claimed to occur in the airways during coughing. This latter figure is a considerable overestimate because of the errors in the measurement of airway cross-sectional area during coughing (Jones *et al.* 1975). When the thickness of the liquid layer was less than 0.5 mm it gained considerable mechanical stability from its adhesion to the airway wall and there was no sign of clearance even at very high flow rates.

The other factor is the viscoelastic properties of the liquid. In general, for a given thickness of lining layer, the more viscous the liquid the more difficult it was to induce strong gas–liquid interaction by increasing air flow, although with polyethylene oxide there was a range of viscosity where gas–liquid interaction increased with increasing viscosity.

Richardson: In the cat the two stimuli used to produce coughing—rubbing the larynx gently with a pledget of cotton wool and giving ammonia directly into the lung—both increased the amount of mucus produced into the trachea. segment by a reflex (Phipps & Richardson 1976).

Sadoul: Some patients with advanced chronic bronchitis are unable to raise sputum by coughing but they have an effective mucociliary clearance because the physical properties of the sputum are not the same in all kinds of patients.

Nadel: And the physical properties of the airways aren't the same either.

Donald: Does deformity of the tracheal or respiratory wall by the pressure pulse of a cough help to loosen the tenacious piece of mucus.

Sadoul: Yes.

Guz: Are the chemists going to tell us what stickiness is?

Silberberg: I think there is no difference in any of the materials in terms of introducing a new surface per unit area. A given number of intermolecular contacts have to be broken and in aqueous systems these are all of about the same magnitude. A macromolecule sticks over a large surface area. Systems which involve macromolecules are therefore more sticky in the sense that moving them, in order to create a fresh surface, will require a much larger force than if the solute were of the same chemical structure but was in the form of individual small molecules. Large molecules also recruit other macromolecules which are nearby and thereby create a further mechanism by which not just one layer of molecules but a whole series of layers may become involved in shearing off the mucus coat. In that sense we may think of mucus as being stickier than water—in actual fact it is probably about the same in terms of a static energy of interaction per unit area. In fact, if cognisance is taken of the fact that surfactant is present in the lung, the energy needed for an additional unit of free surface will be much less than in pure water.

Allison: Is there any simple property which might be related to difficulty in translocating mucus as a result of coughing?

Silberberg: I think it is all a question of molecular size. If a viscoelastic layer is put in contact with a solid support, macromolecular adhesion and simultaneous embedding in the layer create a very strong interaction. If, however, a layer of water is put between the solid support and the viscoelastic material, the material would move much more readily because the flow would occur over a layer which is essentially of lower viscosity and would not require the detachment of the macromolecule from the rigid surface.

Phelps: I wonder, Professor Guz, if sticky is the best word to use? Would it not be better to say that it has to grip but not fix on the surface?

Guz: I still want to know what we ought to be doing to these glands to improve the physics of the secretion.

Allison: One thing that can be done is to stimulate the vagus nerve or use a drug which has the same effect. The other is to use disulphide bond reagents to make the molecules smaller.

Guz: Disulphide bond reagents have been tried for many years but the results are very difficult to evaluate.

J. G. Jones: Most clinicians who work in intensive therapy units believe that if the airways are not moistened patients don't do too well, so they arrange for their patients to breathe aerosolized saline, or they even pour saline into the airways, and the patients get better.

Godfrey: I always wondered about that. The airways are already 100% saturated with water vapour and yet we pump in more water.

J. G. Jones: Let me qualify that. The patients who seem to respond best are those with endotracheal intubation and they seem to be the people who somehow cannot get rid of excess mucus. It may be that putting a mechanical block at the top end of the trachea leads to a build-up of mucus in the large airways which makes the stuff fall back. So if the gas they breathe is not humidified, they get into serious difficulties.

Godfrey: I agree with that.

Silberberg: It seems to me that one needs to increase the thickness of the interciliary fluid layer and if possible lift the mucus off. One way of doing that would be with water, and if you cannot get it from the epithelium directly by some stimulus, you apply it externally, which would probably have the same effect.

Allison: You might also facilitate water flow by increasing ion transport from the epithelium into the periciliary fluid.

Nadel: Clinical experience shows that often the water or saline cannot get in through the airway and it frequently has a deleterious effect. Perhaps, if you really want to get liquid into the periciliary layer, the best way may be to pump it in through the epithelium if you can think of ways of doing it.

J. G. Jones: Professor Silberberg, did you say that the mucus actually takes up water without changing its volume?

Silberberg: No. Mucus does not change its volume nor does it take up water. Most aqueous gels, when put in contact with water, usually swell to a certain equilibrium size. Mucus, however, has the curious property that it does not swell even if its concentration is increased by evaporation of some of the water. It simply stays in the concentrated form.

References

CAMNER, P., PHILIPSON, K. & FRIBERG, L. (1972) Tracheobronchial clearance in twins. *Arch. Environ. Health 24*, 82–87

CLARKE, S. W., JONES, J. G. & OLIVER, D. R. (1970) Resistance to two-phase gas-liquid flow in airways. *J. Appl. Physiol. 29*, 464–471

EDFORS-LUBS, M. L. (1971) Allergy in 7,000 twin pairs. *Acta Allergol. 26*, 249–285

HIGGINS, I. T. T. (1963) Blood groups in miners with coalworkers pneumoconiosis and bronchitis. *Br. J. Ind. Med. 20*, 324

JONES, J. G., FRASER, R. B. & NADEL, J. A. (1975) Prediction of maximum expiratory flow rate from area-transmural pressure curve of the compressed airway. *J. Appl. Physiol. 38*, 1002–1011

LAMB, D. & REID, L. (1972) Quantitative distribution of various types of acid glycoprotein in mucous cells of human bronchi. *Histochem. J. 4*, 91–102

MEYER, F. A. (1976) Mucus structure: relation to biological transport function. *Biorheology 13*, 49–58

PHIPPS, R. J. & RICHARDSON, P. S. (1976) The effects of irritation at various levels of the airway upon tracheal mucus secretion in the cat. *J. Physiol. (Lond.) 261*, 563–581

ROBSON, T., ALLEN, A. & PAIN, R. (1975) Non-covalent forces hold glycoprotein molecules together in mucous gel. *Biochem. Soc. Trans. 3*, 1105–1107

SNARY, D. & ALLEN, A. (1971) Studies on gastric mucoproteins. The isolation and characterization of the mucoprotein of the water-soluble mucus from pig cardiac gastric mucosa. *Biochem. J. 123*, 845–853

SNARY, D. & ALLEN, A. (1972) Studies on gastric mucoproteins. The production of radioactive mucoproteins by pig gastric mucosal scrapings *in vitro*. *Biochem. J. 127*, 577–587

VIRELIZIER, J.-L. (1975) Host defenses against influenza virus: the role of anti-hemagglutinin antibody. *J. Immunol. 115*, 434–439

Criteria for evaluating mucus functions and their disorders in chronic bronchitis

PAUL SADOUL, EDITH PUCHELLE and FRANCOISE GIRARD

Unité de Recherche de Physiopathologie Respiratoire, INSERM U 14, Vandoeuvre-les-Nancy, France

Abstract In chronic bronchitis, disorders of the physical and chemical properties of mucus may contribute to bronchial obstruction. The abnormalities are analysed in sputum collected by physiotherapy. Measurements of the rheological properties (apparent viscosity and strain recovery), content analysis of secretory immunoglobulin A (S-IgA) and of serum albumin, and determination of the transport velocity of sputum on the ciliated frog palate provide reliable indices of the functional capacity of bronchial mucosa. The effectiveness of mucociliary clearance and coughing is analysed in patients by measuring the rate of removal of radioactive particles deposited on proximal airways. Different types of pathological secretions may be observed. In subjects with occasional cough and sputum, the secretions are characterized by a high content of S-IgA and serum albumin, and a high viscosity and low elasticity, reflecting their high degree of cross-linking. In chronic bronchitics, the S-IgA content and viscoelastic properties of sputum decrease as the illness progresses. During infection, purulent sputum exhibits high viscosity and low strain recovery. Such modifications of the rheological properties of mucus may impair mucociliary clearance. The role of the elastic component is predominant. Sputum, characterized by very low strain recovery ($S_R < 4$ units) or conversely by very high strain recovery ($S_R > 15$ units), is transported at a low rate by mucociliary clearance. A marked hyperviscosity ($\eta_0 > 200$ poises (120 N s m^{-2})) also appears as a limiting factor of the mucociliary clearance.

It is generally agreed that excess bronchial secretion is an important factor in the causation of airflow obstruction in patients who have chronic bronchitis. However, the exact nature and the abnormal effects of the mucus in this disease are not well known.

Bronchial secretion has many functions, but the most important appears to be that of trapping inhaled particles and clearing them towards the pharynx. Bronchial secretions humidify the inspired air and maintain an ionic gradient at the mucosal surface (Negus 1961), but they also have a biological protective role against enzymes released into the bronchi either by bacteria or from cellular degradation. Moreover, some of the biochemical constituents of mucus, such as secretory immunoglobulins, may control absorption of antigenic material through mucosal surfaces (Williams & Gibbons 1972) and inhibit their bacterial colonization by preventing the adherence of bacteria to epithelial cells (Walker *et al.* 1972). The disturbance of any of these physiological functions of the bronchial secretions may impair mucus transport and predispose the patient to bronchopulmonary infection.

The study of bronchial secretion in normal subjects presents a problem because it is produced in very small amounts and is rapidly swallowed. Although mucus can be aspirated in laryngectomized subjects, it is not necessarily a correct model for the normal. Sputum collected from patients who have chronic bronchitis is contaminated both by saliva and the degradation products of infection and is certainly not normal, but its collection does allow us to observe the evolution of that disease. To quote Reid (1973): 'In studies of bronchial secretion it is well to compare disease states rather than to worry too much about controls, in the normal sense'.

In the first part of this paper, we attempt to evaluate mucus function and its disorders, and we describe work on the biochemical and rheological characteristics of the sputum in chronic bronchitis. In the second part, we describe the evolution of the pathology of sputum as chronic bronchitis progresses and its consequences on mucociliary function.

RHEOLOGICAL STUDIES

Sputum raised by patients is a very heterogeneous fluid. It can be compared either to a liquid or to a semi-solid gel, since pathological conditions considerably change its biophysical properties. Rheological measurements enable us to ascertain *in vitro* flow and deformation properties under applied stress. Sputum is a non-Newtonian viscous fluid. A single coefficient cannot summarize its viscous characteristics because shear rate and shear stress are not linearly related. Moreover sputum is a thixotropic fluid: if one applies a rate of shear greater than 1 s^{-1} to a sample of sputum in a rotational viscometer, one generally observes a steady decrease in apparent viscosity with time. The scatter of the results published by different authors for the viscosity of sputum, ranging from 0.01 to 10^5 poises (10^{-3} to 10^4 N s m^{-2}), exemplifies the shear-dependence and emphasizes the need for rigid standardization of the techniques. Such a wide variation shows the difficulty of comparing values from different laboratories.

When a force is applied to a flake of mucus, the mucus stores some energy

(Litt 1970). Hwang *et al.* (1969) have noted that the characteristic time of ciliary motion (0.05 s corresponding to about 20 beats/s) is much less than the relaxation time of the mucus (a few seconds to minutes). It is implied that mucus is transported as a solid rather than a liquid under the action of cilia. According to Dulfano *et al.* (1971), the average shear rate corresponding to the frequency of beat of the cilia is of the order of 1 s^{-1}.

A wide variety of rheometric techniques, carefully reviewed by Davis (1973), have been used to study bronchial secretions *in vitro*. These include gravimetric techniques as well as a 'viscometric syringe'. The Ferranti Shirley viscometer is frequently used for studying the rheological properties of sputum. Unfortunately, the rheogram obtained by applying a linear increase followed by decrease in shear rate represents 'a combination of instrument and material effects. The derived parameters do not have any fundamental significance . . . and they cannot be used in a meaningful way to discuss variations in sputum consistency or for correlation with biochemical and histological changes' (Davis 1973).

There are other techniques for measuring parameters such as viscosity, elasticity and relaxation times; several of them are based on oscillatory testing. Commercially available machines such as the Weissenberg rheogoniometer are quite sophisticated and very expensive. They would not be used for evaluating clinical samples. The magnetic microrheometer, the chemical balance, the capillary viscometer and rotational viscometer using the method of constrained elastic recovery after steady flow, have been proposed as relatively simple types of apparatus which give valuable information and are useful for clinical purposes. For rheological measurements of sputum we use a concentric cylinder rheometer which has been modified (Benis *et al.* 1973) to reduce end-effects and to measure strain recovery with a continuous recording. The sample to be tested is introduced between the inner rotating surface and the external fixed surface and the torque imposed on the rotating surface is measured. The applied shear rate is relatively low ($\dot{\gamma}_m = 0.3\ s^{-1}$). Sputum elasticity can be studied after disengagement of the rotating member following the imposition of a steady shear, allowing strain recovery (S_R) to be measured under constrained geometric conditions.

Results obtained in 38 untreated patients suffering from chronic bronchitis are shown in Fig. 1. The absence of correlation between apparent viscosity and strain recovery suggests that these two parameters represent distinctive features characterizing the rheological properties of sputum in patients. A multidimensional statistical analysis has confirmed this finding.

Conditions of sampling must be carefully standardized, for it was demonstrated that sputum produced during 'bronchial toilet' was significantly

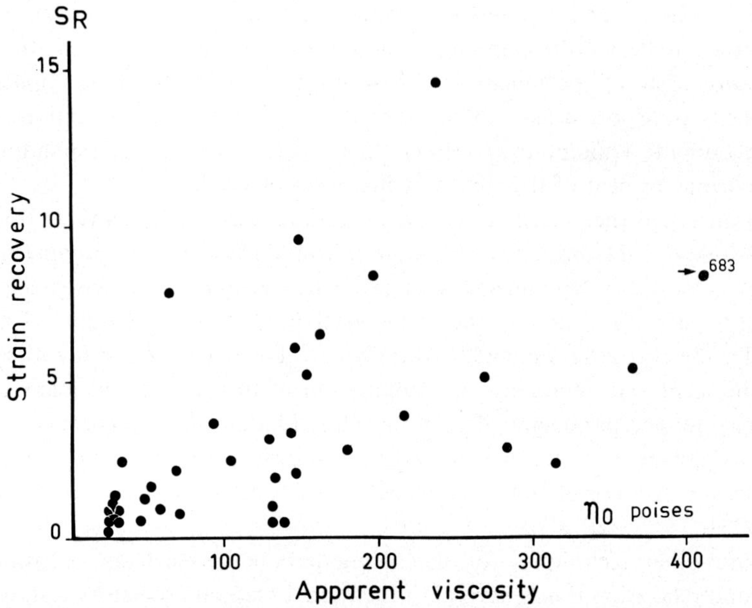

FIG. 1. Relationships between the apparent viscosity (η_0) and the strain recovery (S_R) of sputum collected from 38 patients with chronic bronchitis.

more viscoelastic than that collected later (Puchelle *et al.* 1973*a*). Rheological measurements were made on fresh sputum produced between 10 and 11 a.m. after bronchial toilet, within minutes of production, so that the risks of salivary contamination and enzymic degradation were very low and reproducibility of measurements was satisfactory. In such rigidly standardized conditions, we found that in eight patients studied for one year sputum viscosity and strain recovery were relatively similar (Fig. 2), except for two patients with a decrease in viscoelasticity.

BIOCHEMICAL STUDIES AND RHEOLOGICAL RELATIONSHIPS

Macromolecular components of sputum may be divided into two main groups: proteins and secretory glycoproteins. They play an essential role in bronchial defence, in fibrillar structure, and consequently in the rheological properties of mucus.

Our purpose is not to describe extensively the chemical structure of normal bronchial mucus but to discuss those components which affect the function of bronchial mucosa. Sputum proteins are present in free or combined forms

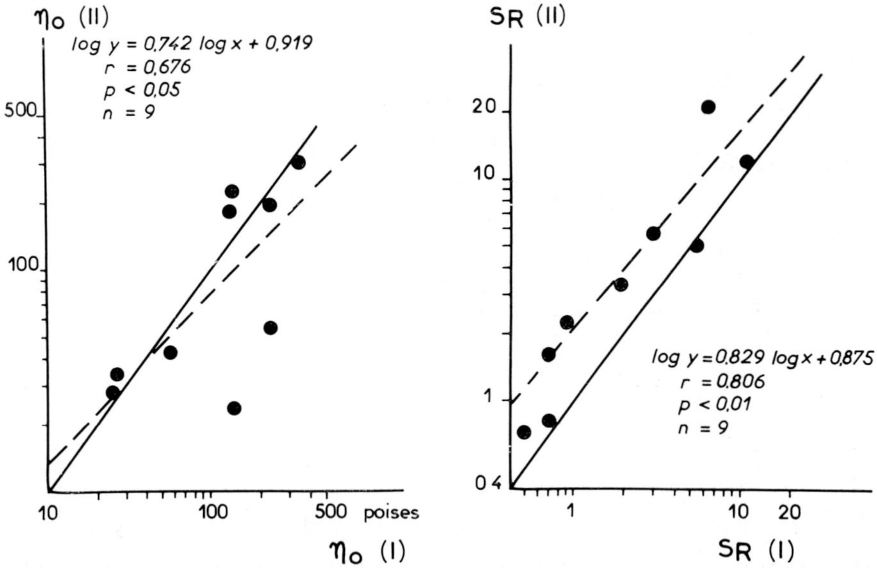

FIG. 2. Comparison of the values of sputum viscosity (η_o) and strain recovery (S_R) in patients with chronic bronchitis within a one-year-period.

and they can be extracted by high power ion-exchange resins (Laine & Hayem 1976). Crossed electrophoresis using antiserum to total serum proteins demonstrates numerous proteins such as serum albumin, α_1-antitrypsin, transferrin and IgA (Fig. 3). The proportions of these various proteins and the complexity of the precipitate patterns vary from one sputum sample to another. During infectious episodes, the diagrams are particularly complex because many serum proteins are present. Monospecific antiserum identifies each one of these proteins and demonstrates, eventually, other complexes. Thus identification in purulent sputum of two electrophoretic forms of α_1-antitrypsin (Fig. 4) that are absent in normal bronchial secretion emphasizes the ability of this glycoprotein to complex with several enzymes (elastases, collagenases) liberated profusely in sputum during cellular lysis (Ohlsson 1971). Other proteins synthesized at the bronchial level, such as IgA, IgG or enzymes like kallikrein, can be found in sputum.

Secretory IgA (S–IgA) represents the more important class of bronchial immunoglobulins and it has protective functions. S-IgA antibodies have specific activity for several viruses and are capable of bacterial agglutination. These proteins also play an important role in determining the viscoelastic properties of sputum. Viscoelasticity is closely related to S-IgA content and

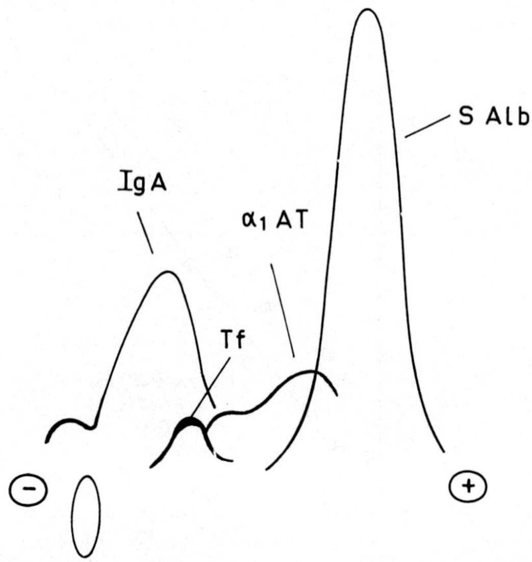

FIG. 3. Pattern obtained from antigen-antibody crossed electrophoresis of sputum using an antiserum to total human serum proteins. IgA, immunoglobin A; Tf, transferrin; α_1 AT, α_1-antitrypsin; S Alb, serum albumin.

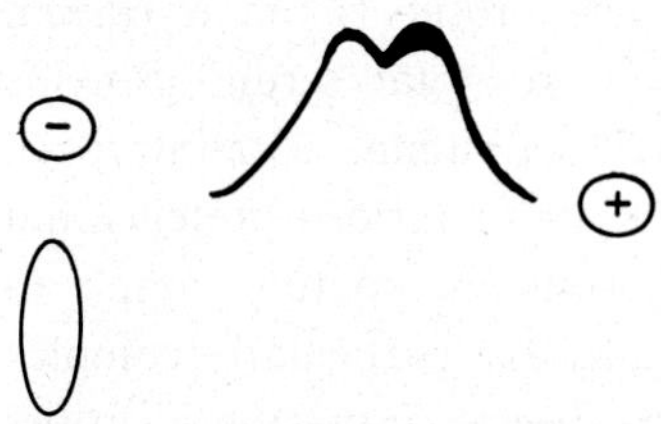

FIG. 4. Typical precipitation pattern obtained from purulent sputum by crossed immuno-electrophoresis, using an antiserum to human anti-α_1-antitrypsin. Two electrophoretic peaks are observed. The slower one represents the complexed form of α_1-antitrypsin with proteases.

viscosity with serum albumin (Table 1). Reducing agents such as *N*-acetyl-cysteine or mercaptoethanol, which break disulphide bonds, reduce the visco-elasticity of sputum. These results suggest the direct influence of protein disulphide bonds in determining the rheological properties of bronchial secretions. The levels of secretory and serum proteins often vary independently in chronic bronchitis. The ratio of S-IgA to serum albumin concentration

TABLE 1

Significance of the correlations obtained between the biochemical constituents and the rheological properties of sputum.

	Apparent viscosity η_0	*Strain recovery* S_R
Proteins		
S-IgA	***	***
Serum albumin	*	N.S.
Mucins		
Dry weight of hydrolysate	***	*
Mucins (galactose + osamines)	***	***
— Sialomucins	*	**
— Sulphomucins	N.S.	N.S.
— Fucomucins	N.S.	N.S.

* $P < 0.05$ ** $P < 0.02$ *** $P < 0.001$ N.S.: not significant. (Data from Puchelle *et al.* 1973*b*.)

furnishes an index of local synthetic activity and of the extent of serum transudation through the bronchial mucosa.

The mucins, glycoproteins of high molecular weight, are the principal element in the fibrillar structure of mucus. The classification proposed by Degand *et al.* (1973) separates the mucins into three categories according to their acidity: fucomucins, sialomucins and sulphomucins. Collection of mucus by bronchial lavage in normal adults confirms the presence of sialomucins and sulphomucins, which are acidic. The mucus of chronic bronchitics contains in addition neutral mucins (fucomucins), reflecting the increased enzymic activity of fucosyltransferase (Lamblin *et al.* 1977). Polyanionic mucins (sialo- and sulphomucins) play an important biological role through their ability to combine with water, proteins and peptides such as kinins. In guinea-pigs, the injection of sialomucin before bradykinin inhibits bronchospasm (Muh *et al.* 1968). The mucins, by their ability to combine with proteins, may modify the rheological properties of bronchial secretions. A close relationship has been observed between mucins (galactose + osamines) and sputum viscoelasticity (Table 1). Sialomucins play an essential role in mucus structure (Puchelle *et al.* 1973*b*).

Some bacterial enzymes are able to modify the function of sialomucins; for example pretreatment with neuraminidase (EC 3.2.1.18) stops them from inhibiting kinin (Muh *et al.* 1968).

Diplococcus pneumoniae neuraminidase lowers viscosity and strain recovery *in vitro* (Puchelle *et al.* 1975). This change was not observed with bovine cervical mucin or with mucus collected from an experimental tracheal pouch, but the chemical composition of both of these substances differs from that of sputum in chronic bronchitis.

The exact model of cross-linking of mucus elements remains controversial. The hypothesis of an electrostatic interaction between the secretory proteins (S-IgA, bronchotransferrin) and the sialic acid of sialomucin was suggested by Degand *et al.* (1973). As well as this mechanism, Meyer (1976) assumed that disulphide linkages between glycoproteins would lead to macromolecule formation. Valuable information on mucus composition was obtained by sophisticated biochemical studies but the methods used cannot be considered as routine. Unfortunately, assays of sialic acid and fucose provide no valid conclusions about mucin equilibrium, and Lopata *et al.* (1974) failed to demonstrate any differences between bronchitis and normal secretions.

ANALYSIS OF MUCUS TRANSPORT

The frog palate offers appropriate conditions for the study of mucus transport, as Sade *et al.* (1970) and King *et al.* (1974) have pointed out. Light aluminium discs will stay on the ciliated mucosa of palates previously depleted of mucus unless fresh mucus is deposited. The observed transport velocity ratio of frog mucus (used as a reference) to patient's mucus offers a valuable index (Puchelle *et al.* 1976*a*). The optimal rheological pattern for mucus transport corresponds to a rather narrow zone for strain recovery (4 to 15 units) and a larger zone for viscosity (25 to 200 poises) (2.5 to 20 N s m^{-2}). Beyond these limits, mucus transport slows down significantly (Fig. 5). These results emphasize the role of the elastic component in mucociliary clearance. They are in agreement with experimental results recently published by Dulfano & Chen (1976).

The efficiency of mucociliary clearance depends not only on biochemical and biophysical characteristics but also on ciliary activity. In chronic bronchitis, ciliated epithelium is severely damaged. Measurement of mucociliary transport *in vivo* will produce further information on the mechanism of bronchial obstruction by secretions.

It is possible to follow the transport of inhaled radioactive particles, although the distribution of these particles in the tracheobronchial tree may be impaired by the bronchial obstruction. Differences in techniques explain the discrepancies in the published results (Toigo *et al.* 1963; Luchsinger *et al* 1968; Thomson & Short 1969). We have proposed a technique for overcoming the difficulties

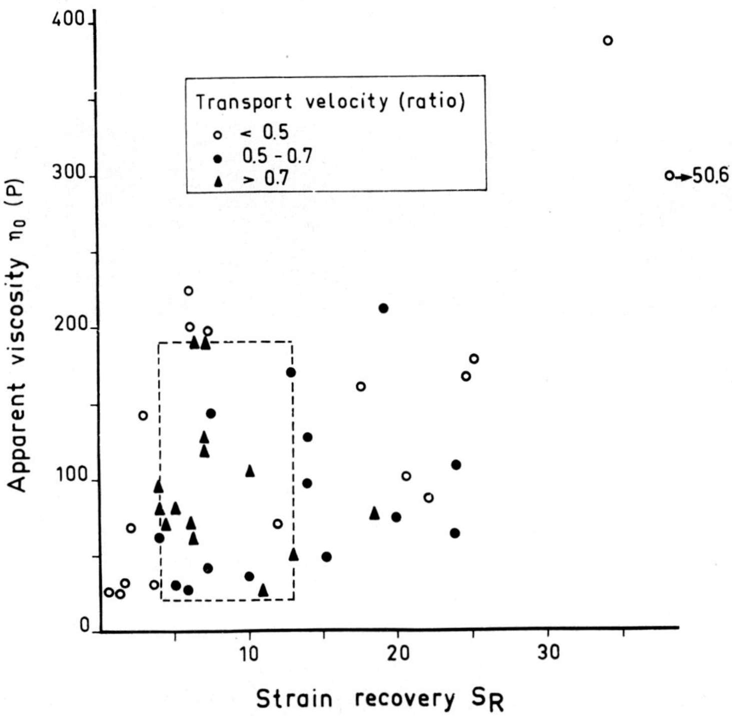

FIG. 5. Relationships between the rheological properties and mucociliary transport velocity of sputum. The range of optimal viscosity and elasticity for mucociliary transport is indicated (broken lines). (From Puchelle *et al.* 1976*a*.)

of distribution. The resin particles (diameter = 8 μm) are dispersed with the aid of a spinning disc generator and deposited in the tracheobronchial tree by rapid insufflation. The particles do not penetrate further than the segmental bronchi. Fig. 6 indicates the progression of mucus flakes. These observations argue in favour of discontinuous transport by the ciliated escalator recently assumed by Yeates *et al.* (1975).

QUALITATIVE MODIFICATIONS OF BRONCHIAL SECRETIONS IN CHRONIC BRONCHITIS

Biochemical and rheological properties of bronchial secretions evolve according to the different stages of the disease.

At an *early stage*, the patient occasionally coughs up sputum without ventilatory disturbances. In such cases Havez *et al.* (1973) have observed a

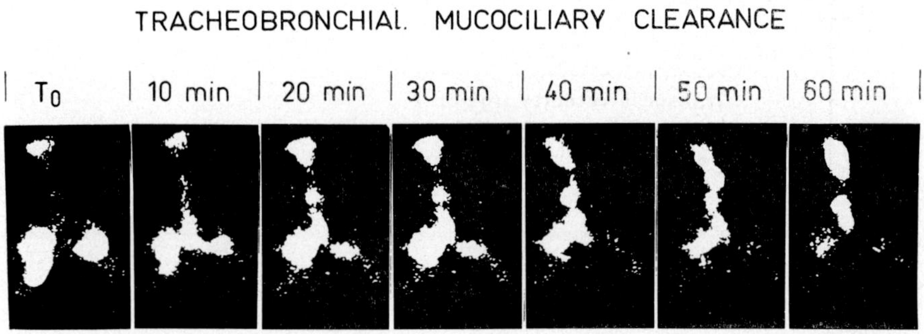

FIG. 6. Sequential scintiphotos taken every 10 min after inhalation of the radioactive (^{99m}TC) aerosol.

high concentration of S-IgA. In four patients coughing up non-purulent sputum (leucocyte counts below 4000 cells/mm^3) S-IgA and serum albumin concentrations were high (Fig. 7). The high protein content reflected bronchial mucosal inflammation as well as its secretory activity. Viscosity was over 100 poises (10 N s m^{-2}) and the strain recovery was very low ($S_R < 4$ units). Such low values may be explained by the highly polymerized structure of the secretions: elongation of the mucoprotein chains is probably limited by numerous strong inter- and intramolecular bonds. Mucus transport evaluated *in vitro* was diminished except for one sample which showed a strain recovery of about 4 units.

In *confirmed chronic bronchitis*, S-IgA tends to decrease. In nine patients S-IgA was significantly lower than normal ($P < 0.05$), as was serum albumin ($P < 0.01$). However S-IgA concentrations varied from one subject to another (range 37.5 to 159 mg/100 ml). In two samples high S-IgA concentrations were accompanied by high strain recovery (30 and 50.5 units).

Mucus transport velocity has been measured on frog palate, and mucociliary clearance was studied *in vivo* after radioactive aerosol inhalation. In only three out of nine patients was mucociliary clearance efficient (relative transport velocity > 1 and radioactive material cleared after 1 hour > 15%). In these three patients, viscosity varied between 50 and 200 poises (5 to 20 N s m^{-2}) and strain recovery between 7 and 10 units. The results obtained *in vivo* confirm the existence of an optimal range of viscosity and strain recovery for mucociliary clearance.

It seems reasonable, therefore, to suggest that, according to the proposal by Meyer (1976) for secretory and serous otitis, two extreme types of secretions, rubber-like and water-like, result in mucociliary abnormalities. The impairment

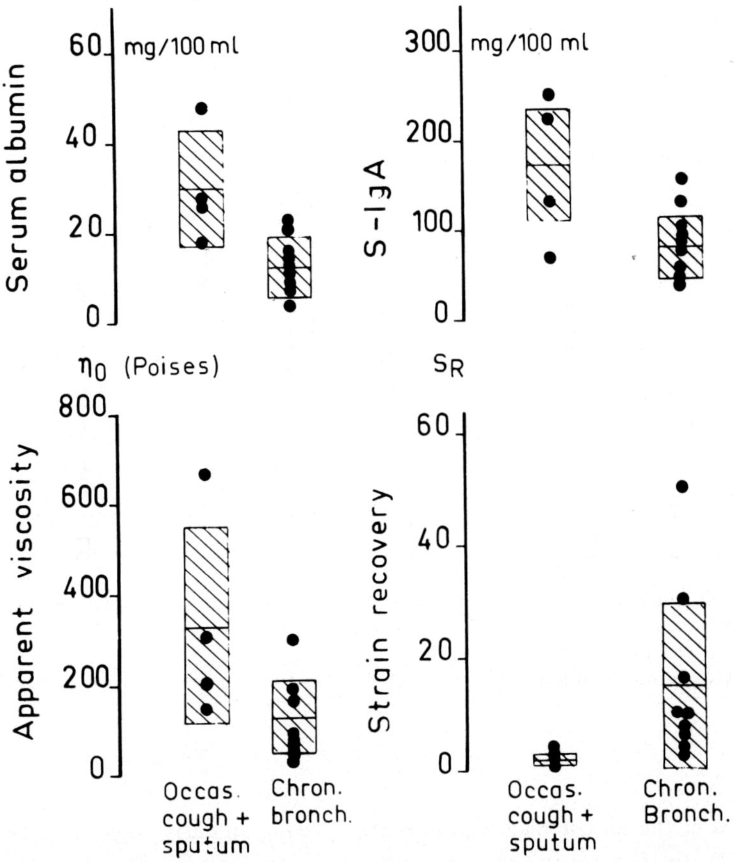

FIG. 7. Comparison of the protein content (serum albumin, S-IgA) and rheological properties (apparent viscosity and strain recovery) of sputum collected from four subjects with occasional cough and sputum and nine patients with chronic bronchitis. Mean values and standard deviations are indicated.

of mucus transport may contribute to airway obstruction. In patients with chronic bronchitis Pham *et al.* (1973) showed in an earlier study that the higher the viscosity of sputum, the more marked were the abnormalities of gas exchange.

During an infectious episode, confirmed by a high leucocyte count in sputum (leucocytes > 5000/mm^3) and a high bacterial concentration (bacteria > 10^8/ml), apparent viscosity was generally increased while the strain recovery diminished (Fig. 8). The dissociated rheological pattern may be secondary to various

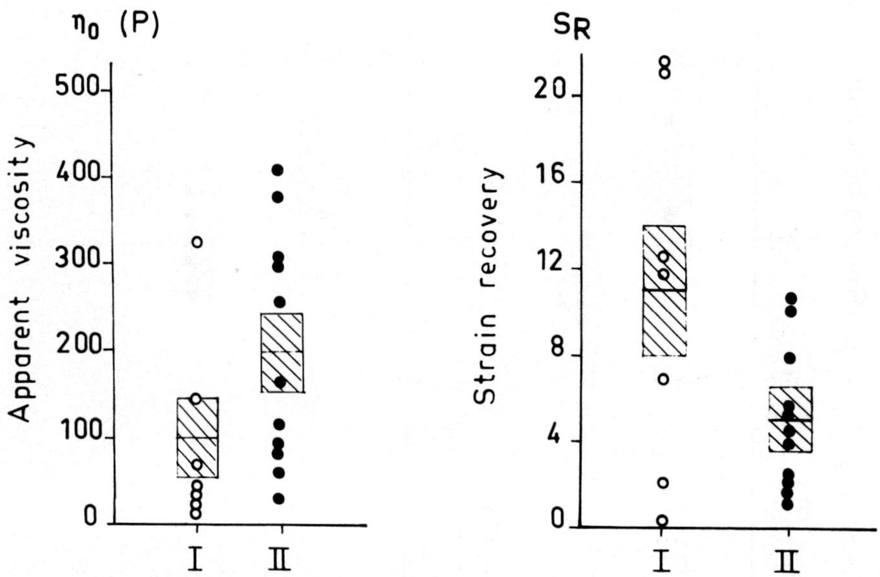

FIG. 8. Values of apparent viscosity and strain recovery of sputum divided into two groups according to the degree of purulence. Mean values and standard errors are indicated.
○ ⩽ 3000 leucocytes/ml sputum $n = 7$.
● < 3000 leucocytes/ml sputum $n = 11$.

modifications of the biochemical equilibrium. During an early stage, we have seen that a sharp increase in secretory and serum proteins may be secondary to an infectious stimulus, but in advanced stages F. Girard (unpublished data) observed no notable increase in sputum proteins during infectious episodes. Similar results have been reported by Medici & Bürgi (1971). The elastic decrease might be due to deterioration of fibrillar structure secondary to bacterial glycosidase activity. Purulent sputum showed a marked slowing down in mucus transport.

Over the years, biochemical and rheological patterns evolve slowly in sputum. Repetitive measurements in the same patients showed that infectious episodes are followed by decreased concentrations of S-IgA (frequently to below 100 mg/100 ml) and by decreased viscoelasticity of mucus, corresponding to a functional decay of the mucosa.

In *advanced stages*, a marked decrease in glandular synthesis (S-IgA < 50 mg/100 ml) is frequently associated with a low viscosity (η_0 < 50 poises) (< 5 N s m^{-2}) and a low strain recovery (S_R < 4). These modifications impair the mucociliary escalator and the efficacy of coughing. In 10 patients observed for 5 to 8 weeks, the S-IgA/serum albumin ratio was low in patients with frequent infectious episodes characterized by high leucocyte counts. These results, in agreement with those of Puchelle *et al.* (1976*b*), suggest that this ratio provides a good index of the defence capabilities of mucosa.

CONCLUSION

With the aid of various investigative methods the functional properties of bronchial secretion in chronic bronchitis can be described.

These properties depend on biochemical composition and on the evolving stages of the disease. In some patients, the decrease in viscosity secondary to mucolytic drugs could be harmful. The physician has to select drugs which are able to modify secretory activity rather than those which simply liquefy the mucus.

The results suggest that in advanced stages of chronic bronchitis, the changes in bronchial secretion may lead to progressive bronchial obstruction which cannot be alleviated either by mucociliary clearance or by coughing.

ACKNOWLEDGEMENT

This work was supported by grants from INSERM ATP 41-76-73 and from the European Economic Community (Luxemburg).

References

Benis, A. M., Puchelle, E. & Sadoul, P. (1973) Adaptation of a concentric cylinder viscometer to the routine measurement of the viscoelastic properties of sputum, in *Rheology of Biological Systems* (Gabelnick, H. L. & Litt, M., ed.), pp. 218–259, C. C. Thomas, Springfield

Davis, S. S. (1973) Techniques for the measurement of the rheological properties of sputum. *Bull. Physio-Pathol. Respir. 9*, 47–90

Degand, P., Roussel, P., Lamblin, G., Durand, G. & Havez, R. (1973) Données biochimiques et rhéologiques dans l'expectoration. I – Définition biochimique des mucines dans l'expectoration. *Bull. Physio-Pathol. Respir. 9*, 199–216

Dulfano, M. J., Adler, K. & Philippoff, W. (1971) Sputum viscoelasticity in chronic bronchitis. *Am. Rev. Respir. Dis. 104*, 88–98

Dulfano, M. J. & Chen, T. M. (1976) Mucus rheology and mucociliary clearance. *Am. Rev. Respir. Dis. 113*, 200

HAVEZ, R., LAINE-BASSEZ, A., HAYEM-LEVY, A. & LEBAS, J. (1973) Données biochimiques et rhéologiques dans l'expectoration. II – Définition biochimique des protéines dans l'expectoration. *Bull. Physio-Pathol. Respir. 9*, 219–233

HWANG, S. H., LITT, M. & FORSMAN, W. C. (1969) Rheological properties of mucus. *Rheologica Acta 8*, 438–448

KING, M., GILBOA, A., MEYER, F. A. & SILBERBERG, A. (1974) On the transport of mucus and its rheologic simulants in ciliated systems. *Am. Rev. Respir. Dis. 110*, 740–745

LAINE, A. & HAYEM, A. (1976) Identification et caractérisation des constituants protéiques de la sécrétion bronchique humaine. *Clin. Chim. Acta 67*, 159–167

LAMBLIN, G., LHERMITTE, M., LAFITTE, J. J., FILLIAT, M., DEGAND, P. & ROUSSEL, P. (1977) Etude comparative des mucines bronchiques purifiées à partir de l'expectoration de sujets atteints de mucoviscidose ou d'autres affections bronchiques chroniques. *Bull. Eur. Physio-Pathol. Respir. 13*, 175–190

LITT, M. (1970) Mucus rheology: relevance to mucociliary clearance. *Arch. Intern. Med. 126*, 417–423

LOPATA, M., BARTON, A. D. & LOURENCO, R. V. (1974) Biochemical characteristics of bronchial secretions in chronic obstructive pulmonary diseases. *Am. Rev. Respir. Dis. 110*, 730–739

LUCHSINGER, P. C., LAGARDE, B. & KILFEATHER, J. E. (1968) Particle clearance from the human tracheobronchial tree. *Am. Rev. Respir. Dis. 97*, 1046–1050

MEDICI, T. C. & BÜRGI, H. (1971) The role of immunoglobulin A in endogenous bronchial defense mechanism in chronic bronchitis. *Am. Rev. Respir. Dis. 103*, 784–791

MEYER, F. A. (1976) Mucus structure: relation to biological transport function. *Biorheology 13*, 49–58

MUH, J. P., LATREILLE, J. P., GUERRIN, F., ROUSSEL, P., DEGAND, P., RANDOUX, A. & HAVEZ, R. (1968) Recherche d'inhibiteurs naturels du bronchospasme à la bradykinine chez le cobaye, in *Hypersécrétion Bronchique*, pp. 193–202, Poinsot, Clichy

NEGUS, V. (1961) Protection of the respiratory tract. *Br. Med. J. 2*, 723–728

OHLSSON, K. (1971) Interaction between human or dog leucocyte proteases and plasma protease inhibitors. *Scand. J. Clin. Lab. Invest. 28*, 225–230

PHAM, Q. T., PESLIN, R., PUCHELLE, E., SALMON, D., CARAUX, G. & BENIS, A. M. (1973) Fonction respiratoire et état rhéologique des sécrétions recueillies pendant l'expectoration spontanée et dirigée. *Bull. Physio-Pathol. Respir. 9*, 293–310

PUCHELLE, E., PHAM, Q. T., CARAUX, G. & ZAHM, J. M. (1973*a*) Etat rhéologique des sécrétions bronchiques chez le bronchiteux chronique. *Bull. Physio-Pathol. Respir. 9*, 143–157

PUCHELLE, E., ZAHM, J. M. & HAVEZ, R. (1973*b*) Données biochimiques et rhéologiques dans l'expectoration. III. Relation des protéines et mucines bronchiques avec les propriétés rhéologiques. *Bull. Physio-Pathol. Respir. 9*, 237–256

PUCHELLE, E., GIRARD, F., HOUDRET, N. & BAILLEUL, V. (1975) Action des neuraminidases de *Diplococcus pneumoniae* et de *Clostridium perfringens* sur les propriétés visco-élastiques des sécrétions bronchiques. *Biorheology 12*, 219–224

PUCHELLE, E., GIRARD, F. & ZAHM, J. M. (1976*a*) Rhéologie des sécrétions bronchiques et transport mucociliaire. *Bull. Eur. Physio-Pathol. Respir. 12*, 771–779

PUCHELLE, E., GIRARD, F., BECK, G., HAYEM, A., BAILLEUL, V. & LAINE, A. (1976*b*) Propriétés rhéologiques et biochimiques de l'expectoration. Rôle de l'infection. *Pathol. Biol. 24*, 93–96

REID, L. (1973) Bronchial secretion. General comments. *Bull. Physio-Pathol. Respir. 9*, 15–30

SADE, J., ELIEZER, N., SILBERBERG, A. & NEVO, A. C. (1970) The role of mucus in transport by cilia. *Am. Rev. Respir. Dis. 102*, 48–52

THOMSON, H. L. & SHORT, M. D. (1969) Mucociliary function in health, chronic obstruction airway disease and asbestosis. *J. Appl. Physiol. 26*, 535–539

TOIGO, A., MARISIO, J. J., MURHALL, H. & LEPPER, M. N. (1963) Clearance of large carbon particles from the human tracheobronchial tree. *Am. Rev. Respir. Dis. 87*, 487–492

WALKER, W. A., ISSLEBACHER, K. J. & BLOCK, K. J. (1972) Intestinal uptake of macromolecules: effect of oral immunization. *Science (Wash. D.C.) 177*, 608–610

WILLIAMS, R. C. & GIBBONS, R. J. (1972) Inhibition of bacterial adherence by secretory immunoglobulin A: mechanism of antigen disposal. *Science (Wash. D.C.) 177*, 691–699

YEATES, P. B., ASPIN, N., LEVISON, M., JONES, M. T. & BRYAN, A. C. (1975) Mucociliary tracheal transport rates in man. *J. Appl. Physiol. 39*, 487–495

Discussion

Silberberg: What are the optimum qualities of the mucus in facilitating transport, and have you plotted the restored velocity ratio against strain recovery?

Sadoul: The optimum qualities are characterized by a viscosity of about 150 poises and a strain recovery of about 6 units. The retardation time, which represents the time taken for the strain to fall $1/e^{th}$ of its initial value after removal of stress, is closely related to viscosity but independent of the magnitude of the strain recovery. In highly viscous sputum, with low mucociliary transport, this retardation time may exceed one minute.

Guz: Could we have strain recovery defined in physical terms?

Sadoul: If you apply a constant stress to the mucus, it will exhibit a primarily elastic response before it flows. This elastic strain is first instantaneous and secondarily retarded. The removal of the stress gives rise to a recoil phenomenon. The difference between the maximal strain and the final strain represents the strain recovery.

Reid: You set up a stress and watch the time it takes for that stress to ease back to zero. It is essentially a time-dependent phenomenon.

Guz: But when Professor Silberberg was talking about the measurement of elasticity, that was time-independent.

Silberberg: No. Time came into those measurements by virtue of the frequency. Suppose we apply a sinusoidal strain. If the material were ideally elastic, the resultant stress would be exactly in phase. If the material were ideally viscous, the stress would be displaced by 90° (maximum stress would occur at zero strain, corresponding, however, to a maximum in rate of strain). Most systems are neither the one nor the other, but lie somewhere in between, and in the type of measurement we have described we can describe this effect by separating the response into two contributions, an elastic part in which energy is only stored and a viscous part in which energy is lost. Professor Sadoul's experiment is essentially the same except that the stress is kept constant and he measured what the strain was doing as a function of time.

When you then take off the stress, the strain recovery is due to the energy that has remained stored in the system. If the material were ideally elastic and stress was applied, it would stay at the initial level of applied strain indefinitely. If the stress is then taken off, the strain immediately returns to zero because all the energy was stored. In the present case part of the energy is lost at a rate which depends on the relaxation time constant of the material itself.

Guz: So strain recovery means the difference between the starting point and where the stress level gets back to.

Reid: In Professor Sadoul's experiment there is uniform strain from the point where the stress is applied to the point where it stops, so what is measured is the strain produced in the liquid and the time it takes to recover when the stress causing it is removed. Graphically, the horizontal is a time axis and the vertical is the stress set up in the liquid. It is a measure of elasticity; it gives one an idea of how long deformity takes to recover and correct itself.

Guz: I never thought of time coming into elasticity.

Silberberg: There are no ideal systems. If you apply a very short pulse of deformation even to a classical liquid like water, you will get an elastic response if the time interval is so short that the molecules have not been given the time they require to move. In all materials time scales are involved for relaxations to take place. If strains are applied over time intervals that are smaller than the time scale of molecular movement they will be elastically recovered. No system is ideally viscous, ideally Newtonian. Neither are systems perfectly elastic. Even a typically elastic material like steel will not indefinitely maintain an applied stress; creep sets in and the material relaxes. Relaxation times may be very long, but no system is ideally elastic. There is no system that will maintain a state of stress for indefinitely long times. Real systems are all viscoelastic. Materials which we readily acknowledge to be viscoelastic merely happen to relax within our normal time scale of minutes and seconds. It is on this basis also that we naturally class water as viscous and steel as elastic.

Davis: Are there any problems with the different methods used for measuring these physical properties that might lead different people to come to different conclusions?

Silberberg: Yes, but in physics there is a range called linear behaviour where things are relatively simple because everything is additive. In that range all methods will give the same information. The advantage of dynamic testing is that you can make things linear by making the amplitude of both the applied stress and applied strain very small. But when you make a large-scale deformation and continuous flow is taking place, the 'remembered' deformations may become very large compared with the dimensions of the structural elements present, and you enter the range of non-linear phenomena.

Davis: When you say 'very small' are those amplitudes appropriate to the sort of deformations that the cilia would apply to this liquid?

Silberberg: It is an arguable point, and it is quite feasible that ciliary deformation is not small enough. But its amplitude can be estimated. Experimentally, moreover, one can test over what range one is in the linear range by changing the amplitude of deformation. As long as the results are amplitude-independent one is in the linear range. If ciliary amplitude therefore falls within this range, linear viscoelastic characteristics will determine the response.

Allison: You use a large amount of material: is it possible to miniaturize the system so as to apply these dynamic measurements in clinical situations?

Silberberg: It is difficult.

Sadoul: You can do it with 0.5 ml.

Silberberg: That is a large amount in terms of the samples one would collect in physiological conditions.

Nadel: But perhaps you could use oscillation techniques to give information on local events.

Allison: Would you recommend this as an operational procedure?

Silberberg: I think it is the best way of doing it.

Davis: Do you encounter the problem of thixotropy when you make or compare dynamic measurements and oscillating measurements?

Silberberg: You can avoid it by working in the linear range. Thixotropy is a typically non-linear phenomenon. But there are more serious complications with mucus; there are irreversible changes. For example, by heating or stirring mucus you can actually break it down and one wants to avoid doing this as much as possible. Hence small deformations are to be preferred and a minimum amount of handling. Time is also against you and you must measure quickly and as closely as possible to the point of secretion. It is for this reason that we tried to measure mucus properties on the epithelium and to put our probe into the mucus as it is welling up.

Nadel: What is the relationship between what comes out of the mouth and the material secreted locally?

Sadoul: You have to be careful to collect the sputum after 'bronchial toilet', when it is already modified by stagnation of the mucus in the bronchial tree. So we take a sample just after bronchial toilet and within 5 or 10 minutes of collection we perform the rheological measurements and do the study on the frog palate simultaneously with the same sample.

Widdicombe: Could we think again about stickiness (see p. 272 *et seq.*)?

Even if you can show a correlation between viscoelastic properties of mucus and either transport or clearance, which you have done very clearly, it does not follow that it is the change in viscoelastic properties of the mucus that causes the change in clearance in man or in transport on the frog's palate. It might be due to a chemical change, in that mucus from different situations may have different chemical constitutions, or it might be due to an action of the chemicals in the mucus on the cilia. Even more likely, the different types of mucus may have a different degree of stickiness, not within the mucus itself but between the mucus and the epithelial layer. I have heard nothing to indicate a relationship between stickiness, if it could be measured, and the viscoelastic properties of mucus, but I would have thought that stickiness between mucus and epithelium is as important as the viscoelastic properties of the mucus itself in terms both of transport and of clearance.

Sadoul: Stickiness is not easy to define because materials can have the same stickiness but different rheological properties. Purulent sputum and mucoid sputum are examples of this.

Widdicombe: It may be the other way around. If you have mucus on an epithelial layer, say in the healthy trachea, you can strip it off extremely easily. But if the trachea is inflamed and damaged the stuff seems to stick extremely hard. As far as one knows, the mucus has not changed its viscoelastic properties much but the stickiness has changed.

Nadel: A similar example comes from the use of an anticholinergic drug in a patient with bronchitis. The patient had no difficulty in coughing up mucus; the problem arose when it got into the back of the throat, which was dry because of the anticholinergic drug. The patient could not get the mucus from the back of his throat out of his mouth, and this has something to do with the interface of the materials.

Reid: We are beginning to see that when people say stickiness, they really mean adhesiveness. In the inflamed trachea which Professor Widdicombe mentioned there was no periciliary layer and no cilia, so adhesiveness becomes a completely different problem. I think we have to go back to the question of adhesiveness in the normal and the relationship between the layers. One simple way is to put secretion on an inclined plane to see whether it 'pours'. If sputum is placed in the bottom of a test tube, which is then tipped, we can see how quickly it flows (Keal 1974). With mucoid sputum there is a close correlation between 'pourability' and viscosity. With purulent sputum there is not such close correlation because purulent sputum is very pourable. This goes back to something that was said earlier, i.e. that some people find it easy to produce sputum when it is purulent. Presumably what happens is that the total 'gob' of secretion which is resting on top of the cilia is surrounded by enough water not to be adhesive but to flow quite well.

Godfrey: We use your test of flowability to demonstrate to medical students the stickiness of asthmatic sputum by inverting the sputum pot above our own heads: usually one gets away with it!

I'd like to thank Professor Sadoul for talking about the other components in the sputum, particularly cells, bacteria, serum proteins and so on. Asthmatic sputum, which is so very sticky, characteristically contains large clumps of degenerating eosinophils. What comes out of dead and dying eosinophils to give it a sticky property?

Allison: DNA: pus is what DNA was originally isolated from, and degenerating leucocytes release lots of DNA.

Godfrey: In that case, does DNAse have any part to play therapeutically?

Allison: DNAse does not attack living cells and is expensive, but would be interesting to try on the viscosity of asthmatic sputum.

Silberberg: Surely we are talking here not only about stickiness but also about 'peelability', or the effort that is required to remove a mucus plaque from the epithelium. Let me illustrate what I mean. Imagine you are applying a piece of Scotch tape to a surface. If you put it down on a smooth surface you can peel it off easily, but if you tried to pull off the whole thing in one go it would not come off very easily. One is thus dependent also upon the flexibility of the layered, sticky material. If it is highly flexible it can be peeled off easily, but if it is very rigid it would have to be lifted off all in one piece. In other words, the removal of mucus from the epithelium depends on the rheological character of the mucus, not just on the forces which attach it to the surface.

Reference

KEAL, E. E. (1974) Criteria for the testing of mucolytic agents. *Scand. J. Respir. Dis. Suppl. 90*, 49–53

Animal models in clinical disease

LYNNE REID

The Children's Hospital Medical Center, Harvard Medical School, Boston, Massachusetts and Department of Experimental Pathology, Brompton Hospital, London

Abstract Hypersecretion of mucus is a feature of several clinical diseases and in some is associated with mucous gland hypertrophy and goblet cell increase. In a variety of species these changes have been produced by irritants, by infection, or by administration of drugs. While the end result may appear the same, differences emerge in the type and amount of glycoprotein secreted and in the amount retained within the cell. Organ culture can be used to ascertain functional activity.

The use of animal models has not only established that these environmental changes cause hypertrophy but indicated some of the intracellular events associated with their development. When new types of granules appear within a cell, they appear first at the apex: a flow chart is offered of the way in which individual cells change and hence the population. The nature of glycoprotein elaborated by a secretory cell can change within hours. A Clara or serous cell can develop into a mucus-secreting or goblet cell. The pattern of reversibility is emerging.

Animal models have contributed much to our understanding of human diseases characterized by hypersecretion of mucus. Experimental studies may be designed to establish that a given agent has an aetiological role or may be primarily concerned to analyse pathogenesis, that is, the way various agents produce structural or functional alteration. In the elucidation of mechanism lies the hope of control.

The secretions aspirated from the airway or coughed up are a mixture of the serum components of tissue fluid—either as transudate or exudate—and the special mucus secretions of the airways. It is with these epithelial or mucus glycoproteins that we are concerned which confer on the secretions the special rheological properties of high viscosity and elasticity (Charman *et al* 1974). Serum yields five times the macromolecular dry weight of mucoid sputum but the sputum is about ten times more viscid at low shear rates. It is excessive secretion of this glycoprotein that is the hallmark of several important diseases. Because the bronchial liquid is such a mixture, its study must be multidisciplinary: histochemical methods (Jeffery, this volume, pp. 5–20; Jones, this volume, pp. 175–188) help us to analyse intracellular events and to relate these to the biochemical analysis of the total secretion (Roberts 1974, 1976).

Organ culture is another method that we have applied to the study of mucus secretion by the bronchial gland in the human and, more recently, in the experimental animal (Trowell 1959; Sturgess & Reid 1972*a*, *b*; Meyrick & Reid 1975; Reid *et al.* 1976). Using Trowell's method, strips of mucosa from human bronchi obtained at surgery can be maintained in culture medium to which radioactive precursors of glycoprotein have been added. After four hours about half the cells have taken up precursor, synthesized and discharged glycoprotein (Sturgess & Reid 1972*a*). Thus the condition of the tissue can be regarded as satisfactory. By the addition of drugs we have been able to study the pattern of control in both the normal and hypertrophied gland (Sturgess & Reid 1972*b*) and, more recently, to analyse separately the control of synthesis, storage and discharge (Coles 1976; Reid *et al.* 1976). Certainly over a period of several hours synthesis and discharge are not coupled but show separate patterns of control. Where we are dealing with such a mixed population of cells the use of organ culture, with study of the cells within the tissue, has the advantage that the various cell types are studied *in situ* and the response of tissue as a whole is considered.

HUMAN DISEASE

Success in the use of animal models of human disease depends in large part on our understanding of the human state. It is necessary to know what features of the pathological picture we want to produce in the laboratory animal.

Chronic bronchitis is defined in terms of hypersecretion of respiratory tract mucus (Medical Research Council 1965). The basic pathological changes are enlargement of the submucosal glands, an increase in the number of goblet cells and their appearance in airways smaller and more peripheral than is normal. With respect to the type of intracellular mucus glycoprotein, acid glycoproteins are relatively increased and, of these, it is the sulphated precursors that are increased, as well as the sialylated form in which the acid is resistant to digestion by sialidase (neuraminidase, EC 3.2.1.18).

Epidemiological studies indicate that the most important single cause of chronic bronchitis is the irritant effect on the airways of tobacco smoking

(Oswald & Medvei 1955). This accords with the common clinical pattern that hypersecretion precedes infection.

In *cystic fibrosis* the patient may, and in fact commonly does, develop these changes of gland hypertrophy and goblet cell increase; but the changes are not present at birth and do not develop if lung infection does not occur or, if it occurs, is virtually cured (Lamb & Reid 1972). In cystic fibrosis there is abnormal susceptibility to pulmonary infection and it seems that in this disease the hypertrophy of mucus-secreting structures follows infection. Here two possible causes—irritation and infection—are suggested for investigation as well as the control pathways concerned in the changes.

Patients with *asthma* may develop these stigmata of chronic bronchitis, but here again the occasional case of long-standing asthma in which these changes do not occur is important evidence that these features of chronic bronchitis are not an essential part of the disease we call asthma (Keal 1971; Keal & Reid 1975; R. Jones, personal communication). Recent chemical studies in our Department by Dr M. T. Lopez-Vidriero indicate the likelihood that gland hypertrophy is virtually always a feature of intrinsic asthma but not of extrinsic asthma. It may be that infection is more common in patients with intrinsic asthma than in those with the extrinsic form (Ciba Foundation 1971).

ANIMAL MODELS

The first requirement for the effective use of animal models to simulate human disease is that the animal be free from pulmonary infection (Reid 1970). The presence of infection may already have produced the changes of chronic bronchitis and so provided a vicarious experiment. For the rigorous conditions of control called for in experiments, it is necessary that the lungs be free from infection. Line-bred laboratory animals free of specific pathogens by no means always meet these criteria, and we have found that histological criteria of cleanness are more sensitive than bacteriological ones.

We have mainly used rats and pigs but since similar changes have been produced in other species (e.g., lamb, Mawdesley-Thomas *et al.* 1971; Mawdesley-Thomas & Healey 1973; dog, Spicer *et al.* 1974), the changes described below are not species-specific.

Our early experiments using sulphur dioxide as an irritant established that goblet cell increase and gland hypertrophy can occur in the absence of infection, and that neither epithelial ulceration nor increased mitotic activity was necessary for goblet cell increase (Reid 1963; Lamb & Reid 1968). Tobacco smoke also produced the stigmata of chronic bronchitis in the rat (Lamb & Reid 1969*a*).

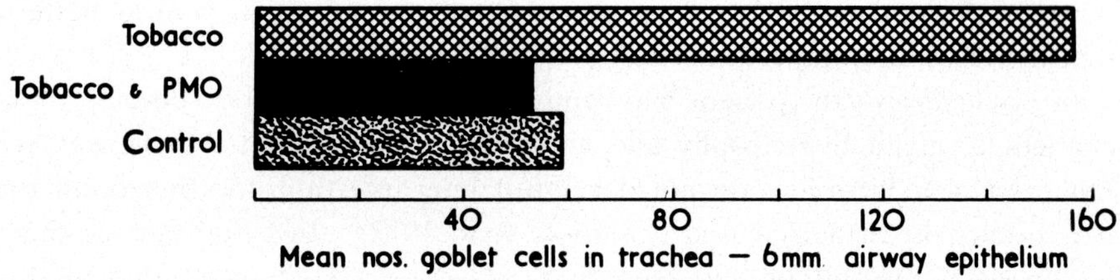

FIG. 1. Goblet cell number in a 6 mm length of trachea taken from animals exposed to (i) smoke from tobacco, (ii) smoke from tobacco to which phenylmethyloxadiazole (PMO) has been added, and (iii) either control or 'sham'-exposed.

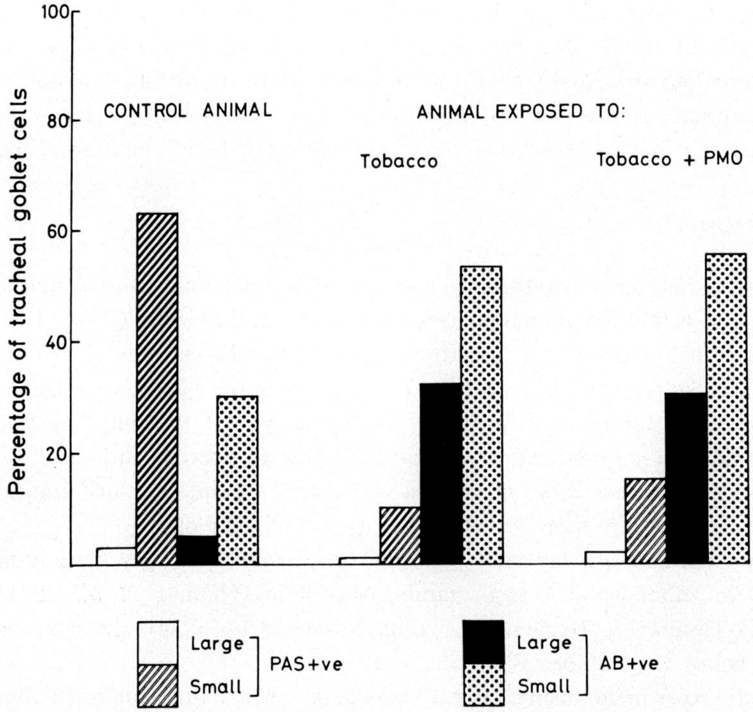

FIG. 2. Distribution of histochemical types of secretory cells in the experimental groups as in Fig. 1. AB+ve—cells staining with Alcian blue, i.e. containing acid glycoprotein. PAS+ve—cells staining with periodic acid–Schiff and containing no identifiable acid radical. 'Small' and 'large' refer to the amount of secretory product within the cell. The histochemical shift is similar in both tobacco groups although only in the 'tobacco alone' is the secretory cell number increased.

As an example of *irritation*, I shall describe a more recent experiment in which rats were exposed to tobacco smoke with or without the addition of an anti-inflammatory agent. In the first experiment rats were exposed to the smoke from 25 cigarettes a day, for five days a week, for periods up to six weeks (Jones *et al.* 1972, 1973). Half the animals received the smoke of cigarettes made from tobacco to which phenylmethyloxadiazole (PMO) had been added (2% by weight). This is an anti-inflammatory agent which used

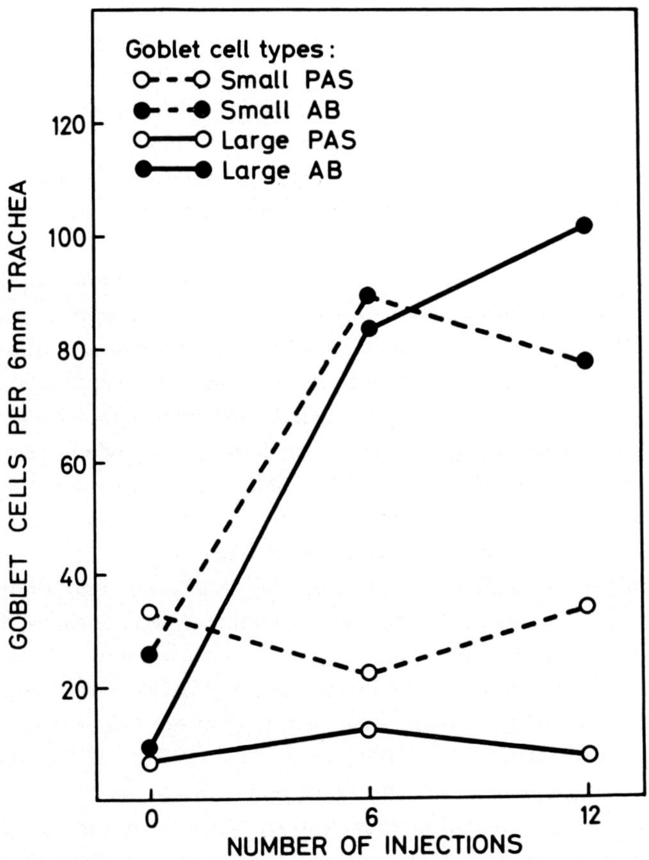

FIG. 3. Increase in number of goblet cells in rat trachea after 6 or 12 injections of isoprenaline sulphate (each 25 mg/100 g body weight); the acid glycoprotein cells (AB+ve) are the ones affected. Pilocarpine produces a similar increase but affects all secretory cell types.

to be included in cough mixtures. From the changes in the trachea it is seen that tobacco alone produces a striking increase in goblet cell number which is 'prevented' by the inclusion of PMO (Fig. 1). By contrast histochemical changes are similar in both groups and significantly different from those in the control animals (Fig. 2). The proportion of goblet cells producing acid glycoprotein is increased. In those animals exposed to tobacco alone this has occurred in a greatly increased cell population; in those exposed to tobacco and PMO the concentration of secretory cells per unit length of trachea is normal. This shift in the type of glycoprotein being packaged for release from the cell seems the most sensitive sign of irritation of airway epithelium.

The normal secretory cell population is made up mostly of cells containing a small amount of secretion; after irritation, it comes to consist mainly of cells containing a large amount of secretion and all granules throughout the cell will include the 'new' acid radical. Cells with discrete granules which probably were separately secreted now have granules with more fragile membranes so that the granules become confluent either before or at the moment of discharge. Clara and serous cells convert to mucus-secreting cells (Jeffery 1973). The PMO does not prevent increase in the amount of retained secretion in the secretory cells.

Several *drugs* have been shown to increase goblet cell number and submucosal gland size. Pilocarpine and isoprenaline sulphate each increase goblet cell number (Sturgess & Reid 1973). The proportion of the various histochemical cell types is normal after pilocarpine but shifts to the acid side after isoprenaline (Fig. 3). These studies were undertaken originally to determine whether isoprenaline increased submucosal gland size as it does salivary gland size. It does, and with a shift to the acid variety. The goblet cell increase was not expected, and these experiments were repeated under germ-free conditions so that the possibility of associated infection could be excluded.

Enzootic pneumonia is an example of an *infection* that is an important economic problem in pig-breeding. Lobar pneumonia was produced experimentally by intratracheal instillation of *Mycoplasma hyorhinis*. Gland hypertrophy developed within three weeks in the piglets (Fig. 4), and a shift in glycoprotein type occurred. (Gland-to-wall ratio: control 0.27 ± 0.008; enzootic pneumonia 0.53 ± 0.026, $P < 0.001$; Jones *et al.* 1975.) The glands of animals in which changes have been induced in these various ways can be studied in organ culture and the structural features related to functional activity. The various patterns that have been identified within a gland that shows hypertrophy are shown in Table 1. These patterns lend further support to the finding in organ culture that the various phases of the secretory cycle are under separate control (Coles 1976; Reid *et al.* 1976).

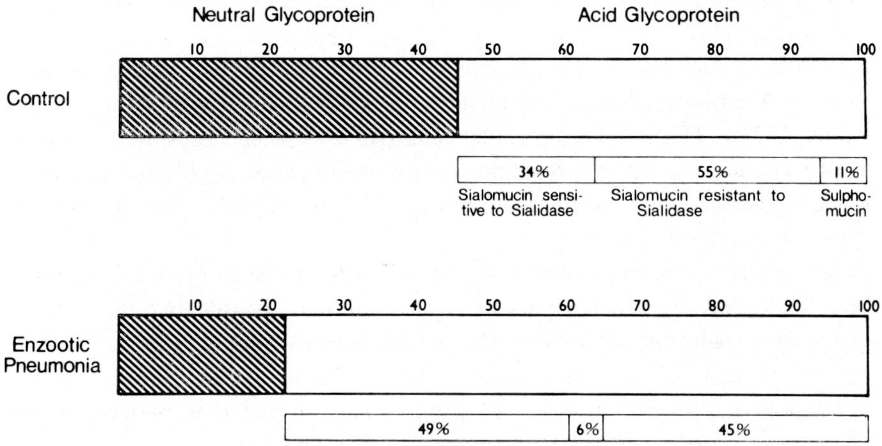

FIG. 4. Neutral and various types of acid glycoprotein (mean values) in mucous cells of the pig bronchial submucosal gland (as % of the total gland area) in control animals and in those with pneumonia after intranasal instillations of *Mycoplasma hyorhinis*.

TABLE 1

Pattern of change in submucosal glands assessed by microscopic examination and organ culture

	Gland-to-wall ratio	*Secretory index in organ culture*	*Amount of retained secretion*
Pilocarpine	↑	↑	Normal
Isoprenaline sulphate	↑	? Normal	↑
Tobacco	↑	↑	↑
PMO	↑	↓	↑

REVERSIBILITY OF MUCUS HYPERSECRETION

A cell, like a factory, can work at baseline activity or 'stimulated' activity. It seems that when an airway is no longer exposed to an irritant, the amount of secretion in the airway falls quickly, probably within hours; that is, the factory remains the same size but output falls. The question that is of interest to us is whether the factory changes its production lines or reduces in size, and how quickly.

Preliminary analysis of follow-up studies suggests that there is reversal, and that the distribution of glycoprotein types shifts back towards the normal (Jones 1977). The number of goblet cells also falls when exposure to tobacco smoke ceases. In the isoprenaline studies, submucosal gland size was back to normal in the pig within three months of stopping administration of the drug (Baskerville 1976).

The return to normal of the goblet cell after tobacco smoke is quicker than we found in earlier experiments after sulphur dioxide but the time of exposure was shorter. It may be that within a given population of cells, shift and return can occur more quickly than when a whole new population has developed that is conditioned and programmed to the new pattern of cell types. The correlation between new goblet cells and mitotic activity suggests that waves of increase in goblet cell number do follow waves of increase in mitotic activity.

GENERAL COMMENTS

It seems, then, that there is experimental support for the theory that gland hypertrophy and goblet cell increase are caused either by irritation without infection or by infection alone.

In the rat, nerves have been found within extrapulmonary airway epithelium (Jeffery & Reid 1973) and submucosal gland that, from their structure, may be either sensory or motor. A nervous reflex from surface epithelium to submucosal gland may occur but, in the rat, goblet cell increase and glycoprotein shift also occur within the intrapulmonary airways that are free of nerves, so a 'direct' or surface effect can occur.

The pattern of secretion by airway epithelial cells is not fixed. The secretion is packaged into granules at the Golgi, but chemical modification to these granules occurs after they have left the Golgi (see also p. 183). Additional enzymes seem to act near the cell apex. With continuing irritation these enzymes are 'turned on' earlier in the course of granule elaboration. The transitional stages within an individual cell can be followed until a stage is reached when all granules in the newly appearing cells are of the new type.

Not only is there a shift in the type of glycoprotein being produced, but in the secretory cell population more cells come to contain a large amount of secretion. So the cell population changes with respect to the type and the amount of glycoprotein within a cell. By using an analogue computer, the proportion of cells at various stages could be analysed. The flow chart shown on p. 184 suggests the way in which individual cells may change to produce the final state.

The similarity in the histochemical nature of the granules in serous and mucous cells and the lower specific activity after organ culture of the serous granules compared with the mucous suggests that the serous cells secrete a weaker solution of a glycoprotein essentially similar to that of the mucous cells (Lamb & Reid 1969*b*, 1970; Meyrick & Reid 1975; Reid *et al.* 1976). It may be that this minor difference is enough to prevent the two polymers from mixing by diffusion, and that they stay apart, the serous product being either the sol in the interstices of the gel or the periciliary liquid layer, while the mucous cell product is represented by the thick gobs of secretion that rest on the airway surface.

In considering the hypersecretory disturbance of airway secretion, a main advantage of the animal model is that the changes that are well established in human disease can be detected at their onset and their pattern and speed of development traced.

ACKNOWLEDGEMENTS

The work reported here was supported in Great Britain by the Medical Research Council, National Coal Board and Tobacco Research Council, and currently by the Council for Tobacco Research, USA.

References

BASKERVILLE, A. (1976) The development and persistence of bronchial gland hypertrophy and goblet cell hyperplasia in the pig after injection of isoprenaline. *J. Pathol. 119*, 35–47

CHARMAN, J., LOPEZ-VIDRIERO, M. T., KEAL, E. & REID, L. (1974) The physical and chemical properties of bronchial secretion. *Br. J. Dis. Chest 68*, 215–227

CIBA FOUNDATION (1971) *Identification of Asthma (Ciba Found. Study Group 38)*, Churchill Livingstone, London

COLES, S. (1976) *The Nature and Control of Glycoprotein Secretion by the Human Bronchial Glands*. Ph. D. thesis, University of London

JEFFERY, P. K. (1973) *Goblet Cell Increase in Rat Bronchial Epithelium Arising from Irritation or Drug Administration – An Experimental and Electron Microscopic Study*. Ph.D. thesis, University of London

JEFFERY, P. K. (1977) Structure and function of airway epithelium, in this volume, pp. 5–20

JEFFERY, P. K. & REID, L. (1973) Intra-epithelial nerves in normal rat airways: a quantitative electron microscopic study. *J. Anat. 114*, 35–45

JONES, R. (1977) Modification of mucus in animal models of disease, in *Mucus in Health and Disease* (Elstein, M. & Parke, D. V., eds.), Plenum Press, London

JONES, R. (1978) The glycoproteins of secretory cells in airway epithelium, in this volume, pp. 175–188

JONES, R., BOLDUC, P. & REID, L. (1972) Protection of rat bronchial epithelium against tobacco smoke. *Br. Med. J. 2*, 142–144

JONES, R., BOLDUC, P. & REID, L. (1973) Goblet cell glycoprotein and tracheal gland hypertrophy in rat airways: the effect of tobacco smoke with or without the anti-inflammatory agent phenylmethyloxadiazole. *Br. J. Exp. Pathol. 54*, 229–239

JONES, R., BASKERVILLE, A. & REID, L. (1975) Histochemical identification of glycoprotein in pig bronchial epithelium: (a) normal and (b) hypertrophied from enzootic pneumonia. *J. Pathol. 116*, 1–11

KEAL, E. E. (1971) Biochemistry and rheology of sputum in asthma. *Postgrad. Med. J. 47*, 171–177

KEAL, E. E. & REID, L. (1975) Pathological alterations in mucus in asthma within and without the cell, in *New Directions in Asthma* (Stein, M., ed.), American College of Chest Physicians, Park Ridge, Illinois

LAMB, D. & REID, L. (1968) Mitotic rates, goblet cell increase and histochemical changes in mucus in rat bronchial epithelium during exposure to sulphur dioxide. *J. Pathol. Bacteriol. 96*, 97–111

LAMB, D. & REID, L. (1969*a*) Goblet cell increase in rat bronchial epithelium after exposure to cigarette and cigar tobacco smoke. *Br. Med. J. 1*, 33–35

LAMB, D. & REID, L. (1969*b*) Histochemical types of acidic glycoprotein produced by mucous cells of the tracheobronchial glands in man. *J. Pathol. 98*, 213–229

LAMB, D. & REID, L. (1970) Histochemical and autoradiographic investigation of the serous cells of the human bronchial glands. *J. Pathol. 100*, 127–138

LAMB, D. & REID, L. (1972) The tracheobronchial submucosal glands in cystic fibrosis: a qualitative and quantitative histochemical study. *Br. J. Dis. Chest 66*, 239–247

MAWDESLEY-THOMAS, L. E. & HEALEY, P. (1973) Experimental bronchitis in lambs exposed to cigarette smoke. *Arch. Environ. Health 27*, 248–250

MAWDESLEY-THOMAS, L. E., HEALEY, P. & BARRY, D. H. (1971) Experimental bronchitis in animals due to sulphur dioxide and cigarette smoke. An automated quantitative study, in *Inhaled Particles III*, vol. 1 (Walton, W. H., ed.) *(Proc. Int. Symp. Br. Occup. Hyg. Soc.)*, Unwin, London

MEDICAL RESEARCH COUNCIL (1965) Definition – classification of chronic bronchitis from clinical and epidemiological perspectives. *Lancet 1*, 776–779

MEYRICK, B. & REID, L. (1975) *In vitro* incorporation of H^3-threonine and H^3-glucose by the mucous and serous cells of the human bronchial submucosal gland: a quantitative electron microscope study. *J. Cell Biol. 67*, 320–344

OSWALD, N. C. & MEDVEI, V. C. (1955) Chronic bronchitis: effect of cigarette smoking. *Lancet 2*, 843–844

REID, L. (1963) An experimental study of hypersecretion of mucus in the bronchial tree. *Br. J. Exp. Pathol. 44*, 437–445

REID, L. (1970) Evaluation of model systems for study of airway epithelium, cilia and mucus. *Arch. Intern. Med. 126*, 428–431

REID, L., MEYRICK, B. & COLES, S. (1976) Glycoprotein synthetic pathways in, and drug effects on, the human bronchial mucosa *in vitro*, in *Organ Culture in Biomedical Research* (Balls, M. & Monnickendam, M., eds.) *(Br. Soc. Cell Biol. Symp. 1)*, pp. 463–480, Cambridge University Press, London

ROBERTS, G. P. (1974) Isolation and characterisation of glycoproteins from sputum. *Eur. J. Biochem. 50*, 265–280

ROBERTS, G. P. (1976) Role of disulfide bonds in maintaining the gel structure of bronchial mucus. *Arch. Biochem. Biophys. 173*, 528–537

SPICER, S. S., CHAKRIN, L. W. & WARDELL, J. R. (1974) Effect of chronic sulfur dioxide inhalation on the carbohydrate histochemistry and histology of the canine respiratory tract. *Am. Rev. Respir. Dis. 110*, 13–24

STURGESS, J. and REID, L. (1972*a*) Secretory activity of the human bronchial mucous glands *in vitro*. *Exp. Mol. Pathol. 16*, 362–381

STURGESS, J. & REID, L. (1972*b*) An organ culture study of the effect of drugs on the secretory activity of the human bronchial submucosal gland. *Clin. Sci. (Oxf.) 43*, 533–543

STURGESS, J. & REID, L. (1973) The effect of isoprenaline and pilocarpine on (a) bronchial mucus-secreting tissue and (b) pancreas, salivary glands, heart, thymus, liver and spleen. *Br. J. Exp. Pathol. 54*, 388–403

TROWELL, O. A. (1959) The culture of mature organs in a synthetic medium. Problems of maintenance of mature organs *in vivo*. *Exp. Cell Res. 16*, 118

Discussion

Kent: Can you give further details about the effects of pilocarpine in organ cultures? What in fact was being measured where you showed increased numbers of goblet cells?

Reid: We measured the number of cells that were discharging radioactive precursor. We used radioactive threonine and glucose.

Kent: Was there any separation of the labelled material? Was it shown to be glycoprotein?

Reid: We have shown that the radioactive precursor is in the mucus glycoprotein.

Kent: I asked because organ culture is more complicated than many other techniques in that the soluble secretions come not only from the subepithelial glands and the goblet cells but a good deal of labelled material also comes from the non-epithelial tissues.

Reid: Yes. We now have micro methods for looking at the harvested mucus. By autoradiography we are looking at the cells and at the position over the organelles of the radioactive precursors. The mucous and serous cells can be separately studied. We avoided epithelium partly for the reasons you mentioned and partly because we felt that it probably did less well in organ culture. But recently Dr Coles (1977), working with superficial epithelium, has shown that in humans, where there is gland hypertrophy, there is also increased uptake and discharge of precursor. We found increased activity in the mucous cells but we cannot yet say anything about the Clara and the serous cells.

Richardson: You said that hypertrophied glands were the stigmata of chronic bronchitis. Thompson & Pavia (1974) have found that when subjects inhaled tagged particles, in bronchitis they penetrated less far into the lung than in the healthy controls. Their view, which is virtually the opposite of yours, is that it is a good thing for chronic bronchitics and people who smoke to have mucous gland hypertrophy to protect their distal (small) airways from damage by noxious agents.

Reid: I don't think there is any contradiction at all; we are talking about this at two levels. Patients with chronic bronchitis are, by definition, those who have a persistent cough, or rather persistent sputum production. Because they have smoked for so long they have developed gland hypertrophy. So there is no contradiction at all. We are identifying the cause of gland hypertrophy but presume that the body thought it was doing a good thing. What is much more interesting is that the body has gone on to produce such a degree of gland hypertrophy and of mucus hypersecretion that this can of itself cause serious disability. Something has happened to stimulate those glands and, if you like, you can call it a protective reaction.

Proctor: You mentioned the idea of aspiration of mucus into the periphery where there is no goblet cell proliferation. Have you any idea of the mechanism? If goblet cells are not proliferating there, the source of mucus is at some distance and one has to visualize the movement of mucus over some length of airway against whatever ciliary activity is going on.

Reid: All I can say is that mucus is sometimes seen out in the alveoli. In some cases of asthma there will still be mucus right out into the alveolar region. This is in status asthmaticus where there is difficult respiration and bronchial constriction. Whether it is a gravitational effect or aspiration I just don't know. The patient has not been able to clear those airways, either because the cilia are lost or because there is such bronchial constriction that they are plugged, or perhaps even because the secretion is particularly viscid.

Proctor: Would this be related to the finding I mentioned (p. 226) of mucus being cleared in the trachea and falling back down the trachea because of some abnormality in cystic fibrosis? Could you have a similar mechanism for asthma.

Reid: It seems not at all unlikely.

Widdicombe: Is it known how much of the muck that is blocking the small airways in status asthmaticus is secreted mucus and how much is transudate, or is it a mixture of the two?

Reid: We do not know in detail in the airways, but we know from viscosity and chemical studies that the highest range of sputum viscosity is in patients with asthma. We also know that in many patients with asthma there is a high serum component and also that in the mucoid sputum from status asthmaticus the DNA content is not particularly high.

Widdicombe: This is sputum from fairly large airways, isn't it?

Reid: Yes, probably. But we have studied plugs of sputum, 2–3 mm in diameter, that had been lavaged from patients with what you might call subacute 'status' or refractory asthma—patients who did not seem to have achieved the maximum response to treatment. We found that what was plugging the small airways was no different chemically from the sputum the patient produced the day before and the day after. And the high viscosity mucoid sputum produced after an attack of asthma—the sort of sputum that can be collected in the wards—does not have a high DNA content either. There has been very little detailed analysis of the effect of DNA. We recently looked at total DNA and assessed the number of cells and the number of fibres. We found that there was very little correlation between the amount of DNA and purulence, or with any of those other features, which fits in with something Professor Sadoul mentioned. If, in a test tube, DNA is added to mucoid sputum it becomes more viscid. We have come to the conclusion that, even in freshly collected sputum, if it is purulent, various things are working in different directions. The presence of DNA, of fibres, of cells, will all tend to increase viscosity of secretions, but these are the sputa that degrade fastest, spontaneously. So even within the airways, over a short time, there will be factors that tend to degrade secretions. Even in fresh purulent sputum one is getting a balance between those factors. It is possible to leave mucoid sputum on the bench for four hours or more and see little change in viscosity.

Nadel: Does isoproterenol (isoprenaline) have any effect on the isolated preparation in culture?

Reid: None of the sympathomimetic drugs had any effect in the human organ culture system over 4, 6 or even 24 hours. So it looks as though in the short term they are not effective (Sturgess & Reid 1972). In animals we can get an effect after six days and Mrs R. Jones has just found an increased effect from isoprenaline at three days (personal communication). But one is dealing with a different time scale. There does not seem to be much of an acute effect on the bronchial glands from the sympathetic system.

Allison: Isoprenaline greatly stimulates DNA synthesis in salivary glands.

Reid: Both pilocarpine and isoprenaline increase the mitotic activity enormously and with isoprenaline we get a lot of superficial cells in division, but it doesn't have that effect in cell culture. Salbutamol (albuterol) has no effect in our animals either, so I wonder how much this is a 'sport' effect of isoprenaline rather than a purely pharmacological one.

Jeffery: Which precursors was Dr Coles using for incorporation into the surface goblet cells, and how long do these precursors take to get from the base of the cell to the apex and be secreted?

Reid: I cannot tell you for goblet cells particularly, but in general in the rat gland the secretory time is about half that of humans.

Jeffery: I am interested in the goblet cells because of our failure to get some of these labels incorporated into the surface goblet cells of the cat.

Reid: I know that Coles (Coles & Reid 1976) had no particular problem with the human goblet cell compared with the gland cell.

Silberberg: What is the significance of the increase in the sulphur-mucin-containing cells after influenza infection?

Reid: If sulphate is the only acid radical it seems to give low viscosity, but this has only been established in one type of fish (Lopez-Vidriero *et al.* 1978). For the human I do not know. When Dr G. Roberts was isolating oligosaccharide side chains he found that the sulphate content of the longer chains was high. But whether this means it is added terminally I don't know. When a cell shifts to sulphation, the sulphate appears first at the apex of the cell, in the granules after they are packaged and about to become Professor Kramer's artifacts. They are apical and will shortly undergo compound exocytosis.

References

COLES, S. J. (1977) Regulation of the secretory cycles of mucous and serous cells in the human bronchial gland, in *Mucus in Health and Disease* (Elstein, M. & Parke, D. K., eds.), Plenum Press, London

COLES, S. J. & REID, L. (1976) The effect of drugs on the incorporation of glycoprotein precursors in goblet cells of normal and hypertrophied airway epithelium, in *Lung Cells in Disease* (Bouhuys, A., ed.), pp. 109–112, North-Holland, Amsterdam

LOPEZ-VIDRIERO, M. T., BHASKAR, K. R., JONES, R., FLETCHER, T. & REID, L. (1978) Biochemical, rheological and histochemical analysis of sulphated glycoprotein from plaice cutaneous mucus *(Pleuronectes platessa L.)*. (in preparation)

STURGESS, J. & REID, L. (1972) An organ culture study of the effect of drugs on the secretory activity of the human bronchial submucosal gland. *Clin. Sci. (Oxf.) 43*, 533–543

THOMPSON, M. L. & PAVIA, D. (1974) Particle penetration and clearance in the human lung. *Arch. Environ. Health 29*, 214–219

Final discussion

CLINICAL ASPECTS

J. G. Jones: Dr Proctor, what is the interpretation of the information you presented on changes in mucus transport with temperature? Is it an effect of temperature on the mechanical properties of the mucus or on the cilia or on the mucus production, or what?

Proctor: Mercke (1974) and Mercke *et al.* (1974) have shown, using *in vitro* preparations, that temperature is one of the factors that influences the rate of ciliary beating and the rate of mucociliary clearance but I have no idea whether this is so *in vivo*, particularly in the human nose. In fact, the design of our study did not permit us to look at the effects of sudden changes in temperature, only at slow changes. I am curious to know the effect of rapid temperature changes on impairment of clearance and we hope to look at that next year. The small changes we noted were probably of little physiological importance.

Godfrey: You had a wide range of nasal clearance in your normal subjects. How many of those with low clearance rates had had colds recently?

Proctor: Now and then we had a volunteer who had had a cold recently. They were easy to pick out because they generally had no clearance at all. With a naturally occurring cold—not the experimentally induced cold—we have some evidence of impaired clearance during the stages when the cold is developing and then almost total loss of clearance, lasting for about two weeks. We have found nothing to account for this tremendous difference of less than 1 mm/min up to about 26 mm/min among apparently normal subjects.

Thurlbeck: I had a change of mind about three concepts related to clinical aspects of mucus in this symposium and I want to make certain that I have changed my mind correctly. Firstly I thought that the difference between the sputum of an asthmatic subject during an attack and an asthmatic who is feeling entirely normal was a quantitative one. Sanerkin & Evans (1965) examined sputum cytology in asthmatics and concluded that the cytological appearance of the sputum of asthmatics who felt entirely well was essentially the same qualitatively as in patients with status asthmaticus. Professor Reid, did you say that the quality of mucus was different in symptomatic compared to asymptomatic asthmatics and that the amount of DNA was different in asymptomatic patients?

Reid: No, because if a patient with asthma is producing sputum he is not normal; he does not produce it between attacks. Normally an asthmatic does not produce sputum persistently like a bronchitic.

Thurlbeck: But if you have a patient with asthma who is not wheezing or acutely ill but is producing a plug, would that plug be the same rheologically and biochemically as a plug in patients in status asthmaticus?

Reid: It would probably be different.

Thurlbeck: My second question concerns mucus hypersecretion, which I think of as being beneficial because it is an inflammatory response. When the airways are injured a train of events occurs—there is a response, which is inflammation, and this results in mucus hypersecretion. If the injury occurred but no mucus hypersecretion resulted, I would assume that the patient would be worse off still. Professor Sadoul suggests that mucus hypersecretion might be bad.

Sadoul: No, I did not say that. At an early stage of the disease, mucus secretion has the ideal composition for improving clearance of particles and mucociliary clearance in general, but after recurrent infectious episodes the secretory IgA decreases, the viscoelasticity decreases and the mucociliary clearance is altered. But it is only at the end of the story that patients are unable to have effective mucociliary clearance and they cannot cough the sputum up properly. Clearance after one hour is roughly the same in some chronic bronchitics as it is in normal non-smokers, but in advanced chronic bronchitics with mucopurulent secretions the mucociliary transport is severely altered. At this stage there are decreases in IgA and changes in the biochemical composition of the sputum, and viscosity as well as strain recovery are decreased.

Allison: Does that answer your question?

Thurlbeck: Yes and no, because we do not have the model of a patient with airway irritation who does not have mucus hypersecretion.

My third problem is this. It seems to me that epithelial function may be more important than the actual mucus itself. Dr Proctor spoke of being able to move an asthmatic mucus plug down a hen trachea, so the function of the epithelium is as important as the nature of the mucus lining that epithelium.

Proctor: I agree with you entirely. It has been known since the latter part of the 19th century that normally functioning ciliary epithelium has an immense capacity for clearing all sorts of materials of immense sizes. What is lacking is evidence that mucus is the villain when there isn't any clearance and I should like to see that proved before I abandoned the idea that when a patient gets into trouble it may be caused by the change in character of the epithelium.

In relation to your first question, I think that teleologically these secretions are a defence mechanism and they are good. When I peel an onion my nose and eyes water immediately and presumably wash away a noxious vapour; when we are exposed to an allergen we have an outpouring of secretion which is aimed at ridding us of something undesirable.

Reid: The question of a long natural history is terribly important. Dr I. Gregg (1968) picked out a group from a general practice who had never come to the doctor for any incident related to the chest. He found that, as a group, all the people with mild and persistent mucus hypersecretion already had a degree of respiratory impairment. So if irritation of the airway is persistent it will not be a case of a normal population of cells secreting fast on just one occasion but the population of cells will have been changed.

Donald: It has been said, but I don't think it has ever been proved, that the bronchitic or the smoker who does not markedly hypersecrete is in greater danger of carcinoma than one who does.

Thurlbeck: Cancer of the lung has in fact been shown to be more likely to develop in bronchitic smokers than in non-bronchitic smokers (Rimington 1971).

Proctor: Macklin (1955) and Hilding (1957) pointed out many years ago that as material is cleared from the lung, wherever two bronchi converge into one there has to be a sharp divergence of the stream to get round the spur, and one is likely to get chronic deposition of small amounts of material in these regions. Recent work with flexible fibre bronchoscopy on identifying occult, very early cancers of the lung indicates that these cancers probably begin near relatively peripheral spurs. What we still do not know is whether one of the harmful effects of smoking is an increased likelihood of chronic deposition of materials in these already somewhat vulnerable regions.

Allison: Is it technically possible to study that point?

Proctor: Not with present techniques. The only technique commonly used today for measuring bronchial clearance is an inhaled aerosol which enables the overall disappearance to be measured but does not yield the information which we get in the nose with the single particle, an exact mapping of the transit along a particular line. I should like to see us develop a technique for measuring tracheobronchial clearance with single particles as we do in the nose; I think it can be done.

We talked earlier about people with a cough and what can be done about it.

There is no evidence that introducing water or mucolytic agents into the airway by means of an aerosol is of help even in patients with tracheostomy or an orotracheal tube. I think humidified air is needed by those people, but there is a big difference between humidified air and water aerosols. There is also some confusion over the fact that tracheotomized patients are often helped by the instillation of actual fluid, especially where they have already developed a dry crust blocking the surface; but that is very different from viscid mucus. If water or saline is poured over a dry crust the patient will often cough it up very promptly. The fluid may act as a substitute for the periciliary fluid that would have been in there if it hadn't dried out.

Widdicombe: Why use water rather than saline? Although we have not been told how easily water can go through the epithelium, I should have thought that saline would be better if you want to loosen up secretions. Is there any evidence that saline is more effective than water?

Proctor: There is no evidence that either helps.

Kent: When water aerosols are given, additional water must be getting into the airways; it has to go somewhere, so presumably the epithelium or some other tissue is having to work that much harder to get rid of it.

Godfrey: Depending on the size of the aerosol particles, much of it would be breathed out again. Very little would actually stay in the airway.

Kent: Is it known how much remains?

Richardson: Yes; several studies have been done on this (e.g. Wolfsdorf *et al.* 1969; Asmundsson *et al.* 1973; Alderson *et al.* 1974). Even using the best particle size and getting subjects to breathe in through their open mouths, it is very difficult to deposit more than 2 ml fluid/h in the airways.

Proctor: And if people breathe through their noses, the fluid never gets past the tip of the nose!

Donald: Is there any evidence that so-called bronchiolytic medicines do any good?

Sadoul: Some of them are noxious because they liquefy the mucus so efficiently that it becomes like water. With samples initially ranging in the rheological zone of optimal transport, the large decrease in viscoelasticity after the addition of a mucolytic agent such as *N*-acetylcysteine may be responsible for a decrease in mucociliary transport.

Guz: What we need are controlled trials.

Reid: I doubt if even controlled trials will help you to match a patient to a particular therapy. There are different stages of a given disease, as well as many diseases.

Sadoul: Mucolytic agents are quite good at improving clearance in some chronic bronchitics but not in other patients, and we do not know why.

Guz: Do you find a correlation between clinical deterioration—that is, the patient finding it difficult to bring up sputum—and what you find on the frog palate?

Sadoul: Yes. My chemist has predicted to me several times that a patient would die in the near future because of the changes in the viscous property and the viscoelasticity. In a few cases she was right and the patient died within a six-month or one-year period because he could not raise sputum either by mucociliary clearance or by coughing.

Reid: How many of those patients were in heart failure?

Sadoul: I do not know; some might have been.

Nadel: In defining the viscoelastic properties of mucus we need to differentiate between the hydration and the cross-links and the physical properties of this material that has to be transmitted up the airway. There is strong evidence that the material has to have a somewhat limited range of properties in order to store energy and impart it up the airway. Professor Sadoul told us that the material he was studying had very wide differences in its properties, so when we talk about mucus and secretions we are talking about two different things that interact and are coupled through the cilia. The quality and thickness of the periciliary layer are likely to be important in mucociliary clearance. I will separate, in this discussion, the water that interacts with the mucoproteins and the periciliary layer that allows transmission. There is no evidence of what happens to the water, but techniques are available for studying in its own milieu the interaction of the sol layer and the airway epithelium. Is it possible to study the fluid interactions *in vivo*?

The distribution of the fluid may be different in various areas. Does fluid near gland openings differ from the remainder of the epithelial surface? There are the therapeutic possibilities of modifying the sol layer by actions on ion pumps. If the sol layer is inadequate, you can turn the chloride pump on with terbutaline or other agents such as acetylcholine and histamine. Halides (e.g. bromide, iodide) affect analogous pumps from the same progenitor systems in the gut. What are their effects on airway ion pumps? Does potassium iodide act on ion pumps?

Vascular and airway luminal osmolarity and ion contents could also have a marked effect on these pumps. There might be specific materials released locally and circulating in the blood which block the ion pumps in specific diseases such as asthma and cystic fibrosis. In addition to characterization of effects on ion pumps, techniques are available for studying the effects on total mucociliary clearance *in vivo*. You can look at gross clearance as Dr Proctor described, or at the local properties for which Professor Silberberg has devised techniques.

Douglas: Could you fit into this scheme some of the old remedies that are used to activate secretion?

Nadel: Ipecacuanha! Airways are very sensitive to stimulation by SO_2, dust, mechanical factors, histamine and a very large number of agents. As a result of the stimulus acetylcholine is released and that causes secretion. Ipecac, by stimulating sensory nerve endings (perhaps in the gut), might reflexly stimulate glandular secretion.

Richardson: Perry & Boyd (1941) discovered that when they gave ipecacuanha into the stomach of rabbits it increased the output of respiratory tract fluid but when they gave the substance intravenously it was ineffective. They concluded that it worked by a reflex initiated by stomach afferent nerves.

Widdicombe: Don't you think, Professor Nadel, that the interaction between mucus and receptor sensitivity is very important?

Nadel: Yes. One question that arises is why a tiny particle of dust stimulates sensory nerve endings, in the airways, and I think it is relevant to the stimulation of mucus secretion as well.

Silberberg: What intrigues me is the extent to which the mucus layer covers the surface. If one is beginning to think in terms of islands of mucus rather than a continuous blanket, this could have considerable bearing on the whole question of the physiological state of the epithelium.

Reid: May I go back to the question of the number of layers? We have seen the electron microscope picture of something that is literally part of the cell surface; there is a perivillous layer and a periciliary layer, and whether they are the same or not we do not know; then there is a superficial or continuous glycoprotein sheet, although even that may not be homogeneous, since it is a mesh of fibres with other substances caught between them, so perhaps it is not as smooth as a sheet. Then there is something really viscid and like a raft or gob.

Silberberg: If the stimulus comes to epithelium, does it have to penetrate a mucus layer or would it make immediate contact with the interciliary fluid and the tips of the cilia? In other words, is there a layer which protects cilia from immediate contact with air?

Reid: I would think so. The cilia are still part of the *milieu interne*.

Richardson: When you sprinkle carbon dust on the open trachea, for the first minute or so it remains where it landed, and then it starts to move. Perhaps it first of all settles at the tips of mucus-free cilia and stays there until some mucus comes along, collects it and shifts it up the airway.

Silberberg: Have you studied that as a function of size of the particles?

Richardson: No.

Nadel: One possibility here is that the particle stimulates the local production of mucoprotein.

Allison: That happens in the frog.

Silberberg: You can see this quite easily on the frog palate since this epithelium is very rich in glands.

Nadel: In an isolated preparation, what is the coupling mechanism?

Allison: Presumably it is nervous, and could be investigated with blockers.

Donald: It has been claimed that iodides are only effective or produce more fluid if the subject is sensitive to iodine. Is that true?

Richardson: Falliers *et al.* (1966) tested the effects of giving iodide to asthmatic children. They found that children treated with the drug needed less steroids and had improved lung function tests.

Douglas: There seems to be some therapeutic advantage in activating vagal reflex secretion. Can you potentiate that locally, by using anticholinesterases?

Nadel: Those reflexes are often markedly potentiated in the presence of disease. Certainly they are potentiated in so-called reactive bronchitics and in some asthmatics. As far as I know this has not been studied in bronchial secretion but it has been studied in animals and in humans for bronchomotor tone, and there is a potent feedback system in the cholinergic nervous system for smooth muscle. That would provide a diffuse response. Earlier, I described an interaction of 5HT and vagal efferent nervous effects (p. 150). Locally released 5HT might potentiate the effects of normal vagal impulses.

Silberberg: Is it known what chemical messenger is responsible for starting secretion in these cases? Can you inhibit it and stop secretion? Can you, for example, prevent goblet cells from discharging?

Nadel: You can inhibit the chloride pump by furosemide, so one of the logical things to do is to test the effect of furosemide on gland secretion and on mucociliary clearance.

Allison: Might your anti-inflammatory drugs be inhibiting the release of secretions rather than their accumulation in the cells?

Reid: Yes, we know that butazolidine reduces uptake as well as discharge (Coles *et al.* 1978).

Allison: Speaking as a general pathologist, I do not find it very helpful to regard these chronic events as being merely inflammatory. By chronic inflammation we mean a sustained infiltration of leucocytes. One feature of an inflammatory process is increased vascular permeability with the appearance of mediators, exudation of serum constituents and other changes. Would you agree?

Reid: Yes. There is acute secretion from the normal airway; in chronic bronchitis there is a hypertrophied system that is hypersensitive to drugs.

From organ culture we know that the hypertrophied gland is hypersensitive to a given stimulus, and from studies of total sputum we know that there is a serum component.

Thurlbeck: We need to modify our concepts, because we are dealing with recurrent episodes of irritation rather than just one episode. Every time one inhales when smoking a cigarette, irritants result, so there are many repeated episodes of insult. You can interpret the response as being inflammation.

Allison: There are interesting possible links, however. For example, the factor in cystic fibrosis serum which stops the movement of cilia is now thought by some investigators to be the complement cleavage product, C3A. Work in my laboratory has shown that some complement cleavage products will stimulate cells; for example C3b stimulates secretion of enzymes and complement cleavage products by macrophages. Some of these inflammatory mediators may stimulate mucus-secreting cells also.

Davis: The chloride ion content of sputum from patients with cystic fibrosis is less than normal (Matthews *et al.* 1963). If the 'factor' in cystic fibrosis inhibits the ion pumps in airway epithelium as it does in sweat glands (Mangos 1973), the movement of chloride into the airway secretions would be reduced. The associated water movement would be less and the secretions would become sticky. On the other hand, patients in status asthmaticus, who produce mucus plugs, are severely dehydrated (Ambiavagan & Jones 1967). Since the submucosal fluid is likely to be hypertonic, water secretion resulting from ion transport across the epithelium would decrease (Diamond & Bossert 1968) and the airway would form thicker mucus.

Proctor: There is considerable doubt now whether the so-called C.F. factor influences cilia at all or whether the influence is purely on mucus secretion with an indirect effect on cilia.

J. G. Jones: It has been suggested that one might stimulate the vagus to switch on the interciliary fluid pump in patients. Perhaps we are already doing that, and pouring saline and putting suction catheters into the airway may work because it is in fact stimulating vagal receptors and switching on the pump. It is not just adding water to the mucus but switching on the pump that may promote clearance of mucus.

Donald: Can you do this without also getting a vagal motor effect?

Nadel: Yes, because terbutaline turns this chloride pump on but it also inhibits bronchomotor contraction. In fact it may be possible to potentiate the effect of the cholinergic stimulus on the pump. Both acetylcholine and terbutaline seem to increase chloride secretion but they act antagonistically on the bronchomotor system.

References

ALDERSON, P. O., SECKER-WALKER, R. H., STROMINGER, D. B., MARKHAM, J. & HILL, R. L. (1974) Pulmonary deposition of aerosols in children with cystic fibrosis. *J. Pediatr. 84*, 479–484

AMBIAVAGAN, M. & JONES, E. S. (1967) Resuscitation of the moribund asthmatic. *Anaesthesia 22*, 375–391

ASMUNDSSON, T., JOHNSON, R. F., KILBURN, K. H. & GOODRICH, J. K. (1973) Efficiency of nebulizers for depositing saline in human lungs. *Am. Rev. Respir. Dis. 108*, 506–512

COLES, S. J., LEVINE, L. & REID, L. (1978) Secretory activity of the rat laryngeal gland in organ culture: the effect of tobacco smoke and anti-inflammatory agents. (in preparation)

DIAMOND, J. M. & BOSSERT, W. H. (1968) Functional consequences of ultrastructural geometry in 'backwards' fluid-transporting epithelia. *J. Cell Biol. 37*, 694–702

FALLIERS, D. J., MCCANN, W. P., CHAI, H., ELLIS, E. F. & YAZDE, N. (1966) Controlled study of iodotherapy for childhood asthma. *J. Allergy 38*, 183–192

GREGG, I. (1968) A study of the causes of progressive airways obstruction in chronic bronchitis, in *Current Research in Chronic Respiratory Diseases (11th Aspen Conf.)*, pp. 235–248, Karger, Basel

HILDING, A. C. (1957) Ciliary streaming in the bronchial tree and the time element in carcinogenesis. *N. Engl. J. Med. 256*, 634–640

MACKLIN, C. C. (1955) Lung fluid, alveolar dust drift, and initial lesions of disease in the lungs. *Can. Med. Assoc. J. 72*, 664–665

MANGOS, J. A. (1973) Microperfusion study of the sweat gland abnormality in cystic fibrosis. *Tex. Rep. Biol. Med. 31*, 651–663

MATTHEWS, L. W., SPECTOR, S., LEMM, J. & POTTER, J. L. (1963) Studies on pulmonary secretions. The over-all chemical composition of pulmonary secretions from patients with cystic fibrosis, bronchiectasis and laryngectomy. *Am. Rev. Respir. Dis. 88*, 199–204

MERCKE, U. (1974) The influence of temperature on mucociliary activity. *Acta Oto-Laryngol. 78*, 253–258

MERCKE, U., HAKANSSON, C. H. & TOREMALM, N. G. (1974) The influence of temperature on mucociliary activity. *Acta Oto-Laryngol. 78*, 444–450

PERRY, W. F. & BOYD, E. M. (1941) A method for studying expectorant action of animals by direct measurement of the output of respiratory tract fluid. *J. Pharmacol. Exp. Ther. 73*, 65–77

RIMINGTON, J. (1971) Smoking, chronic bronchitis and lung cancer. *Br. Med. J. 2*, 373–375

SANERKIN, N. G. & EVANS, D. M. (1965) The sputum in bronchial asthma: pathognomonic patterns. *J. Pathol. Bacteriol. 89*, 535–541

WOLFSDORF, J., SWIFT, D. L. & AVERY, M. E. (1969) Mist therapy reconsidered; an evaluation of the respiratory deposition of labelled water aerosols produced by jet and ultrasonic nebulizers. *Pediatrics 43*, 799–808

Chairman's closing remarks

A. C. ALLISON

Division of Cell Pathology, MRC Clinical Research Centre, Harrow

In summing up this meeting I shall start by discussing briefly what I have gathered from the meeting about the chemistry of respiratory tract mucus and the process of secretion. The basic constituents of mucus are protein chains and sugar side chains, and, for the moment at least, we are all seduced by the model which we might call the multiple bottle-brush model of Masson, modified by Silberberg. Models are useful mainly as a guide for further research, so first of all we need information on whether this model is correct, secondly whether it is general, and thirdly what chemical differences in mucins correspond to the histochemical differences which have been described. Although some work has been done on the chemical basis of these histochemical reactions, we still know very little about it and I believe that it is time for the histochemists and the chemists to get together. For example, there are ways of separating components of respiratory tract mucus and there is no difficulty, when you have this material in a test tube, in fixing it and staining it to see which of the staining reactions corresponds to the individual chemical components.

Broadly speaking, then, mucus contains multiple polypeptide chains with sugar side chains, and we can be fairly confident about where these are likely to be synthesized. One thing we should like to know is whether, in the secretory granules, the material is fully polymerized or whether it is in some precursor form which is polymerized later. Clearly, disulphide bonding is important and we discussed the possibility that sugar chains also join the polypeptide chains together.

A few points about the synthesis. We know that proteins are synthesized on polyribosomes, and when the proteins are packaged for secretion the polyribosomes are attached to membranes of the rough endoplasmic reticulum. There is an interesting enzyme catalysing disulphide interchange reactions which might be relevant in this situation. It has been studied by Anfinsen in Bethesda and by Rabin at University College, London (Rabin *et al.* 1971). The enzyme is associated with the rough endoplasmic reticulum and normally is made inaccessible by the ribosomes attached to the endoplasmic reticulum. When these ribosomes are detached the enzyme is exposed and you can measure its activity by its capacity to renature proteins such as ribonuclease which have been denatured so that the disulphide bonds are in the wrong place; when the denatured ribonuclease is exposed to the enzyme catalysing disulphide interchanges it will recover activity. Ribosomal association with membranes is very hormone-dependent. For example, in male rats, female sex hormones in low concentrations produce detachment of ribosomes, and vice versa. We discussed briefly the progestational hormones which change the nature of the cervical mucus and are thought to be one of the major ways in which the contraceptive pill works. It is possible that one aspect of control of mucin secretion might be at the level of the ribosome and disulphide interchange. It would be interesting to know whether the interchain disulphide bonding takes place at the time of synthesis or later, and it is conceivable that a comparable enzyme exists at the cell membrane and that it could bring about polymerization to form macromolecules at that stage.

What is likely to happen next? We know that the polypeptide chains pass through the membranes of the endoplasmic reticulum to get into the Golgi-associated endoplasmic reticulum, and in many cases this is achieved by their having a special hydrophobic piece on the end of the chain which is then clipped off, the so-called pre-prohormones. In general, as Professor Kramer reminded us, the processes of sequential addition of sugars and of transfer of sulphate are likely to happen in the Golgi system. Professor Phelps warned us that some of these transferases are not membrane-associated and might be able to migrate within cells, but many of the transferases appear to be associated with Golgi membranes. It looks as though the levels of particular nucleotides in the cell are of special importance in controlling transferase activities, although these may not be limiting.

To come to packaging, this begins with the formation of very small condensing vacuoles in the vicinity of Golgi-associated endoplasmic reticulum. In certain secretions, for example immunoglobulins, such microvesicles migrate to the plasma membrane and fuse with it, and this occurs in the absence of specific transport systems. Colchicine or cytochalasin, for example, which affect microtubule structure and microfilament activity respectively, have no effect on the rate of synthesis or release of immunoglobulins. In other cases, including mucus secretion, the final secretory granules are much bigger than the condensing vacuoles, so it seems likely that there is controlled membrane fusion, to give first relatively large secretory granules from condensing vacuoles;

a pause follows, with storage of this material, and then later, as a result of a specific trigger, another membrane fusion phenomenon occurs, resulting in discharge of mucus from the cells.

We know very little about the intracellular translocation of secretory granules in mucus-secreting cells. In some other cell types agents disrupting microtubules can inhibit the release of secretions, for example procollagen in fibroblasts. It would be quite easy to establish, particularly in the kind of organ cultures that Professor Reid was referring to, whether colchicine or vinblastine disturbs the accumulation of secretory granules near the apex of the cells.

Incidentally, these cells start by being nearly round and then acquire polarity, and we know this type of polarity in other cell types is dependent on normal microtubular structure. One would imagine that, where there is a recently divided precursor cell, in the absence of microtubule formation it would not be able to form its usual columnar differentiated form. This again could be investigated experimentally.

On the question of the fusion of the secretory granule membrane and plasma membranes, Professor Douglas reminded us of the importance of calcium in a variety of release phenomena and of the many ways in which local increases in calcium concentrations can be achieved. We do not yet know whether the same is true in mucus-secreting cells but there are experiments that could be done. For example, preliminary work of Kim Balfre has shown that the calcium ionophore A23187 can induce release of mucus, and these experiments could be done with suitable controls to show that the cells remain viable. They can be done in the presence of EGTA, which is a specific extracellular calcium chelator, and if A23187 still stimulates mucus secretion it is likely that calcium is being released from an intracellular pool. If A23187 is inactive in the presence of EGTA, one can add calcium or barium or strontium. If you need an extracellular source of calcium, this will tell you that the main calcium permeability event takes place in the plasma membrane. It seems probable that what is happening is the sequential fusion of the plasma membrane with the granule membrane and of the granule membranes with one another, and this is one of the features of certain types of secretion but not of others. The membranes around mucus-containing granules seem ready to fuse, so that any small stimulus can do this, such as perfusion with Tyrode solution, as Professor Kramer described.

We should also like to know how events occurring at the base of the cell, where there are nerve endings and where certain drugs are apparently active, finally bring about this secretory event, and how it can be controlled, for example by anti-inflammatory agents.

Now we come to the surface of the respiratory epithelial cells. On the surface of the ciliated cells two major specialized components are present, the cilia with their beautiful arrangement of microtubules which provides their motile power, and the microvilli, which have two distinctive features. One is their finger-like projections, which have a large amount of surface membrane over them which greatly increases the area of the apical plasma membrane. In the intestine and the kidney this is associated with reabsorption, and we discussed the possibility that reabsorption of materials is also occurring in the respiratory tract. The other feature of microvilli is that they have central regions consisting of microfilaments. From intestine fairly pure fractions of isolated microvilli can be obtained for studying their properties, as Mooseker & Tilney (1975) have done, and it might be possible to do the same with respiratory epithelium. This would be interesting for several reasons. One would like to know, for example, whether the plasma membrane covering microvilli has ion-transporting ATPases, or enzymes that catalyse disulphide interchanges, transglycosylation and so forth.

I want to revert to the phenomenon of transglycosylation and mention again the experiments done at Johns Hopkins (Roth 1973). If there are two apposed cells, sugar chains stick out of the plasma membranes: they can be carbohydrate moieties of either glycolipids or glycoproteins. Evidence has been produced for the presence of so-called transglycosylating enzymes in the plasma membranes of these cells. The enzymes are thought to catalyse the formation of cross-links between cells that are involved in cell adhesion. If this enzyme exists in the plasma membranes of respiratory epithelial cells, some cross-linking of polypeptide chains of mucus might also take place there.

The glycolipids and glycoproteins of the plasma membrane of respiratory epithelial cells may have long carbohydrate chains, forming part of the glycocalyx. The glycocalyx, in turn, interacts with the material in the perivillous layer and it would be interesting to know whether there are any local differentiations—how thick it is, and so on. Relatively specific staining techniques can now be applied. There is specialization of this material on the tips of the cilia, as Anderson & Hein (1977) have shown in the rabbit oviduct. They stained the apical filamentous glycocalyx or ciliary crown with polycationic ferritin which is basic and sticks to acidic groups of glycoproteins. The ciliary crown provides a polyanionic mass which might be able to interact with the mucus rafts directly or through ions, as discussed below.

We mentioned the presence of the different layers above the epithelial cells. It is clearly important to distinguish between the superficial layer, or sheet, or whatever you choose to call it (I think it is convenient to call all of them layers), the layer which lies around the microvilli, and the periciliary layer.

We do not know whether these last two are distinct. We can be fairly sure that the inner layers are composed not just of water and ions, but also of macromolecules which contribute to their staining properties. Obviously, it would be interesting to isolate the inner layers to see whether their chemical composition and physical properties differ from those of the mucus layer. It might be technically possible to do so because sometimes layers shear off quite conveniently, but it would be difficult. Information about the histochemical reactions, or the histochemical identification of the individual components, would help us to know the composition of the inner layers. The relative lack of electron-density in this region as opposed to the mucus layer, which Professor Iravani pointed out, may suggest that macromolecular concentrations are low, but other interpretations are not excluded.

How is the mechanical energy in the cilia linked to the motion of the particles? (And here I should like to plead a small semantic point. It might be useful to refer to this as *translocation* of particles, simply because *transport* is used for several other processes such as transport across the plasma membrane.) It is instructive to go back to the theory of colloids, namely, that there is a double layer of ions associated with the surfaces of many cells and charged macromolecules (see Allison & Valentine 1960). Divalent ions are much more effective than univalent; a layer of divalent ions probably exists above the polyanionic material near the surface of the cilia and also beneath the mucus layer; the interaction of cilia and the mucus layer may be mediated by the overlapping ionic layers. It would be easy to remove the divalent ions with chelating agents such as EDTA to see whether this has any effect on translocation.

There is obviously a great deal more that needs to be done. This meeting has usefully summarized available information on respiratory tract mucus and, I hope, indicated areas which are most readily open for further exploration.

References

ALLISON, A. C. & VALENTINE, R. C. (1960) Virus particle adsorption. III. Adsorption of viruses by cell monolayers and effects of some variables on adsorption. *Biochim. Biophys. Acta 40*, 400–410

ANDERSON, R. G. W. & HEIN, C. E. (1977) Distribution of anionic sites on the oviduct ciliary membrane. *J. Cell Biol. 72*, 482–492

MOOSEKER, M. S. & TILNEY, L. B. (1975) Organisation of an actin filament-membrane complex. Filament polarity and membrane attachment in the microvilli of intestinal epithelial cells. *J. Cell Biol. 67*, 725–743

RABIN, B. R., BLYTH, C. A., DOHERTY, D., FREEDMAN, R. B., ROOBOL, A., SUNSHINE, G. & WILLIAMS, D. J. (1971) in *Effects of Drugs on Cellular Control Mechanisms* (Rabin, B. R. & Freedman, R. B., eds.), pp. 27–47, Macmillan, London

ROTH, S. (1973) A molecular model for cell interactions. *Q. Rev. Biol. 48*, 541–563

Index of contributors

Entries in **bold** *type indicate papers; other entries refer to discussion contributions*

Indexes compiled by William Hill

Subject index